ATHLETIC & ORTHOPEDIC
INJURY
ASSESSMENT

A CASE STUDY APPROACH

David C. Berry, Ph.D., ATC, EMT-B
SAGINAW VALLEY STATE UNIVERSITY

Michael G. Miller, Ed.D., ATC, CSCS
WESTERN MICHIGAN UNIVERSITY

Leisha M. Berry, MSPT, ATC

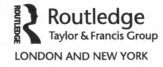

Routledge
Taylor & Francis Group

LONDON AND NEW YORK

Library of Congress Cataloging-in-Publication Data

Berry, David.
  Athletic and orthopedic injury assessment : a case study approach / David Berry,
Michael G. Miller, Leisha Berry.
    p. cm.
  Includes bibliographical references and index.
  ISBN 978-1-934432-01-3
  1. Sports injuries—Diagnosis—Case studies. 2. Musculoskeletal system—Wounds
and injuries—Case studies. I. Miller, Michael G. II. Berry, Leisha. III. Title.
  [DNLM: 1. Athletic Injuries—diagnosis—Case Reports. 2. Musculoskeletal
System—injuries—Case Reports. 3. Sports Medicine—methods—Case Reports.
QT 261 B534a 2010]
  RD97.B49 2010
  617.1'027—dc22

                                                                2010022836

First published 2011 by Holcomb Hathaway, Publishers, Inc.

Published 2017 by Routledge
2 Park Square, Milton Park, Abingdon, Oxon OX14 4RN
711 Third Avenue, New York, NY 10017, USA

Routledge is an imprint of the Taylor & Francis Group, an informa business

Copyright © 2011 by Taylor & Francis

ISBN 978-1-934432-01-3 (pbk)

Contents

O rthopedic assessment is an essential link to becoming a successful clinician. Being able to competently diagnose an injury allows a clinician to determine the appropriate clinical rehabilitation required for the patient, plan an appropriate prevention program to reduce the likelihood of re-injury, and help avoid negative repercussions. Without an accurate diagnosis or understanding of the pathophysiology or pathomechanics involved with an injury, there may be significant consequences, with the potential for disability or death.

Unfortunately, cognitive and psychomotor competencies are often taught and assessed as fragmented pieces rather than as a whole. This fragmentation places students at a disadvantage because they may not develop the ability to systematically acquire and interpret needed information and to make clinical connections between classroom theory and reality. To use a jigsaw puzzle as an analogy, students may possess all the necessary pieces (learned components of an injury assessment) to put together the puzzle (complete an injury assessment), but they may lack the ability to actually put those pieces together. The pieces are meaningless unless they can be systematically joined to form a complete image.

A systematic approach can help readers learn how to make these connections—to put the pieces together. By repeatedly and logically applying the various skills and knowledge they have learned in their courses, students can become skilled at combining and applying the key information needed to guide their physical examination and to determine the correct clinical diagnosis. The case studies in *Athletic and Orthopedic Injury Assessment: A Case Study Approach* are meant to foster this approach. Each case study and its corresponding questions are aimed at fostering the continued development and refinement of independent learners who understand injury evaluation as part of a whole system. The case study questions and answers are designed using an evidence-based approach to ensure clinical decisions are based on the best available evidence (at the time of writing), clinical expertise, and patient preferences rather than on anecdotal practice.

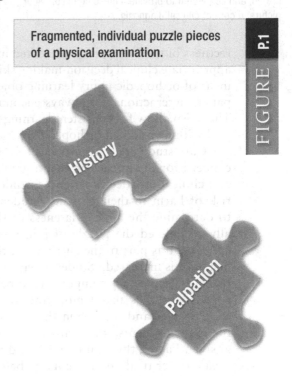

Fragmented, individual puzzle pieces of a physical examination.

FIGURE P.1

This book uses the higher-level thinking required of the National Athletic Trainers' Association Executive Committee for Education (NATA-ECE) clinical proficiencies.[5] The proficiencies have been written using the higher levels of Bloom's taxonomy: comprehend, apply, analyze, synthesize, and then evaluate. This book follows this learning process by allowing students to step into the role of an evaluating clinician as they acquire and interpret information and attempt to make rational, evidence-based, and ethical clinical decisions. By thoroughly reading the scenarios and answering the corresponding questions, readers must comprehend the content of the cases, analyze the data and actions, synthesize the information, and then evaluate the situation and their own reactions. Through this process, readers combine classroom theory (knowledge and comprehension) with clinical reality (application).

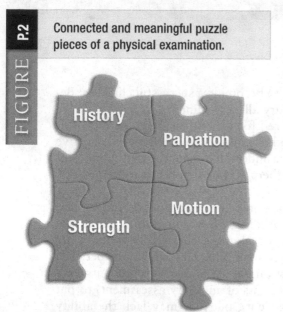

FIGURE P.2

Connected and meaningful puzzle pieces of a physical examination.

History

Palpation

Motion

Strength

Physical examination information must be acquired, interpreted, and connected to provide a meaningful complete picture: a correct clinical diagnosis.

WHY USE CASE STUDIES?

As an educational strategy used in a variety of professional preparation programs, case studies create a safe, simulated learning environment. Students learn to acquire, analyze, and judge the correctness of the information presented in the case, and react to and communicate the appropriate clinical decision-making skills. Case studies help to demonstrate achievement of orthopedic injury learning objectives and expose students to situations and patient interactions not always encountered during clinical education experiences. They also allow for consistent learning and ensure that all students have a chance to deal with a variety of orthopedic injuries.

Case study analysis provides for "safe experimentation and reflection without concern for the impact on real organizations or clients."[4] Using classroom theory and clinical practice experiences, students can make clinical decisions without any risk of harm to their patients. Students can then reflect upon these experiences, to determine the appropriateness of their actions and whether or not they actually completed the puzzle of injury evaluation. When these reflective behaviors are taught as part of the curriculum, the potential to change professional practice behavior is increased.[2] Students learn how to engage in lifelong self-assessment and reflection, necessary components to becoming a competent professional.[1,6]

Case studies also demonstrate that in some situations there may be no clear, easy answer and that often there is not one correct answer. This is a challenge for many students, and many clinicians, who may seek a clear, black and white answer. Facing this reality and building the skills needed to deal with these gray areas are critical components of being ready to face the complicated world of real patients.

HOW TO USE THIS BOOK

W e hope that *Athletic and Orthopedic Injury Assessment: A Case Study Approach* will be an integral part of the educational and clinical component of an athletic training education program. Much of the information presented should be a review of content taught in individual academic or clinical courses; however, new information may be presented to further enhance the learning and problem-solving experiences. These case studies can be used in a variety of courses and settings including:

- upper and lower body assessment
- clinical/practicum
- test preparation
- capstone courses or seminars, as a way of bridging the gap between "snapshots" of content and actually applying or integrating all course content
- clinical settings, as a way to show mastery of the subject matter.

The more than 130 case studies in this text are grouped into chapters by area of the body, but the chapters or even cases do not need to be used in this order. All of the cases are intended to address the goal of "learning over time," in which readers must demonstrate not only the correct decisions to be made, but also what not to do in a given situation. Finally, the case studies may be useful in preparing for the Board of Certification national certification examination. The computer-based examination utilizes case scenarios both in the multiple choice and testlet questions. Students are required to read, acquire, and interpret information presented on an examination, and then make appropriate clinical decisions based on their knowledge. The questions following each case ask readers to assess the injury and also to comment on the actions of the characters in regard to professional behaviors, ethics, communication skills, and other tools needed to function as a clinician.

The answers to the first two cases of each chapter are included in Appendix A of this book. These will give readers an idea how to formulate their answers and will assist students who may need examples to stimulate their thinking. A companion book, *Athletic & Orthopedic Injury Assessment: Case Responses and Interpretations*, is available, including suggested answers to all case questions in this book. An electronic version of this companion book is available to instructors who adopt this casebook. For instructors preferring a print version, copies are available for purchase (and you will also have the option to make printed copies available to your students). Instructors can find more information about this companion book at www.routledge.com/9781934432013 (see the information page for this book) or by contacting your sales representative via email or phone. A PowerPoint presentation is also available upon adoption. The presentation will assist you in your class discussion by providing:

- a list of case participants
- a copy of the case questions
- images to support answers
- main points from the anatomical reviews
- suggestions regarding ligamentous and special tests

All of the above will provide a quick reference as you work through the case questions and answers with your students.

USING THE CASE STUDIES AS A LEARNING TOOL

In this text, the written cases are a combination of actual experiences encountered by the authors during their professional careers, modifications of case reports found in the literature, and fictional situations created to simulate what a clinician may experience. The cases typically contain enough information to allow students to identify the patient's clinical diagnosis. Occasionally information may be omitted, or inaccurate, or designed to create professional or ethical dilemmas, thus forcing students to challenge the clinical competence and decision-making skills of the clinician in the case. Some case studies provide clear objectives, asking students to address only one concern, while others are written using a variety of qualitative and quantitative information to allow students to learn and practice how to systematically approach a situation and make appropriate decisions. Finally, some cases will require students to think beyond the injury assessment process and incorporate other educational competencies, professional behaviors, ethics, communication skills, and other athletic training tools necessary to function as a professional.[6]

The cases can be assigned to individual students, teams, or a class to promote student-to-student exchanges and peer learning[4] through role playing. Role playing deals with problems or situations where students must analyze and interpret information, act out the problem or situation, and then reflect and discuss the consequences of these actions.[3]

We recommend a modification to the "WHAT" framework as one method of assisting students in becoming reflective clinicians.[2] It encompasses three phases: "What," "So What," and "Now What."

- "What" begins with a careful reading of a case study. This phase also includes the reader returning to the case and describing in his or her own words exactly what has just occurred and how he or she would have handled the situation. This response, often in the form of a clinical decision, can be expressed either verbally or in a written format.
- The "So What" phase comes after an individual has identified what happened and responded to the situation. The So-What is an opportunity for an individual to examine his or her own feelings regarding the case, determine the effects of what the case's clinician did or did not do to handle the situation, and finally, determine if these decisions, actions, or responses are in line with those of others and, more important, learn from these actions or decisions.
- The "Now What" phase takes what has been learned and allows one to apply it to his or her professional practice by asking "What can or should I do differently when I am confronted with this particular situation?"

The following are additional suggestions intended to help you use the case studies to improve student learning and bridge classroom theory and clinical practice experiences so students can make the appropriate clinical decisions.

1. Begin by reading through the case scenarios. They are divided into sections according to joints. If students are unfamiliar with some of the medical abbreviations, a list of acronyms and terms is included in the book's Glossary.

2. Select the case scenarios most appropriate for your class. (Although the cases in this book are unnamed so as not to reveal the diagnosis, each chapter of the companion answer book opens with a quick reference list of the cases and the con-

ditions they address.) Cases can be assigned to individuals or as group homework assignments, in-class group discussions, or acted out through role playing.

3. If cases are assigned as homework, be sure to assign the cases several days prior to the due date as many cases require students to evaluate the current literature to determine the best evidence-based practice. Written assignments provide an opportunity for you to assess students' abilities to analyze, interpret, and synthesize the case; make clinical decisions; and evaluate the literature. It also is a chance for students to practice writing skills and time-management skills.

4. Review the answers provided in the companion answer book prior to class. While every effort has been made to provide accurate information, changes in best practices may occur over time. Also, previous education and clinical experiences and certainly geographical location may impact the end result or handling of the case. Adjust or modify your answers accordingly; differences of opinion are good—they help students understand that they will not be working in a vacuum.

5. Review the answers with your students. The companion PowerPoint will help with this process by allowing you to present case questions to your students as you and your class discuss the cases and work through the answers. The PowerPoint also allows you to share related art from the *Case Responses and Interpretations* companion book, such as photographs showing correct testing procedures and actual injury locations. Ask students to reflect on your answers, their answers, and their clinical experiences. Ask them to determine why they did or did not answer a question a certain way. Ask them to identify what they learned from the assignment.

6. If you opt for a group discussion, focus on bridging the classroom theory with clinical practice. For example, ask them what makes this case different from reality if they have had the opportunity to experience a similar case. Again determine why students did or did not answer a question a certain way. Have them identify what they learned from the assignment and how this may change their practice behaviors. Ask how they would handle the situation after reading the case and taking part in the discussion.

7. If role playing is used, assign the cases several days prior to class so students are able to learn their roles. (Since there is no formal script, students will need time to prepare.) Role playing can be conducted in several different formats. A basic form includes allowing a student to act the part of the patient in the case while another student (or students) acts as the clinician(s). Consider providing the "actors" with the clinical diagnosis so they can then research and elaborate on any information lacking in the case. Encourage them to really "play the part"; the more they engage in the role the more lifelike it will be. This is an opportunity for you to assess their clinical decision-making, application, communication, and interpersonal skills. Have the non-acting students critique the other students' application skills. Challenge them to identify alternative approaches to handling the situation.

8. Feel free to modify or add questions as needed to help focus on other athletic training cognitive and psychomotor skills. (A list of suggested additional questions is provided in Chapter 1 of the companion book.) The case questions should be a jumping-off point for your lectures or classroom discussions. For example, in the rotator cuff impingement case study in Chapter 4, the answers focus only on injury evaluation, so you may decide to:

- Add an additional paragraph on initial care and then have students follow up with a rehabilitation plan.
- Add additional questions focusing on the use of therapeutic modalities.
- Create a writing assignment based on the case.

If you wish to offer possible modifications or other suggestions, please feel free to contact us via our publisher at info@hh-pub.com. Constructive feedback, suggestions, and comments are always welcome. Enjoy the case studies, and remember we are all in this together, educating students.

ACKNOWLEDGMENTS

We would like to thank the following individuals, who reviewed this book at various stages and offered suggestions for improving it: Joel Beam, University of North Florida; Joel Bloom, University of Houston; Ray Castle, Louisiana State University; Andrew Doyle, Indiana Wesleyan University; David Draper, Brigham Young University; Joe Gallo, Salem State College; Paul Geisler, Ithaca College; Brian Hughes, Central Missouri State University; Tamerah Hunt, The Ohio State University; Pat Lamboni, Salisbury University; James Leone, Bridgewater State College; William Lyons, University of Wyoming; Mary Meier, Iowa State University; William Pitney, Northern Illinois University; Christopher Rizzo, University of New England; Jeff Roberts, San José State University; Julie Rochester, Northern Michigan University; James Scifers, Western Carolina University; Benito Velasquez, University of Southern Mississippi; Rhonda Verdegan, University of Wisconsin–Stevens Point; Janet Wilbert, The University of Tennessee at Martin; and Ericka Zimmerman, University of Charleston West Virginia. The book is better as a result of their constructive comments, and we appreciate their help.

Our sincere thanks to those individuals who contributed case studies to this book; their names are credited on the opening pages of those cases. We would like to thank the athletic training students who over the years have offered their insight in the development of these case studies. Thanks, too, to those who either provided images or participated in the photo shoots including Joel Bass, Landon Deru, and Nikki Pappas. Many thanks to those at Holcomb Hathaway: Lauren Salas and Colette Kelly, who believed in and supported this project; Gay Pauley, whose professionalism and patience was invaluable; and the rest of the staff and freelancers. Finally, to our family and friends, thank you for your support and understanding throughout this project.

References

1. Branch W, Paranjape A. Feedback and reflection: Teaching methods for clinical settings. *Acad Med.* 2002;77:1185–1188.

2. Driscoll J. Reflective practice for practice. *Senior Nurse.* 1994;13(7):47–50.

3. Joyce B, Weil M. *Models of Teaching* (8th ed.). Boston, MA: Allyn and Bacon; 2009.

4. National Athletic Trainers' Association. *Athletic Training Educational Competencies* (4th ed.). Dallas, TX: Author; 2006.

5. Salmons J. Case methods for online learning [electronic version]. 2006, *E-learning Magazine.* Available at: http://www.elearnmag.org/subpage.cfm?section=tutorials&article=11-1. Accessed July 19, 2010.

6. Westberg J, Jason H. Fostering learners' reflection and self-assessment. *Fam Med.* 1994;26(5):278–282.

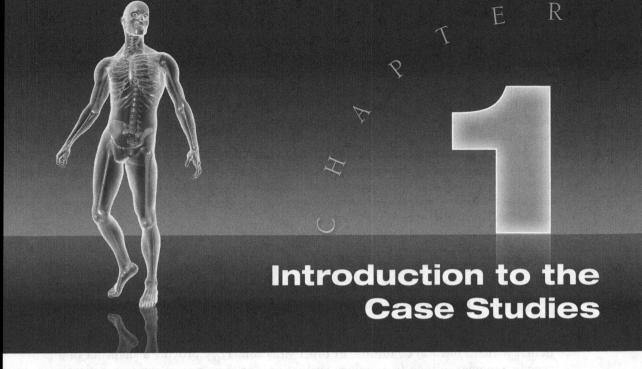

CHAPTER 1

Introduction to the Case Studies

INTRODUCTION

C ertified athletic trainers are qualified and credentialed health care professionals who assist in (1) the prevention of injuries and illnesses; (2) the recognition,
evaluation, and diagnosis of injuries and illnesses; (3) the immediate care of
injuries and illnesses; (4) the treatment, rehabilitation, and reconditioning of injuries
and illnesses; (5) the administration of the health care system; and (6) professional
development.[1] The National Athletic Trainers' Association Executive Committee for
Education (NATA-ECE) also emphasizes the need for proper recognition and management of orthopedic injuries through their support of numerous learning objectives
(cognitive and psychomotor competencies) and outcomes (clinical proficiencies) in
the area of orthopedic clinical examination and diagnosis.[3] These learning objectives and outcomes help prepare you to become competent and effective health care
clinicians. The NATA educational materials have been written using the higher levels of Bloom's taxonomy scale, which includes comprehending, applying, analyzing,
synthesizing, and then evaluating. These are skills that will help you make rational
clinical decisions. This text uses a case-study approach to assist you in the learning
process by allowing you to step into the role of an evaluating clinician and put your
knowledge into practice.

Being able to competently diagnose an injury is critical for allowing a clinician
to determine the appropriate clinical rehabilitation required for an injured patient.
Without an accurate understanding of the pathophysiology or pathomechanics involved in the injury, it may also be difficult for the clinician to plan an appropriate
prevention program to reduce the likelihood of re-injury. Finally, there may be times
when incorrectly diagnosing an injury may have significant repercussions (e.g., death
or disability). Therefore, it is important to have the chance to practice diagnostic

skills and learn to make thoughtful, evidence-based decisions. The case studies in this book provide this chance because they allow for "safe experimentation and reflection without concern for the impact on real organizations or clients."[4] You can use theory and experience from clinical practice to make clinical decisions without any risk of harm to actual patients. Case studies allow you to then reflect on these experiences, determining the appropriateness of your actions and connecting the information you have learned about injury evaluation.

The case studies can also be useful if you are preparing for the Board of Certification national certification examination. In the exam, you will be called on to read, acquire, and interpret information presented in scenarios similar to those in this book and then to make appropriate clinical decisions based on your knowledge. These case studies will accustom you to that format.

WHAT IS A CASE STUDY?

A case study has been described as a "description of an actual situation, commonly involving a decision, a challenge, an opportunity, a problem, or an issue faced by a person (or persons) in an organization."[2] Case studies used in the health care setting are fictional, researched, or actual encounters with a particular patient, medical condition, or other situation. They provide a snapshot of a specific moment in time (e.g., injury evaluation); or they may examine a patient's condition from the onset of the condition to its resolution (e.g., case reports in peer-reviewed journals).

The case studies in this book are meant to simulate what you may encounter in the real world and to assist you in learning how to make appropriate clinical decisions using a step-wise approach. As Woolever[6] suggests, there is no right approach to clinical decision making and each practitioner will approach a case slightly differently using various methods and acquired data. However, he does provide four strategies to improve the likelihood of making the correct decision.[6] These strategies include the following steps:

1. Determine your probabilities. What is the likelihood the patient has a specific diagnosis, based on his or her signs, symptoms, history, physical examination, and so on?

2. Gather data by further evaluating the patient, gathering additional history, taking vital signs, and performing a physical exam.

3. Update your probabilities, including the pre-test probability of any tests or procedures a practitioner may perform. Carefully collect and interpret additional data from these procedures and any other diagnostic tests.

4. Consider a treatment to see whether it crosses your treatment threshold. If it does, consider the patient's context before moving forward. If you don't have enough information to convince yourself to cross the threshold, consider other options, which may include gathering additional data or watchful waiting.

If you would like more guidance, the University of California, San Diego School of Medicine also addresses the concept of clinical decision making and offers two case examples of the step-wise approach to this process (http://meded.ucsd.edu/clinicalmed/thinking.htm).

HOW TO USE THIS BOOK

E ach of the case chapters examines a different region of the body (e.g., head and face, cervical spine, and so forth). These chapters open with an anatomical review to focus your attention on the particular anatomical area and to provide you with a brief recap of the major structures, if needed. You will then find that each case focuses on a particular injury or injuries. For the first two cases of each chapter, the answers have been included in the answer appendix of the book. This is to provide you with examples of how the questions can be answered and to get your mind moving if you don't know how to begin.

The cases found in this text are based on real incidents encountered by the authors during clinical practice, on case studies found in research and articles, and on some fictional situations developed from research. Be aware that some of the actions taken by the practitioners in the case studies are incorrect and that sometimes a clear answer will not be readily available. You will be asked to analyze situations that go beyond the injury assessment process; address issues in professional behavior, ethics, and communication; and exercise other skills necessary to function as a clinician. (See Appendix B for the Board of Certification's Standards of Professional Practice.)

The following directions are intended to help you get the most out of the book and to guide you through the learning process.

1. Begin by reading all the way through the case study once or twice. Reading the cases at least twice will allow you to begin to gather a better sense of the situation. Most cases will begin with an opening paragraph that sets the scene for the injury. A history and physical examination will then follow, typically providing enough information to guide the injury evaluation process. Remember, however, that sometimes not all of the information is complete or accurate. It is your job to analyze the case critically and determine what is missing, incomplete, or inaccurate. Some cases provide diagnostic imaging results, immediate care, or rehabilitation techniques to assist in the process. A glossary of commonly used abbreviations and terms is available at the end of this book.

2. Read through the case again, highlighting the information you believe is key. Restate to yourself what has occurred and how and what you would have done in this situation. The use of different-colored highlighters may help you categorize the information you have analyzed and interpreted. This process can assist you in piecing together segments of information to make correct clinical decisions. For example, use yellow for correct actions and decisions made by the athletic trainer and for clinically relevant information in the case, orange for incorrect actions, pink for questionable actions and decisions, blue for information and terms you are not familiar with, and green for ethical or legal dilemmas. A sample case is shown in Figure 1.1, with different patterns indicating the various colors.

   The highlighting will help you organize the information in the case and plan your course of action. You can clearly review all of the clinically relevant information, such as Madison's explanation of how she jammed her index finger, her discomfort level, the position of her second DIPJ, and what was revealed during DIPJ extension. You will be aware of everything you need to review, such as myotomes and dermatomes. You will also be reminded of Tyler's incorrect decision to manipulate the joint and of his ethically questionable decision not

| FIGURE | 1.1 | Sample case study with highlighting (patterns stand in for colors on this black and white version). |

Madison, a 12-year-old basketball player and avid video gamer, was at the local athletic club playing in a youth league basketball tournament. As she moved down the court her teammate passed the ball to Madison when she was not paying attention. Realizing the pass was for her, Madison attempted to catch the ball off the tip of her fingers but missed. She immediately grabbed her finger and began crying. The referee called a time out and her coach went to see what was wrong. Her coach recognized her finger was deformed and immediately placed ice on her finger. He called the front desk and requested further medical care. Tyler, a certified strength and conditioning coach and certified athletic trainer who worked for the athletic club, was asked to evaluate Pam's finger.

History: As Tyler begins his history he notes that Madison is supporting her left index finger. Madison explains to Tyler that the basketball "jammed" her index finger. Further questioning by Tyler reveals that when the ball struck the index finger of the involved hand, the finger was straight. Madison denies any popping or unusual sounds; however, she rates her pain 7/10.

Physical Examination: On physical examination Madison presents with moderate-to-severe discomfort. Madison's second DIPJ appears to be in a flexed position and Tyler tries to manipulate the joint. No swelling or ecchymosis is present at this time. Tyler determines Madison is point tender on the dorsum of the DIPJ. Passive range of motion is WNL, while MMT reveals 0/5 during DIPJ extension. Tyler's assessment of the collateral ligament stability is unremarkable. Neurologically Madison's myotomes and dermatomes are intact.

Tyler decides not to call Madison's parents and explains to her what has occurred and the required immediate and follow-up care. Madison completes some necessary paper work and goes home.

         = yellow   = orange   = blue   = green

to call Madison's parents. The highlighting allows you to take all aspects into account when formulating your own response to the case.

3. If you are working in pairs or small groups, compare your actions and/or decisions with those of your partners. If differences arise, determine why these differences occurred, and discuss the different interpretations of the case.

4. After highlighting and reviewing the case study, answer the questions as if you were the athletic trainer in charge. When necessary, be critical of the decisions made by the athletic trainers in the case studies. They will not be offended if you tell them they were wrong or their decisions were inappropriate.

5. Be sure to answer the questions completely; some questions contain multiple parts. There may be several interpretations involved in answers, so write down everything you think would be pertinent or acceptable. When asked to document the results of the physical examination, consider using the SOAP note format (see Appendix B).

TABLE 1.1	Select listing of evidence-based medicine resources.[5]
BIBLIOGRAPHIC DATABASES	
PubMed (MEDLINE)	http://www.ncbi.nlm.nih.gov/entrez/query.fcgi
SPORT Discus (sports medicine/fitness)	http://www.sportdiscus.com/
CINAHL (nursing/allied health)	http://www.cinahl.com/index.html
EMBASE (international biomedical)	http://www.embase.com/
GENERAL EVIDENCE-BASED MEDICINE RESOURCES	
Cochrane Library	www.cochrane.org
SportsMed Update	www.sportsmedupdate.info
ACP Journal Club/Best Evidence	http://www.acpjc.org/?hp
UpToDate	http://www.uptodate.com
PEDro	http://www.pedro.fhs.usyd.edu.au/
Hooked on Evidence	http://www.apta.org/hookedonevidence/index.cfm
Evidence-Based Medicine Online	http://ebm.bmjjournals.com
Bandolier Evidence-Based Health Care	http://www.jr2.ox.ac.uk/bandolier/extra.html
Centre for Evidence-Based Medicine	http://www.cebm.net/index.asp
BestBETs	http://www.bestbets.org/

Reprinted with permission.

6. Many questions may require you to evaluate and review the current literature in order to determine if your clinical actions or decisions, or the actions of the case's clinician, follow the best evidenced-based practice currently available (Table 1.1). This allows you to determine the effects of what you did and whether you are following the standard of care. Consider using the references in each chapter as a starting point.

7. Review your answers with your instructor, and examine your responses to the case before and after you learned his or her answers. Determine whether or not you handled the situation correctly. If not, reflect on what you can learn from your actions or decisions and what you can do to avoid making the same mistake(s).

8. Now, take all that you have learned and apply it to your professional practice by asking, "What can I do differently if I am confronted with this particular situation?" or "How can I improve my patient outcomes?"

9. One last piece of advice: Don't wait until the last minute to complete your assignment, because not all of the answers are readily available.

Enjoy and learn from the case studies!

REFERENCES

1. Board of Certification. *Board of Certification Role Delineation Study.* 5th ed. Omaha, NE: Board of Certification; 2004.

2. Mauffette-Leenders LA, Erskine, JA, Leenders MR. *Learning with Cases.* London, Ontario, Canada: Ivey Publishing; 1997.

3. National Athletic Trainers' Association. *Athletic Training Educational Competencies.* 4th ed. Dallas, TX: National Athletic Trainers' Association; 2006.

4. Salmons J. Case methods for online learning [Electronic Version]. *E-learning Magazine;* 2006.

Available from: http://www.elearnmag.org/subpage.cfm?section=tutorials&article=11-1. Accessed May 25, 2007.

5. Steves R, Hootman JM. Evidence-based medicine: What is it and how does it apply to athletic training? *J Ath Train.* 2004;39(1):83–87.

6. Woolever DR. The art and science of clinical decision making [Electronic Version]. *Family Practice Management.* 2008;15(5):31–38. Available from: http://www.aafp.org/fpm/2008/0500/p31.html. Accessed April 20, 2010.

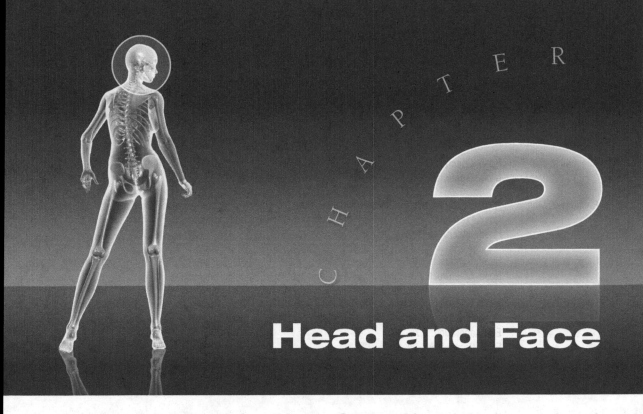

2

Head and Face

INTRODUCTION

I n this chapter we will examine the clinical evaluation and management of 19 different head and face pathologies using a combination of on-field and off-field scenarios. The cases are primarily traumatic events that commonly occur while engaging in athletics and/or physical activity. We believe these cases, several of which are based on actual cases seen in our clinical practice over the years, are a good representation of athletic injuries and illness that can occur to the eye, ear, nose, jaw, and brain. Keep in mind that some of the cases presented in this chapter, as in many of the chapters, intentionally include inappropriate actions or mismanagement by the clinician.

The area of the head and face includes the ear, eye, nose, mouth, teeth, tongue, and jaw. An acute trauma sustained to the head and face is often the result of a direct blow from athlete-to-athlete contact, a playing apparatus (e.g., sticks, standards, the ground), or a high velocity projectile (e.g., ball or puck).[1-6,9-15] Epidemiological studies conducted by the Injury Surveillance System of the National Collegiate Athletic Association (NCAA) from the 1988–1989 athletic season through the 2003–2004 season demonstrate that of all the reported injuries sustained during games and practices, concussions top the list as the most prevalent of all head and facial injuries. Nasal fractures were the second most common of all reported head and facial injuries. Athletes in all 15 NCAA sports reported were at risk.

Of the 15 reported sports, women's field hockey appears to place athletes at the greatest risk for head and facial trauma,[11] with women's lacrosse a close second (Table 2.1). In women's field hockey, injuries classified as above-the-neck accounted for almost one quarter (24%) of all injuries sustained during a game. A majority of the injuries result from contact with a stick or ball. Trauma occurred to the head (41.2%), nose (20.9%), face (18.5%), eye (7.5%), mouth (5.8%), teeth (2.4%),

TABLE 2.1	Head and face competition and practice injuries across 15 NCAA sports.[1–6,9–15,20,21]		
SPORT	COMPETITION INJURIES	PRACTICE INJURIES	MECHANISM OF INJURY
Baseball	Head, Concussion: 3.3% Nose, Fracture: 1.0%	Head, Concussion: 1.6% Nose, Fracture: 1.1%	Player contact, other contact (wall, balls, ground)
Basketball, Men	Head, Concussion: 3.6% Nose, Fracture: 1.7% Head, Laceration: 1.0%	Head, Concussion: 3.0% Nose, Fracture: 1.5%	Player contact, other contact (standards, balls, ground)
Basketball, Women	Head, Concussion: 6.5% Nose, Fracture: 1.7%	Head, Concussion: 3.7% Nose, Fracture: 1.2%	Player contact, other contact (standards, balls, ground)
Field Hockey	Head, Concussion: 9.4% Nose, Fracture: 5.2% Eye, Laceration: 1.7% Face, Contusion: 1.7%	Head, Concussion: 3.4%	Player contact, other contact (sticks, balls, ground)
Football	Head, Concussion: 6.8%	Head, Concussion: 5.5%	Player contact, other contact (balls, blocking dummies, ground)
Gymnastics	Head, Concussion: 2.6%	Head, Concussion: 2.3%	Contact with an object (such as apparatus or floor)
Ice Hockey, Men	Head, Concussion: 9.0% Chin, Laceration: 1.6%	Head, Concussion: 5.3%	Player contact, other contact (pucks, boards, dummies, ice)
Ice Hockey, Women	Head, Concussion: 21.6%	Head, Concussion: 13.6%	Player contact, other contact (pucks, boards, dummies, ice)
Lacrosse, Men	Head, Concussion: 8.6%	Head, Concussion: 3.6%	Player contact, other contact (balls, sticks, or the ground)
Lacrosse, Women	Head, Concussion: 9.8% Nose, Fracture: 2.5% Head, Laceration: 1.3% Eye, Contusion: 1.2%	Head, Concussion: 4.6% Nose, Fracture: 2.2% Eye, Contusion: 1.3%	Player contact, other contact (ball, sticks, ground)
Soccer, Men	Head, Concussion: 5.8% Head, Laceration: 1.5% Nose, Fracture: 1.2%	Head, Concussion: 1.8%	Player contact, other contact (balls, goals, ground)
Soccer, Women	Head, Concussion: 8.6% Nose, Fracture: 1.1%	Head, Concussion: 2.2%	Player contact, other contact (balls, goals, or the ground)
Softball	Head, Concussion: 6.0% Nose, Fracture: 1.0%	Head, Concussion: 2.8% Nose, Fracture: 1.3%	Player contact, other contact (ball, bases, fence, ground)
Volleyball	Head, Concussion: 4.7%	Head, Concussion: 2.0%	Player contact, other contact (balls, standards, floor)
Wrestling	Head, Concussion: 4.8% Nose, Fracture: 1.0%	Head, Concussion 2.5%	Player contact, other contact (match, benches)

temporomandibular joint (2.4%), and ear (1%). Note that the only facial protection required of all collegiate field hockey players is a mouth guard. In women's lacrosse, mouthguards and protective eyewear are the only required protection.[24]

In high school, rare injuries and conditions (defined as eye injuries, dental injuries, neck and cervical injuries, and dehydration) accounted for 3.5 percent of all high school athletes' injuries during the 2005–2006 and 2006–2007 school years.[18] Eye and dental traumas were the most commonly seen in baseball and boys' and girls' basketball, probably resulting from a lack of head or facial protection. Common eye injuries included contusions, lacerations, and abrasions (12.8%, $n = 5$), with one injury resulting in a loss of peripheral vision. Common dental injuries were tooth avulsions, fractures, and luxations. Only three injured athletes were wearing applicable protective mouthguards.

ANATOMICAL REVIEW

Head

The human head consists of the skull and brain. Trauma sustained to the head can result not only in tearing of the outermost layer of protective tissue (the scalp) but also in a skull fracture and/or trauma to the brain.

Skull

The skull, which is wider posteriorly than anteriorly, is comprised of 22 flat or irregular-shaped bones joined together by an irregular-shaped immovable joint (the joint of the mandible, which is commonly known as the jaw, is the exception). The skull can be divided into two specific areas: the cranium section and the facial section (Table 2.2). The cranium (brain case) consists of eight bones and protects the brain and brain stem (Figure 2.1). The facial skeleton is comprised of the remaining 14 bones.

The outmost protective covering of the skull is the scalp. This is a very resilient, highly vascular structure that functions to help absorb impact forces if the skull strikes the ground or is struck with an object (projectile, stick) or by another person.

TABLE 2.2	Bones of the skull.
CRANIUM	**FACIAL**
Frontal bone	Inferior nasal conchae (right and left)
Ethmoid bone	Lacrimal (right and left)
Occipital bone	Mandible
Sphenoid bone	Maxilla (right and left)
Parietal bone (right and left)	Nasal (right and left)
Temporal bone (right and left)	Palatine (right and left)
	Vomer
	Zygomatic (right and left)

FIGURE   2.1   Lateral view of the skull.

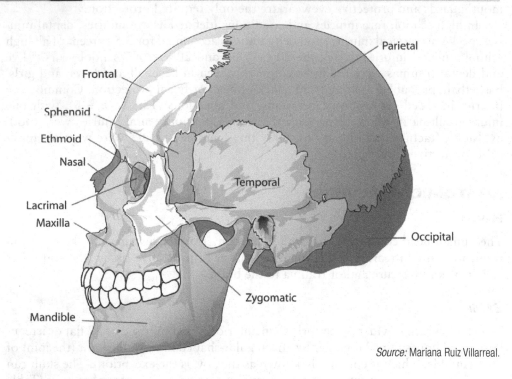

Parietal

Frontal

Sphenoid

Ethmoid

Nasal

Temporal

Lacrimal

Maxilla

Occipital

Zygomatic

Mandible

Source: Mariana Ruiz Villarreal.

Brain

The brain, which is housed and protected by the cranium, consists of the cerebrum, diencephalon (which includes the thalamus and hypothalamus), cerebellum, and brainstem (which includes the midbrain, pons, and medulla) (Table 2.3). Specific structures called sulci and fissures divide parts of the brain into lobes. An athlete who is struck in the head may present with signs and symptoms and/or deficits in function specifically associated with trauma to a particular lobe.

TABLE   2.3   Structures and functions of the brain.[17,23]

STRUCTURE	FUNCTION
Cerebrum	
Frontal	Considered the emotional control center and home to one's personality. Responsible for cognition (intelligence, problem solving, memory), expressive language, motor planning and function, mathematical calculations, motivation, self-insight, and regulation of emotions.
Occipital	Responsible for interpretation of visual stimuli from the optic pathway.
Parietal	Responsible for sensory detection, perception, and interpretation.
Temporal	Responsible for hearing, comprehension of language, and long-term memory.

TABLE	2.3	Continued.

Diencephalon

Thalamus	Receives sensory information from the sensory organs and relays the information to the appropriate parts of the cerebral hemispheres.
Hypothalamus	Responsible for regulating the autonomic nervous system, releases hormones from the pituitary gland, regulates temperature, hunger, thirst, fatigue, and circadian rhythm.
Epithalamus	Responsible for the secretion of melatonin and regulating food and water intake.
Subthalamus	Responsible for regulating movements produced by the skeletal muscles.
Cerebellum	Responsible for unconscious awareness of the body's position in space (proprioception). Accomplishes this by receiving information from joint and muscle receptors, interpreting and making decisions about how to adjust the body for coordinated, precise control of movement and balance.

Brainstem

Midbrain	Plays a role in the automatic reflexive behaviors dealing with vision and hearing.
Pons	Acts as the relay station between the spinal cord, cerebellum, and the cerebrum. Mediates mostly unconscious motor function (e.g., shifting weight balance). Assists in sleep and arousal control and regulates respiration rate.
Medulla oblongata	Acts to carry descending motor messages from the cerebrum to the spinal cord and ascending sensory messages from the spinal cord to the cerebrum. Also contains the respiratory, vasomotor (blood vessel), and cardiac centers controlling breathing, blood pressure, and heart rate, as well as reflex activities such as coughing, gagging, swallowing, and vomiting.

The brain is divided into right and left cerebral hemispheres by a longitudinal fissure. The cerebrum is further divided into four regions, based on their location within the cranium (frontal, parietal, temporal, and occipital) (Figure 2.2), and is responsible for voluntary muscular activities, sensory perceptions (temperature, touch, pain, pressure), special senses (sight, sound, smell, and taste), and the higher brain functions such as memory, learning, and emotions. The cerebellum controls the coordination of voluntary muscular motions. In the brainstem, the pons controls respiration rate, and the medulla oblongata controls functions such as heart rate, breathing, and blood pressure (Figure 2.3).

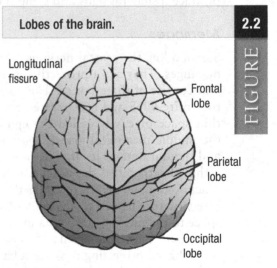

Lobes of the brain.   **2.2**

FIGURE

Longitudinal fissure

Frontal lobe

Parietal lobe

Occipital lobe

Source: AMA Physician Resources.

2.3   Lateral view of the brain.

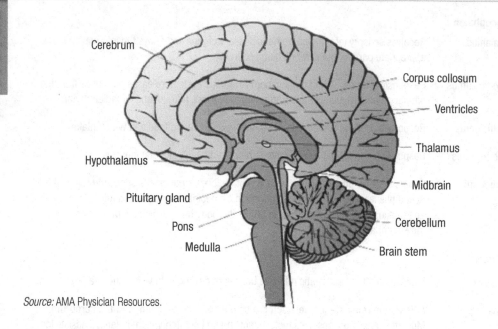

Cerebrum

Corpus collosum

Ventricles

Thalamus

Hypothalamus

Midbrain

Pituitary gland

Pons

Cerebellum

Medulla

Brain stem

Source: AMA Physician Resources.

Cranial nerves

Originating on the brain are 12 pairs of cranial nerves (CN) numbered from anterior to posterior. Considered part of the peripheral nervous system, the cranial nerves provide sensory and motor innervations for the head, neck, and face. Trauma to the brain resulting in intracranial bleeding and increased intracranial pressure will alter the function of any affected cranial nerves, and this can be detected through a complete cranial nerve neurological examination (Table 2.4). Most cranial nerve lesions produce ipsilateral signs and symptoms.

Meninges

Surrounding the central nervous system (CNS) are special structures known as the meninges. They are a protective membrane surrounding the brain and spinal cord and consist of three layers. The outer layer is called the dura mater. It surrounds the entire CNS and is separated from the outside cranial and skeletal bones by a thin space or cavity called the epidural space. Also located in the dura mater is the middle meningeal artery, the main blood arterial supply to the cranial bones and the dura mater itself. The next layer is located beneath the dura mater and is a thin sheath called the arachnoid mater. The space between the dura mater and arachnoid mater is referred to as the subdural space. The arachnoid mater is a delicate structure named for its spider-like filaments passing through the subarachnoid space to the final layer, the pia mater, the innermost layer of the meninges. The pia mater attaches to the brain and spinal cord and follows the contours of the surface of the brain, projecting into the sulci and fissures. The space between the arachnoid and pia mater, the subarachnoid space, is where the cerebral spinal fluid (CSF) is

TABLE	2.4	Cranial nerve functions and examinations.[17,23,26]	

NERVE	NUMBER	FUNCTION	EXAMINATION
I	Olfactory	Smell	■ Have the patient close his eyes, then present an odor.
II	Optic	Visual acuity; pupillary reflex to light; peripheral vision	■ For visual acuity, use a Snellen chart. ■ For peripheral vision, use a finger or penlight and ask the patient to acknowledge when she sees the object in her peripheral vision.
III	Oculomotor	Eyeball movements up, down, medially, and laterally; pupillary reflex to light	■ For eye movement, ask the patient to follow a pen or finger while making an H movement. ■ For pupillary reflex, shine light into patient's pupils (direct and consensual light reflex).
IV	Trochlear	Eyeball movements downward and in toward the nose	■ For eye movement, ask patient to follow pen or finger while making an H movement.
V	Trigeminal	Mastication and sensation	■ For mastication, ask patient to clench teeth and move jaw side-to-side. ■ For sensation, ask patient to close eyes, apply gentle touch, warmth, cold, or pinprick to uninvolved side of forehead, cheek, jaw, and chin. Repeat on involved side.
VI	Abducens	Eyeball movement laterally	■ For eye movement, ask patient to follow pen or finger while making an H movement.
VII	Facial	Facial expression, taste receptors on anterior 2/3 of tongue	■ For facial expression, ask the patient to raise eyebrows, smile (show teeth), frown, and puff out both cheeks. ■ For taste, have patient close eyes, then present sweet, salty, and sour solutions to outer and lateral tongue.
VIII	Vestibulocochlear	Hearing and balance	■ For hearing, ask patient to close eyes and say "left" or "right" when a sound is heard as clinician snaps fingers together very near to, yet not touching, each ear. ■ For balance, perform a Romberg test with patient's eyes open and closed.
IX	Glossopharyngeal	Swallowing and taste receptors on posterior 1/3 of tongue	■ For swallowing, ask patient to swallow and say "Ah." ■ For taste, have patient close eyes, then present sweet, salty, and sour solutions to outer and lateral tongue.
X	Vagus	Speaking and swallowing/ gag reflex	■ For speaking, ask patient to speak clearly. ■ For swallowing/gag reflex, use Q-tip to assess the gag reflex by touching patient's posterior pharyngeal wall.
XI	Spinal accessory	Shoulder shrug (sternocleidomastoid and trapezius)	■ Ask patient to shrug shoulders as strongly as possible while resisting motion.
XII	Hypoglossal	Tongue movement	■ Ask patient to stick out tongue and move it side to side.

contained. The CSF is a clear, colorless fluid circulating between the ventricles of the brain and central canal of the spinal cord. The watery fluid allows the brain to float and acts as a buffer against external forces applied to the head. Trauma such as skull fracture may cause the CSF to leak out of the nose (rhinorrhea) and ears (otorrhea) along with blood.

Face

The facial skeleton consists of nine bones, four of which are paired (nasal, zygomatic, maxilla, and palatine) and one which is unpaired, the mandible.[23] In athletics, structures such as the nasal bone are commonly injured with a direct blow to the face. Protective equipment such as mouthguards and nasal guards help minimize injury.

Nasal

The nose consists of two distinct components, the external nose and the nasal cavity, and is responsible for the following functions: (1) respiration, (2) olfaction (smell), (3) filtration of dust, (4) humidification of inspired air, and (5) reception of nasal secretions.[23,29] The external nose projects antero-inferiorly as it joins the forehead inferiorly via the nasal bridge. The support framework for the external nose is mostly cartilaginous, except for the superior bony part of the nose, which consists of the nasal bone.[23,29] The nose varies in shape and size, based on differences in the nasal cartilage. The two external openings, known as the nares, are separated from each other by the nasal septum.

The nasal cavity is the space between the nostrils and the posterior nasal septum, and it turns into the nasopharynx, the area where air passes through the posterior choanae.[23,29] It is divided into two halves by the nasal septum, and each half consists of a floor, roof, and two walls. The roof of the nasal cavity consists of the frontal and nasal bone, ethmoid and sphenoid. The floor is formed by the maxilla and the plate of the palatine bone. The walls of the nasal cavity include the medial wall, formed by the cartilaginous nasal septum, and lateral wall, formed by the superior, middle, and inferior conchae and the vertical plates of the palatine bones. The superior and middle conchae are part of the ethmoid bone. The nasal cavity is lined with a mucous membrane and hair follicles designed to trap and filter dust particles while warming and moistening the air before it passes to the upper respiratory tract and to the lungs.

The septum is very flexible and has the ability to spring back into shape when compressed. But despite the septum's flexibility, the nose is still vulnerable to trauma simply because of its location.[23,29] Direct trauma can result in damage to the cartilage, nasal bone, soft tissues, and even to the skull, which can result in a leakage of CSF.[29]

Eye

The eye consists of the orbit, the eyeball, and CN II, called the optic nerve. The orbit, or eye socket, is a bony recess located within the skull, and it functions to protect the eye and its associated structures. It also acts as a site of muscle attachment for the eye muscles.[23] The outer or periphery of the orbital opening is the orbital margin. The superior half of the orbital rim is the supraorbital margin and is formed by the frontal bone. The inferior half is the infraorbital margin and is formed laterally by the zygomatic bone and medially by the maxilla. The lateral orbital margin is formed by the frontal and zygomatic bones; the medial orbital margin is formed by the frontal bone and the maxilla. The facial bones form the lateral and medial walls, orbital floor (inferior), and orbital roof (superior). The strongest of these structures is the lateral wall, which consists of the zygomatic and sphenoid bones. The weakest is the medial wall, comprised of the lacrimal, ethmoid, maxilla, and sphenoid bones. This is followed by the floor (inferior wall) of the orbit, which consists of the maxilla, part of the zygomatic bone, and the palatine bone. Weakness of the medial and inferior walls may result in blow-out fractures of the orbit with a sudden increase in intra-orbital pressure (blow to the eye by an object larger than the orbit).

The content of the orbit consists of the optic nerve and the eyeball, a fluid-filled globe that also contains muscles and blood vessels (Figure 2.4). Working together with the optic nerve, the structures of the globe allow for visual acuity, motility, and protection against dirt and debris.[23] The structures of the eye are found in Table 2.5, and the muscles of eye motility are found in Table 2.6.

FIGURE 2.4   Structures of the eyeball.

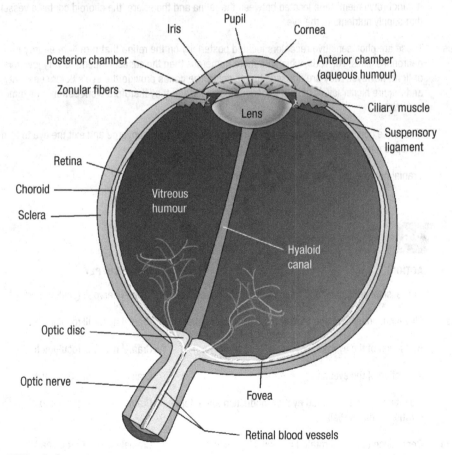

Source: Wikimedia Commons.

TABLE	2.5	Structure and function of the eye.[23,27,28]

STRUCTURE	FUNCTION
Sclera	Known as the "white of the eye," this is the tough, outer envelope of the eye (except for its anterior one sixth, which is the cornea) that becomes continuous with the sheath of the optic nerve.
Cornea	Transparent tissue of the anterior sixth of the outer wall of the eye, continuous with the sclera. The cornea is the chief refractory structure of the eye.
Pupil	Dark circular aperture in the center of the iris. The pupil allows light rays to enter the eye by dilating or constricting.
Iris	The pigmented contractile tissue surrounding the pupil.
Conjunctiva	The mucous membrane surrounding the anterior surface of the eyeball and the inside surface of the eyelids. The conjunctiva is the site of bacterial or viral infections known as conjunctivitis.
Lens	A transparent, concave/convex, elastic structure located behind the iris that serves to sharpen and focus near and distant objects upon the retina.
Retina	A thin and delicate light-sensitive membrane. The retina forms the innermost layer of the eyeball.
Choroid	A dark brown membrane located between the retina and the sclera, the choroid contains vessels that supply nutrients to the eye.
Rods and Cones	These are photosensitive receptors located posteriorly on the retina that turn light energy into neuronal signals. The rods, which are more numerous than the cones, respond to very low levels of light; however, they are not sensitive to color. The cones provide the eye's color sensitivity and require higher levels of light to generate signals, and they therefore work better in daytime conditions.
Optic disc	This is the point where the axons of the retina's ganglion cells converge and exit the eye to form the optic nerve.
Optic nerve	Cranial nerve II, the nerve of sight, is connected to the retina.

TABLE	2.6	Muscles acting on the eye.[23]

MUSCLE	ACTION	NERVE SUPPLY
Inferior rectus	Depression, adduction, and lateral rotation of the eyeball	Cranial nerve III (oculomotor)
Superior rectus	Elevation, adduction, and medial rotation of the eyeball	Cranial nerve III (oculomotor)
Medial rectus	Adduction of the eyeball	Cranial nerve III (oculomotor)
Lateral rectus	Abduction of the eyeball	Cranial nerve VI (abducens)
Inferior oblique	Elevation of medial rotated eyeball, abduction and lateral rotation of the eyeball	Cranial nerve III (oculomotor)
Superior oblique	Depression of medial rotated eyeball, abduction and medial rotation of the eyeball	Cranial nerve IV (trochlear)

Ear

The ear consists of three distinct components: the external ear, the middle ear, and the inner ear. As a whole, the ear is responsible for hearing and balance.[23,25] The external ear contains the pinna (or auricle) and the external auditory canal. Together, these structures collect and conduct sound to the tympanic membrane (eardrum). The middle ear contains air, three small bones known as auditory ossicles (malleus, incus, and staples), a nerve, and two small muscles. The middle ear and external ear are separated by the tympanic membrane (a semitransparent membrane that moves in response to air vibrations passing through the external auditory canal).[23,25] The middle ear is also connected to the nasopharynx via the pharyngotympanic tube (Eustachian tube), which is responsible for equalizing pressure on either side of the tympanic membrane (Figure 2.5). The inner ear contains the vestibulocochlear organs responsible for hearing and balance. The cochlea is considered the organ of hearing; the semicircular canals and the vestibule are the organs of balance.

Oral cavity

The oral cavity includes the lips, cheeks, gingivae, teeth, tongue, and palate.[23] The lips surround the mouth, creating an external border of the oral cavity. They are attached to the gingivae (gums) via the labial frenula, which can be irritated with an improperly fitted mouthguard.[8] The cheeks form the lateral wall of the oral cavity and work in conjunction with the lips, acting as an oral sphincter that moves

---

| FIGURE | 2.5 | Structures of the ear. |

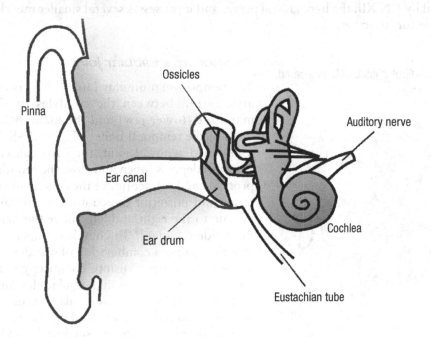

TABLE	2.7	Structure and function of a tooth.

STRUCTURE	FUNCTION
Root	Anchor of the tooth. Fixes the tooth to the tooth socket via the periodontal ligament and cenentum, a layer of bone-like mineralized tissue covering the dentin of the root and neck of a tooth.
Neck	Portion of the tooth between the root and the crown.
Crown	Portion of the tooth that projects from the gingivae and is covered with enamel, or an artificial substitute for that part.

food between the spaces of the lips and check into the oral cavity.[23] The gingivae, a fibrous tissue covered with a mucous membrane, is attached to margins of the alveolar process (tooth sockets) located on the mandible and maxilla and to the teeth themselves.[23] Thirty-two teeth (4 incisors, 2 canines, 4 premolars, and 6 molars per row), equally divided into upper and lower rows, allow for cutting, tearing, crushing, and grinding of food. Each tooth consists of three components (Table 2.7) and is made of dentin (hard calcified substance), enamel (a hard, inert substance covering the dentin of the tooth), and the pulp cavity, which houses the connective tissue, blood vessels, and nerves of the tooth.[23,27]

The palate forms the roof of the oral cavity and the floor of the nasal cavity.[23] The anterior two thirds of the palate is known as the hard palate and the posterior third is known as the soft palpate. The final structure is the tongue, a mobile muscle attached to the floor of the mouth (via the lingual frenulum) and is responsible for mastication (chewing), taste, swallowing, speech, and oral cleaning. The tongue is innervated by CN XII, the hypoglossal nerve, and it possesses several smaller muscles responsible for its action.

FIGURE 2.6 Temporomandibular joint. TMJ is located within the circle.

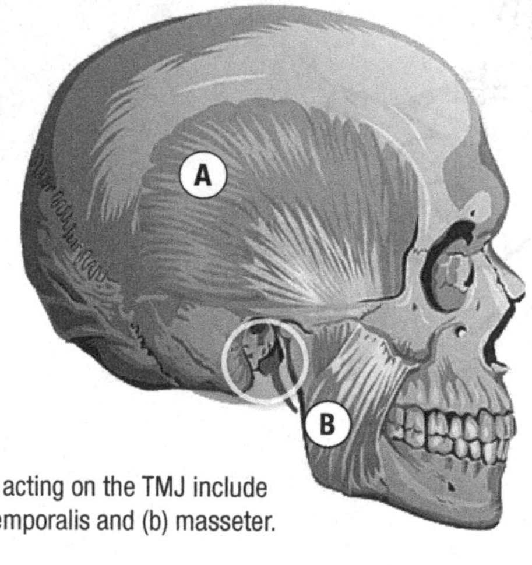

Muscles acting on the TMJ include the (a) temporalis and (b) masseter.

Temporomandibular joint

The temporomandibular joint (TMJ) is the articulation between the condyles of the mandible (lower jaw) and the mandibular fossa of the temporal bone[23] (Figure 2.6). As a modified synovial joint, the TMJ can elevate and depress (open and close the mouth), protrude and retract (move the chin in an anterior and posterior direction), and laterally deviate to the right and left (move the mandible side-to-side).[19] To completely open the mouth requires a combination of mandibular depression and protrusion; completely closing the mouth requires mandibular elevation and retrusion. Normal mandibular depression and protrusion can be assessed by asking the patient to place as many stacked knuckles into the oral cavity as possible (knuckle test), with two being the minimum number of knuckles to indicate a properly functioning TMJ.

The TMJ is surrounded by a fibrous joint capsule that is thickened laterally, forming the temporomandibular ligament. It is further stabilized by the stylomandibular and sphenomandibular ligaments. The TMJ also possesses an intraarticular disc that divides the joint cavity into a superior and inferior compartment.[23] These discs act to increase the congruence of joint and serve as shock absorbers. They are attached to mandible condyles and move with the condyles during movement of the jaw. Muscles acting on the TMJ are located in Table 2.8.

SPECIAL TESTS

M any of the cases in this chapter use different special or neurological assessment procedures to help determine the clinical diagnosis. Although the details on how to perform each and every special and neurological test are beyond the scope of this section, Table 2.9 does provide a list of some of the more common testing procedures used when evaluating head and facial injuries. Refer to Table 2.4 for procedures used to assess the cranial nerves. For a more thorough review, please refer to your favorite evaluation text or journal article(s).

TABLE 2.8	Muscles acting on the temporomandibular joint.		
MUSCLE	**ORIGINS**	**INSERTIONS**	**ACTIONS**
Lateral pterygoid	Superior head: infratemporal surface and intratemporal crest of the wing of sphenoid Inferior head: lateral surface of the lateral pterygoid plate	Neck of mandible, articular disc and joint capsule	Protrudes and depresses mandible bilaterally, unilaterally produces side-to-side movement
Medial pterygoid	Deep head: medial surface of lateral pterygoid plate and palatine bone Superficial: maxilla tuberosity	Surface of medial ramus of mandible	Elevates mandible, protrudes mandible bilaterally, alternates to grind
Masseter	Inferior border and medial surface of zygomatic arch	Lateral surface of ramus of mandible	Elevates and protrudes mandible, deep fibers retract
Temporalis	Temporal fossa, deep surface of the temporal fascia	Coronoid process of the mandible, anterior border of the ramus of the mandible	Elevation, side-to-side grinding movement of the mandible

TABLE 2.9	Special tests of the head and face.
SPECIAL TEST	**FUNCTION**
Fluorescent dye and cobalt blue light	Detection of a corneal abrasion or laceration
Pupillary reaction	Detection of mechanical or neurological deficits of oculomotor nerve (CN III)
Visual acuity	Detection of damage or pressure on the optic cranial nerve (II)
Eye tracking	Detection of damage or pressure on the oculomotor (III), trochlear (IV), or abducens (VI) cranial nerve
Otoscope	Detection of fluid, inflammation, trauma, and foreign objects in the ears, nose, or oral cavity
Tongue blade	Detection of a mandibular fracture
Maxillary fracture	Detection of maxilla fracture
Halo	Detection of CSF leakage
Standardized Assessment of Concussion (SAC)	Objective tool for assessing an athlete's mental status during the acute period after a concussion; measures orientation, immediate memory, concentration, and delayed recall
Neuropsychological testing	Paper-and-pencil or computerized testing to quantify deficits in memory and cognition
Graded symptoms check list	Tools used as part of a concussion assessment to identify an athlete's signs and symptoms following injury
Romberg	Detection of cerebellum dysfunction and damage to the vestibulocochlear cranial nerve (VIII)
Balance Error Scoring System (BESS)	Assesses balance and coordination; uses 3 stance positions and tests on both a firm and a foam surface with the eyes closed and open; scored based on errors performed by the patient

REFERENCES

1. Agel J, Dick R, Nelson B, Marshall SW, Dompier TP. Descriptive epidemiology of collegiate women's ice hockey injuries: National Collegiate Athletic Association Injury Surveillance System, 2000–2001 through 2003–2004. *J Athl Train.* 2007;42(2):249–254.

2. Agel J, Dompier TP, Dick R, Marshall SW. Descriptive epidemiology of collegiate men's ice hockey injuries: National Collegiate Athletic Association Injury Surveillance System, 1988–1989 through 2003–2004. *J Athl Train.* 2007;42(2):241–248.

3. Agel J, Evans TA, Dick R, Putukian M, Marshall SW. Descriptive epidemiology of collegiate men's soccer injuries: National Collegiate Athletic Association Injury Surveillance System, 1988–1989 through 2002–2003. *J Athl Train.* 2007; 42(2): 270–277.

4. Agel J, Olson DE, Dick R, Arendt EA, Marshall SW, Sikka RS. Descriptive epidemiology of collegiate women's basketball injuries: National Collegiate Athletic Association Injury Surveillance System, 1988–1989 through 2003–2004. *J Athl Train.* 2007;42(2):202–210.

5. Agel J, Palmieri-Smith RM, Dick R, Wojtys EM, Marshall SW. Descriptive epidemiology of collegiate women's volleyball injuries: National Collegiate Athletic Association Injury Surveillance System, 1988–1989 through 2003–2004. *J Athl Train.* 2007;42(2):295–302.

6. Agel J, Ransone J, Dick R, Oppliger R, Marshall SW. Descriptive epidemiology of collegiate men's wrestling injuries: National Collegiate Athletic Association Injury Surveillance System, 1988–1989 through 2003–2004. *J Athl Train.* 2007;42(2):303–310.

7. American Academy of Neurology. Practice parameter: the management of concussion in sports (summary statement). Report of the Quality Standards Subcommittee of the American Academy of Neurology. *Neurology.* 1997;48:581–585.

8. Berry DC, Miller MG. Athletic mouthguards and their role in injury prevention. *Athl Ther Today.* 2001;6(4):52–56.

9. Dick R, Ferrara MS, Agel J, Courson R, Marshall SW, Hanley MJ. Descriptive epidemiology of collegiate men's football injuries: National Collegiate Athletic Association Injury Surveillance System, 1988–1989 through 2003–2004. *J Athl Train.* 2007;42(2):221–233.

10. Dick R, Hertel J, Agel J, Grossman J, Marshall SW. Descriptive epidemiology of collegiate men's basketball injuries: National Collegiate Athletic Association Injury Surveillance System, 1988–1989 through 2003–2004. *J Athl Train.* 2007;42(2):194–201.

11. Dick R, Hootman JM, Agel J, Vela L, Marshall SW, Messina R. Descriptive epidemiology of collegiate women's field hockey injuries: National Collegiate Athletic Association Injury Surveillance System, 1988–1989 through 2002–2003. *J Athl Train.* 2007;42(2):211–220.

12. Dick R, Lincoln AE, Agel J, Carter EA, Marshall SW, Hinton RY. Descriptive epidemiology of collegiate women's lacrosse injuries: National Collegiate Athletic Association Injury Surveillance System, 1988–1989 through 2003–2004. *J Athl Train.* 2007;42(2):262–269.

13. Dick R, Putukian M, Agel J, Evans TA, Marshall SW. Descriptive epidemiology of collegiate women's soccer injuries: National Collegiate Athletic Association Injury Surveillance System, 1988–1989 through 2002–2003. *J Athl Train.* 2007;42(2):278–285.

14. Dick R, Romani WA, Agel J, Case JG, Marshall SW. Descriptive epidemiology of collegiate men's lacrosse injuries: National Collegiate Athletic Association Injury Surveillance System, 1988–1989 through 2003–2004. *J Athl Train.* 2007;42(2):255–261.

15. Dick R, Sauers EL, Agel J, Keuter G, Marshall SW, McCarty K. Descriptive epidemiology of collegiate men's baseball injuries: National Collegiate Athletic Association Injury Surveillance System, 1988–1989 through 2003–2004. *J Athl Train.* 2007;42(2):183–193.

16. Guskiewicz KM, Bruce SL, Cantu RC, et al. National Athletic Trainers' Association Position Statement: management of sport-related concussion. *J Athl Train.* 2004;39(3):280–297.

17. Gutman S. *Quick Reference Neuroscience for Rehabilitation Professionals.* Thorofare, NJ: Slack Inc; 2001.

18. Huffman EA, Yard EE, Fields SK, Collins CL, Comstock RD. Epidemiology of rare injuries and conditions among United States high school athletes during the 2005–2006 and 2006–2007 school years. *J Athl Train.* 2008;43(6): 624–630.

19. Levangie PK, Norkin CC. Joint Structure and Function: A Comprehensive Analysis. Philadelphia, PA: FA Davis; 2001.

20. Marshall SW, Covassin T, Dick R, Nassar LG, Agel J. Descriptive epidemiology of collegiate women's gymnastics injuries: National Collegiate Athletic Association Injury Surveillance System, 1988–1989 through 2003–2004. *J Athl Train.* 2007;42(2):234–240.

21. Marshall SW, Hamstra-Wright KL, Dick R, Grove KA, Agel J. Descriptive epidemiology of collegiate women's softball injuries: National Collegiate Athletic Association Injury Surveillance System, 1988–1989 through 2003–2004. *J Athl Train.* 2007;42(2):286–294.

22. McCrory P, Meeuwisse W, Johnston K, Dvorak J, Aubry M, Cantu RC. Consensus statement on concussion in sport 3rd international conference on concussion in sport held in Zurich, November 2008. *J Athl Train.* 2009;44(4):434–448.

23. Moore K, Dalley A. *Clinically Oriented Anatomy.* Baltimore, MD: Lippincott Williams & Wilkins; 2005.

24. National Collegiate Athletic Association. *2009–10 NCAA(r) Sports Medicine Handbook.* Indianapolis, IN: National Collegiate Athletic Association; 2009.

25. Reynolds T. Ear, nose and throat problems in accident and emergency. *Nurs Stand.* 2004;18(26):47–55.

26. Schultz SJ, Houglum PA. *Examination of Musculoskeletal Injuries.* Champaign, IL: Human Kinetics; 2005.

27. Starkey C, Ryan J. *Evaluation of Orthopedic and Athletic Injuries.* Philadelphia, PA: FA Davis; 2002.

28. Steadman's Concise Medical Dictionary. *Steadman's Medical Dictionary.* Philadelphia PA: Lippincott Williams & Wilkins; 2001.

29. Weller MD, Drake-Lee AB. A review of nasal trauma. *Trauma.* 2006;8(1):21–28.

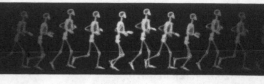

T om, a 19-year-old collegiate baseball player, was struck in the face by a fastball pitch while at bat. The umpire immediately called time and summoned Mary, the certified athletic trainer covering the game.

ON-SCENE ARRIVAL

When Mary arrives, Tom is in obvious discomfort, rolling around on the ground in pain, holding his face. A primary assessment reveals no immediate threats to Tom's life. A rapid assessment of Tom reveals trauma to his left eye. His vital signs are: blood pressure 122/78, a radial pulse of 88 and strong, and respiration of 14 and regular.

HISTORY AND PHYSICAL EXAMINATION

Back on the bench, Tom is alert, cooperative, and in severe discomfort. He states that the baseball hit him in the left eye. He complains about poorly localized pain within and around the eye (Figure 2.1.1) (i.e., orbit) and hypoesthesia to the cheek and teeth. Mary questions Tom about his vision and determines the presence of diplopia. Mary questions Tom about any past or previous ocular injury or illness, which he denies.

FIGURE **2.1.1**

The location of pain falls along the line where Tom is pointing.

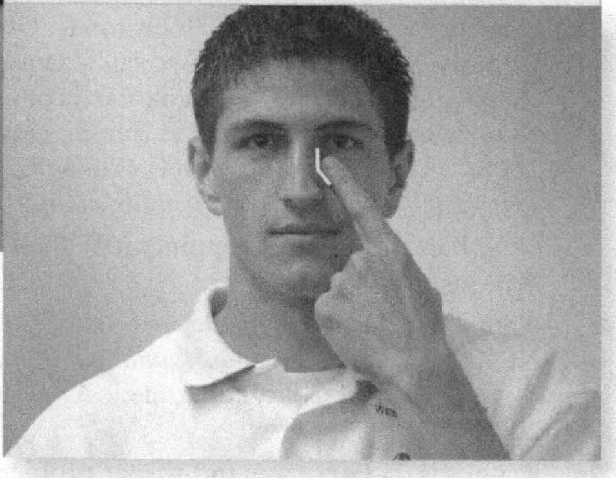

While Mary is collecting Tom's history, she notices Tom's left eye is beginning to swell and appears to be sunken inferiorly. A small laceration is also noted along the superior orbital margin. The left infra-orbital and medial orbital margin is point tender with no apparent gross deformity. An assessment of extra-ocular movement demonstrates limited ability to gaze upward and pain when attempting to do so.

After completing the evaluation Mary decides it is necessary to remove Tom from the game and immediately refers him for further medical management.

? QUESTIONS   CASE 2.1

Please answer the following questions based on the above case information.

2.1/**1.**   Based on the information presented in the case, determine (a) the differential diagnoses and (b) the clinical diagnosis.

2.1/**2.**   Based on the clinical diagnosis, identify the harmful effects of being struck in the eye with a blunt force object larger than the diameter of the orbit.

2.1/**3.**   If Tom had also presented with changes in visual acuity and/or vision loss, what would be the clinical implication, and how could a clinician assess these changes?

2.1/**4.**   During Mary's observation of the eye, suppose she notices subconjunctival hemorrhaging and a shallow anterior chamber in combination with the above signs. What steps should Mary take to manage this situation?

2.1/**5.**   Based on the information presented in the case, what if anything would you have done or added to help guide the physical examination?

2.1/**6.**   After completing the physical examination, Mary documented her findings and sent a copy of the report to the administration office. Please document your findings as if you were the treating clinician. If the case did not provide information you believe is pertinent to the clinical diagnosis, please feel free to add this information to your documentation.

Sherrie, a 20-year-old collegiate field hockey player, reported to the university athletic training room before practice one afternoon. In two years of playing field hockey, Sherrie had never complained about any problems and had never been hurt. Tamara, the certified athletic trainer responsible for the care of the field hockey team, knew something must be seriously wrong if Sherrie was seeking her out.

HISTORY

Sherrie's chief complaint (CC) is left-eye pain. Sherrie states that, "My eye has been killing me since last night; it feels like I have something in there." Tamara asks Sherrie why she did not report to the athletic training room last night after practice if her eye hurt that bad. Sherrie replies, "It didn't bother me until later in the night, but when I woke up this morning, that's when I realized it really hurt. In fact, it feels like there is something still in my eye right now. It is so bad that I am having problems seeing." Sherrie also reports photosensitivity when in brightly lit rooms. She denies any previous history of eye trauma or illness, aside from myopia.

PHYSICAL EXAMINATION

Tamara begins her physical exam by observing the soft tissue around Sherrie's left eye, which appears red and watery. Tamara notes that Sherrie is having a difficult time keeping her left eye open during the exam and complains of pain with extraocular muscle movement. Her visual acuity, tested using a Snellen chart, is limited, though Sherrie is not wearing her contacts because of the ocular pain.

Tamara decides it would be best to place an eye patch on Sherrie's left eye and refers her to one of the team physicians for further examination.

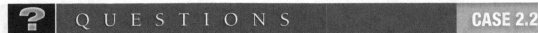

Please answer the following questions based on the above case information.

2.2/**1.**   Based on the information presented in the case, determine (a) the differential diagnoses and (b) the clinical diagnosis.

2.2/**2.**   Based on the information presented in the case, what type of physician should Tamara refer Sherrie to and why?

2.2/**3.**   Tamara asked Sherrie several history questions to guide the physical examination. Based on the clinical diagnosis above, identify three to five specific history questions you as the evaluating clinician may have asked.

2.2/**4.**   There is one mechanism of injury common to the case's clinical diagnosis that typically occurs outside of participating in athletics. Identify this MOI and discuss how it causes the clinical diagnosis.

2.2/**5.**   (a) Overall, do you believe Tamara adequately evaluated Sherrie's condition, given the information provided in the case? (b) What, if any, tests or procedures were omitted that could have helped in establishing the clinical diagnosis? (c) Describe how these test(s) are performed.

CASE 2.3

uesday morning clinic hours were going well for Shelia, the certified athletic trainer at Eastern Hawaii College. She was preparing to eat her muffin for breakfast when Peter, a 20-year-old wrestler, arrived complaining of a problem with his right eye. Shelia had noticed that he was at practice Friday, but when Shelia left Friday afternoon, no one reported any apparent injuries or illnesses.

HISTORY

Shelia begins her evaluation of Peter by asking him about his current CCs. Peter states, "My right eye has been bothering me since late Saturday night. It is itchy and burning, and I am constantly wiping tears out of my eye." When questioned about sensitivity to bright lights and pain, Peter responds that he has none. Peter informs Shelia that when he awoke, his right eye was crusted over and that he had difficulty opening his eye.

PHYSICAL EXAMINATION

As the physical exam begins, Peter is alert and cooperative and appears to be suffering only minor discomfort to his right eye at the time. Shelia notes he is wearing glasses this morning, rather than his contacts. She also identifies conjunctival redness, swelling, and some mild tenderness around the eyelid (Figure 2.3.1), along with some mucopurulent discharge emanating from his right eye. A boil-like lesion with a yellowish center is also located along the base of the right eyelash. The right eye exam is unremarkable. The remainder of his face and head exam reveals no signs of injury or illness.

After completing her exam, Shelia immediately decides to call the University's team physician from the treatment area to get his opinion of the situation. While she is on hold, she writes up her notes and eats her muffin. When the physician comes to the phone, she agrees that Peter should be seen immediately because of the discharge emanating from his eye.

FIGURE 2.3.1

Peter's location of pain and conjunctival redness.

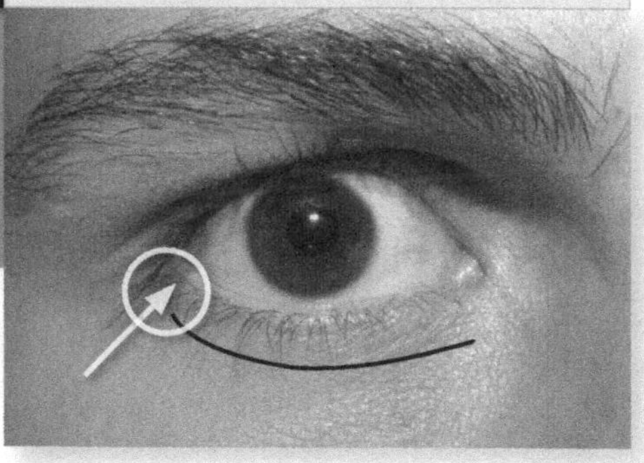

Palpation of Peter's eye was performed without gloves and Peter's pain is along the line.

? QUESTIONS   **CASE 2.3**

Please answer the following questions based on the above case information.

2.3/**1.** Based on the information presented in the case, determine (a) the differential diagnoses and (b) the clinical diagnosis.

2.3/**2.** Based on the case, it is possible that Shelia should have spent more time evaluating Peter's eye. What type of functional and special tests, if any, would you have performed and why?

2.3/**3.** Based on the clinical diagnosis, explain whether you would expect Peter to have difficulty opening the affected eye.

2.3/**4.** The yellow discharge noted during the inspection indicates what possible types of infection?

2.3/**5.** What is/are the most common methods of contracting the above clinical diagnosis?

2.3/**6.** What behavior of Shelia's makes this case very disturbing?

CASE 2.4

A 15-year-old male adolescent named Larry presented to Bud, the certified athletic trainer at a local roller hockey game. Larry's CC was "eye pain." While playing in a roller hockey game, Larry was struck in the face with the blunt end of a hockey stick. He stated he was wearing his helmet; however, he was not wearing a face shield.

HISTORY

Larry complains of severe eye pain and tenderness around his eye. He says that he is able to see out of his left eye but not his right eye. There is no reported loss of consciousness. Larry walked up to the first-aid tent with assistance from his coach.

PHYSICAL EXAMINATION

During the physical examination Larry is alert, cooperative, and in moderate-to-severe discomfort. His right eye is already beginning to swell shut. Bud notes a large area of ecchymosis developing over the right peri-orbital region. Larry has tenderness over the inferior orbital region and attempts to open his eye with much apprehension but without much success. The eye's anterior chamber appears deepened and presents with what appears to be a teardrop-shaped pupil. A small-to-moderate amount of blood is also readily visible in the anterior chamber of the eye (Figure 2.4.1). Larry is able to sense light from the right eye, but his vision is markedly decreasing. A cursory examination of visual acuity reveals Larry's ability to correctly identify the number of Bud's fingers being held up at a distance of two feet. His left-eye exam is unremarkable. The remainder of the face exam reveals no signs of injury.

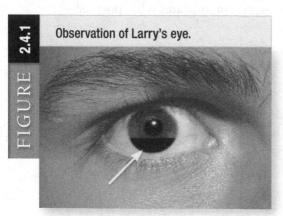

FIGURE 2.4.1

Observation of Larry's eye.

Arrow points to blood visible in the eye.

Bud, along with Larry's coach, decides to call Larry's parents so that he can be immediately transported to the hospital. Bud decides it would be best to have Larry remain in a supine position while his parents and emergency medical services (EMS) are called. The coach hands Larry a bottle of water to quench Larry's thirst while Bud is finishing up the evaluation.

Please answer the following questions based on the above case information.

2.4/**1.** Based on the information presented in the case, determine the likely clinical diagnoses and identify the difference between them.

2.4/**2.** Based on the information presented in the case, discuss the manner in which Bud assessed Larry's visual acuity and why he chose to assess it this way.

2.4/**3.** If this athlete were evaluated in the athletic training room, discuss how Bud should then assess visual acuity and how the results should be interpreted?

2.4/**4.** Overall, do you believe that Bud adequately assessed Larry's condition? What if anything would you have done differently as the evaluating clinician?

2.4/**5.** If Larry's eyelid was too swollen to open, what strategies could you use to evaluate the eye, if any?

2.4/**6.** Do you believe Bud managed the current situation appropriately? What if anything would you have done differently?

A 27-year-old male intramural soccer player reported to a free sports medicine clinic at the local hospital on Monday afternoon. He was worried about what he described as "blurred vision and little floating dots in my right eye."

HISTORY

Chris, a soccer player, explains that he was playing in a club tournament over the weekend and was struck in the face with a soccer ball. He reports that he was initially seen by the athletic trainer and the physician covering the event and was cleared of any head or facial injuries. However, changes in his vision began to occur during the last 24 hours. He states that he is able to see out of his left eye but not his right eye. He reports no loss of consciousness and no signs of post-concussion syndrome (PCS).

PHYSICAL EXAMINATION

Chris is alert and cooperative and in minimal discomfort. He opens and closes his right eye with no difficulty. He is able to sense light with the right eye, but his vision is markedly decreased and he complains of little black dots floating across his field of vision. A visual acuity test reveals 20/50 in the right eye and 20/10 in the left eye. Normal light-touch sensation over his right and left cheeks is noted. His left eye (non-involved) exam is unremarkable. The remainder of his face and head demonstrates no signs of injury. The athletic trainer covering the clinic decides to immediately refer this athlete to the eye clinic for further evaluation.

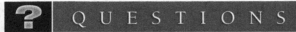

Please answer the following questions based on the above case information.

2.5/**1.** Based on the information presented in the case, (a) determine the clinical diagnosis, and (b) identify the hallmark symptom reported in this case.

2.5/**2.** Describe the etiology of the clinical diagnosis.

2.5/**3.** What type of physician should the athletic trainer refer this athlete to and why?

2.5/**4.** The mechanism of injury in this case was a direct blow causing a jarring force in the head. Identify another potential MOI for this condition that is not related to an athletic injury.

2.5/**5.** As the evaluating clinician, imagine a patient presenting with the same MOI but with immediate changes in visual field and sudden onset of one large floater. What pre-hospital care would be necessary?

CASE 2.6

Dan, a 21-year-old collegiate wrestler, presented to Dr. Cost at the university's open sports medicine clinic with a CC of ear pain and tenderness to the upper earlobe.

HISTORY

Dan explains to Dr. Cost that his coach has not been enforcing the headgear rule during wrestling practice this year, and as a result of this, most of the team has avoided wearing them, including himself. After a series of questions, Dr. Cost determines that Dan is suffering from moderate ear pain and tenderness around his left auricle. What concerns Dr. Cost, however, is the slight hearing loss Dan reports in his left ear.

FIGURE 2.6.1

Observation of Dan's left ear.

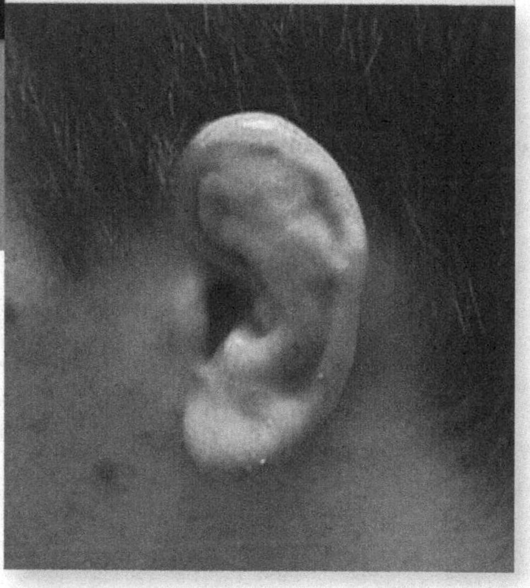

Source: www.uwec.edu. Used with permission.

PHYSICAL EXAMINATION

Dan is alert, cooperative, and in moderate discomfort. His left external ear appears violently red. Dr. Cost notes a large area of effusion around the area of the left auricle (Figure 2.6.1). Upon palpation Dan's left ear is tender and feels both smooth and hard. He is able to hear from the left ear but with some minor-to-moderate loss noted compared with the right. His balance is unremarkable. Normal light-touch sensation over his left and right cheeks and temple area is noted. His right-ear exam is unremarkable. The remainder of his face and head are without signs of injury and/or illness. Dr. Cost decides she is going to manage this in the clinic today.

Please answer the following questions based on the above case information.

2.6/**1.** Based on the information presented in the case, determine the clinical diagnosis and its etiology.

2.6/**2.** During Dr. Cost's inspection of the ears, she noted swelling of the external ear structures. In addition to examining the external ear, Dr. Cost also evaluated the middle and inner ear. Explain the most appropriate procedure for evaluating the middle and inner ear.

2.6/**3.** Dr. Cost asked several history questions to guide the physical examination. Identify three to five history questions Dr. Cost or a clinician may have asked in order to properly evaluate this case.

2.6/**4.** How do you think Dr. Cost is going to manage this case?

2.6/**5.** What supplies will a certified athletic trainer need to lay out to assist the physician based on the question above?

2.6/**6.** What, if any, steps will the team's athletic trainer need take to prevent this from occurring in the future.

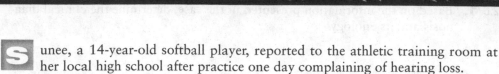

2.7

Sunee, a 14-year-old softball player, reported to the athletic training room at her local high school after practice one day complaining of hearing loss.

HISTORY

Sunee explains to Melanie, the athletic trainer, that over the last couple of weeks her hearing has progressively gotten worse and she has begun noticing some ringing in the ears. In fact, she mentions that she has had to move to the front of the class in order to hear her teachers. Melanie questions Sunee about any previous hearing loss or any trauma to the head. Sunee denies any history of hearing loss or being struck in the head or even experiencing any other trauma within the last couple of days.

FIGURE 2.7.1

Examination of Sunee's left ear with an otoscope.

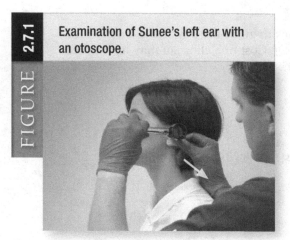

Arrow indicates the direction of pull on the pinna.

PHYSICAL EXAMINATION

Sunee is alert, cooperative, and presents with no significant signs of discomfort. Melanie notes nothing unusual in her observations of the external ear structures. An examination of the external auditory canals (Figure 2.7.1) reveals a yellowish substance packed tightly within the canals. An assessment of hearing using air conduction demonstrates a slight hearing impairment in the left ear. The remainder of her head and face are without signs of injury or illness. Melanie decides that in order to properly and safely manage this athlete she needs to be referred to the team physician.

? QUESTIONS

Please answer the following questions based on the above case information.

2.7/**1.** Based on the information presented in the case, determine the clinical diagnosis and its pathophysiology.

2.7/**2.** What, if any, other clinical problems may this condition cause?

2.7/**3.** Describe how Melanie was able to identify the yellowish substance packed in the ear canal and the technique she used.

2.7/**4.** What, if any, neurological tests should Melanie have completed and documented?

2.7/**5.** What is the best approach to manage this clinical diagnosis?

CASE 2.8

Nada, a 41-year-old recreational swimmer, presented to the community hospital's free athletic training clinic Monday morning with CCs of otalgia and difficulty hearing on the left side. After completing some paperwork, Nada was brought into an examination room.

HISTORY

Leisha, the staff athletic trainer on-call, begins questioning Nada about her ear. A review of the swimmer's past medical history reveals a recent bout of pneumonia (*Staphylococcus aureus*) two weeks earlier. Leisha further questions Nada and learns that she routinely cleans her ear canals with cotton applicators after practice. She also complains of mild-to-moderate pruritus. Pain is rated at 5/10.

PHYSICAL EXAMINATION

Nada is alert, cooperative, and in minor-to-moderate discomfort. A visual observation of the external structures reveals a mild otorrhea (scant white mucus) from the external auditory canal. Tenderness is noted during traction of the pinna. An internal exam of the ear canal using an otoscope demonstrates a red, severely inflamed auditory canal, littered with moist, purulent debris. A Weber's test is negative. Her right ear exam is unremarkable. The remainder of the head and face are without signs of injury or illness.

Leisha decides that the best course of action is to refer the patient to the on-call physician for treatment.

Please answer the following questions based on the above case information.

2.8/**1.** Based on the information presented in the case, determine the clinical diagnosis and its pathophysiology.

2.8/**2.** Define *otalgia* and *pruritus* and state the clinical diagnosis in laymen's terms.

2.8/**3.** Identify three to five history questions Leisha could have asked to properly evaluate this condition.

2.8/**4.** Traction of the pinna is used to differentiate between which two medical conditions?

2.8/**5.** If the otorrhea presented as a bloody discharge, especially in the presence of granulated tissue, what medical condition would Leisha now be concerned about?

2.8/**6.** If, during the external auditory canal evaluation, Leisha visualized a tympanic membrane that appeared red and inflamed, what condition is potentially present?

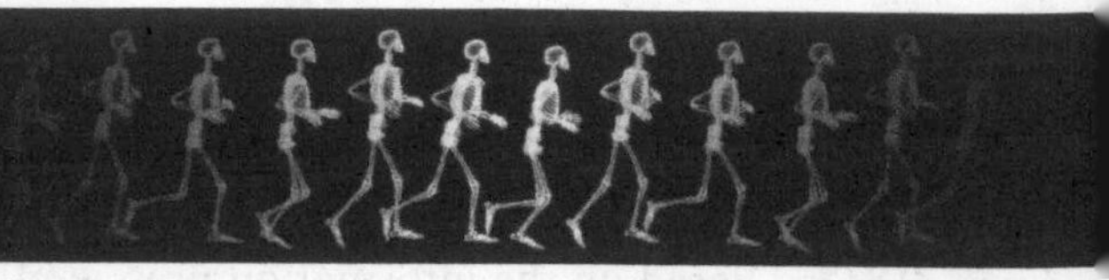

Sara, a 17-year-old volleyball player, was struck in the face while trying to block a volleyball spike during the first match of the high school volleyball season. Samantha, the certified athletic trainer covering the event, jogged onto the court to assess Sara. Samantha was aware that Sara has no past history of facial trauma or head injuries.

ON-SCENE ARRIVAL

When Samantha arrives, Sara is conscious and appears to be in obvious discomfort. A primary assessment reveals no immediate threats to Sara's life. Her nose has a steady stream of moderately bright blood streaming from both nostrils and Sara immediately begins complaining of facial pain and tenderness (Figure 2.9.1). Taking the appropriate blood precautions, Samantha eventually controls the hemorrhaging and performs a cursory head evaluation that is unremarkable.

PHYSICAL EXAMINATION

Sara is brought to the sideline for a more in-depth evaluation. A moderate area of effusion is noted over the bridge of the nose and over the right zygomatic arch area. Tenderness (Figure 2.9.1) and crepitus is noted over the bridge of the nose, along the zygomatic arch and lateral rim of the right eye. A visible deformity of the nasal bridge is present, along with a palpable step-off deformity along the zygomatic arch.

FIGURE 2.9.1

Sara's location of pain and tenderness.

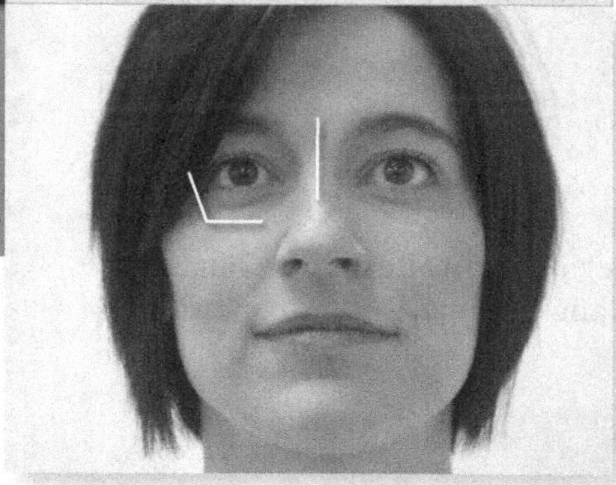

The location of pain falls along the lines.

During the sideline assessment Sara begins complaining of difficulty breathing from her nose. Normal light-touch sensation over her right cheek and nasal structures is noted. Her hemorrhaging is under control; however, she is still having difficulty breathing from her nose. Her vision is also declining in the right eye because of peri-orbital swelling. The remainder of her facial structures and head is unremarkable. Ten minutes after the initial injury, Sara is alert, and her vital signs are: pulse 72, respiration 16, and blood pressure 100/70.

Sara's coach discusses the possibility of returning Sara to the game with Samantha, and after some persuasion, Samantha fits Sara with a face shield and allows her to return to play.

Please answer the following questions based on the above case information.

2.9/**1.** Sara is clearly suffering from a nasal fracture. However, she also presents with another injury. Please identify this potential injury and discuss the injury's MOI.

2.9/**2.** What is the medical term for a bloody nose?

2.9/**3.** What is the difference between bright red blood and dark red blood when dealing with a nosebleed?

2.9/**4.** Why did Sara begin to have difficulty breathing?

2.9/**5.** What, if any, tests should Samantha have performed?

2.9/**6.** Overall, do you believe that Samantha handled the situation appropriately? If not, what would you have done differently as the evaluating clinician?

2.9/**7.** Using an algorithm, briefly outline the evaluation procedures you would take during an on-field and sideline assessment of the clinical diagnosis.

CASE 2.10

John, a 35-year-old recreational ice hockey player, was struck in the neck with a puck as he slid across the ice trying to block an opponent's shot. He was in a quadruped position when the certified athletic trainer, Artie, arrived on scene.

ON-SCENE ARRIVAL

John is dyspneic and having difficulty communicating with Artie. Within 30 seconds Artie has calmed John down and reassures him enough so that John can weakly verbalize his CCs of pain and the inability to swallow.

HISTORY AND PHYSICAL EXAMINATION

John is alert, producing a coughing sound and is in moderate-to-severe discomfort. Artie is aware that John has no past history of neck or facial trauma. There appears to be a minor tracheal shift to the right. He is point tender with crepitus over the larynx and hyoid. John has increased anterior neck pain when swallowing. His respirations are rapid (Table 2.10.1(a)), and he is dyspneic.

Artie stabilizes John's neck and requests the emergency medical technicians (EMTs) onto the ice. Artie and the EMTs work together to administer supplemental oxygen via a nasal cannula mask at 15 L/min, spine board him, and transfer him onto a stretcher for transport.

During transport to the hospital, John's vital signs begin to change (Table 2.10.1(b)). Eventually John loses consciousness, becomes cyanotic, and begins to spit up frothy blood. The EMTs stop and request advanced life support to assist in managing John's airway and breathing.

TABLE	2.10.1	John's vital signs.

(a) On-Ice

VITAL SIGNS	FINDING
Pulse	122, regular and bounding
Respiration	21, labored
Blood pressure	132/86
Skin	Hot and moist
Mental status	Alert

(b) Transport

VITAL SIGNS	FINDING
Pulse	146, regular and thready
Respiration	25, shallow and labored
Blood pressure	120/76
Skin	Pale, cool, and clammy
Mental status	Declining

Please answer the following questions based on the above case information.

2.10/**1.** Based on the information presented in the case, determine the differential diagnoses.

2.10/**2.** In addition to the throat, what other anatomical structures should Artie assess during the physical examination?

2.10/**3.** Define "dyspneic."

2.10/**4.** Had the puck struck the anterolateral neck, which anatomical structures should an athletic trainer be concerned about and why?

2.10/**5.** During transport John began spitting up frothy blood. (a) Why was this not identified earlier in the assessment? (b) How could Artie have checked for blood in the throat during his initial assessment?

2.10/**6.** Did Artie appropriately manage the current situation? What if anything would you have done differently?

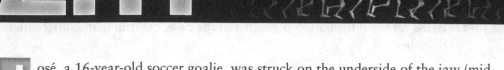

J osé, a 16-year-old soccer goalie, was struck on the underside of the jaw (mid-line) as he attempted to block a shot (Figure 2.11.1). Amy, the certified athletic trainer covering the game, raced onto the field to assess José, who was not moving.

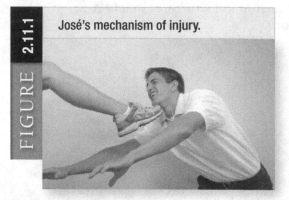

FIGURE 2.11.1

José's mechanism of injury.

ON-SCENE ARRIVAL

As Amy arrives on the scene, José appears to be breathing, but is unconscious. Within a few seconds (3 to 5) he regains consciousness and begins supporting his jaw.

HISTORY

José has difficulty speaking due to his intense pain but is able to communicate his CCs of lower jaw pain and the inability to open his mouth. Amy asks one of José's teammates how long he was unconscious. The teammate says, "He looked out of it right after he was hit, probably 10 or maybe 15 seconds." José has no past history of facial trauma or concussions.

PHYSICAL EXAMINATION

José appears semi-alert and in severe discomfort. There is observable deformity of the mandible and malocclusion (Figure 2.11.2). He is point tender over the anterior-lateral aspect of the left mandible, with immediate swelling. Amy asks José to open and close and move his jaw side-to-side. He refuses because of the intense pain.

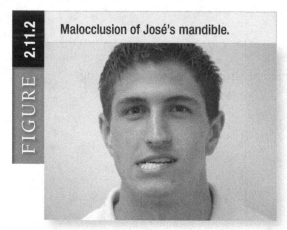

FIGURE 2.11.2

Malocclusion of José's mandible.

His breathing and pulse rate appear to be increasing as the physical exam continues. Amy's examination of the cervical spine is unremarkable; however, she decides to stabilize the neck and jaw for safety.

While waiting for EMS, Amy notices José becoming cyanotic. This is followed by a loss of consciousness. When the EMTs arrive, they work with Amy to maintain José's airway to ensure adequate breathing and spine board him as quickly and safely as possible. His vital signs en route to the hospital are: blood pressure 100/66, respiration rate 18, and heart rate 132.

| ? | QUESTIONS | CASE 2.11 |

Please answer the following questions based on the above case information.

2.11/**1.** Based on the information presented in the case, determine (a) the differential diagnoses and (b) the clinical diagnosis. (c) What if any secondary trauma/condition may José be suffering concurrently?

2.11/**2.** In addition to the mandible, what other bony anatomical landmarks should Amy have assessed/palpated during her physical examination?

2.11/**3.** If you were the evaluating clinician, what if anything would you have done differently?

2.11/**4.** Identify and describe how to perform a special test used to assist in determining the clinical diagnosis.

2.11/**5.** What is the possible explanation for why Amy did not perform the special test identified in question 4, and what is the sensitivity of this test?

2.11/**6.** An athlete sustaining this type of injury is also at risk for developing a concussion. Discuss how and why concussion occurs and how a clinician can prevent concussion as well as the clinical diagnosis injury from occurring.

CASE **2.12**

S am, a 28-year-old recreational ice hockey player, was warming up without his helmet before an ice hockey league game. He was on the ice stretching when a teammate's pass went awry, striking Sam in his face in a downward direction under the left eye. He fell to the ice holding his face. Mike, the certified athletic trainer covering the event, made his way to Sam in order to assess him.

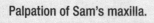

FIGURE 2.12.1

Sam's location of pain, which falls along the line.

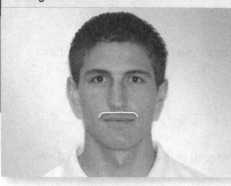

HISTORY

As Mike arrives at Sam's side, he notes that he has an intact airway and is breathing. He also notes a steady stream of blood flowing from his nose. With extreme difficulty Sam says, "I never saw the puck until it was too late, and it struck me in the nose and face just above my upper jaw." His CCs are pain, tenderness along the mid-portion of the face (Figure 2.12.1), and the feeling that his upper jaw is moving.

PHYSICAL EXAMINATION

Sam is alert, semi-cooperative, and in severe discomfort. He has no known past history of facial trauma. His nose does not appear to have any gross visible deformities; however, the upper central incisors appear to be in a forward position relative to the lower incisors. During palpation of the maxilla, crepitus is noted over the maxillary arch, along with movement of the upper central incisors and hard palate (Figure 2.12.2).

FIGURE 2.12.2

Palpation of Sam's maxilla.

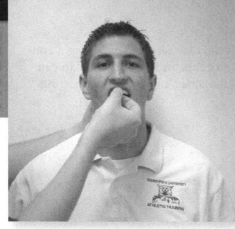

Sam continues to have minor hemorrhaging from both nostrils. The hemorrhaging is eventually controlled.

Further evaluation reveals minor-to-moderate areas of effusion and ecchymosis along the alveolar process. Normal light-touch sensation over Sam's right and left cheek and nasal structures is noted. The remainder of his facial structures appear to be unremarkable.

Emergency medical services are called, and Sam is placed on a spine board and transported to the hospital. His vital signs 10 minutes after the initial injury are: pulse rate 88; blood pressure 122/86; respiration rate 16 and normal; and mental status is alert, semi-cooperative, and in severe discomfort.

Please answer the following questions based on the above case information.

2.12/**1.** Based on the information presented in the case, determine (a) the differential diagnoses and (b) the clinical diagnosis.

2.12/**2.** The trauma sustained to the facial structures in this case is classified using the LeFort system. Identify Sam's fracture type based on the information provided in the case above and your knowledge of the common mechanism of injury.

2.12/**3.** If Sam presented with pain and tenderness along the bridge of the nose and the zygomatic arch, bilateral subconjunctival hemorrhaging, abnormal skin sensitivity, and mobility of the maxilla, what further fracture classification is most likely to represent his signs and symptoms?

2.12/**4.** If Sam reported a direct blow to the nasal bridge or upper maxilla and presented with facial elongation or flattening of the face, diplopia, movement of the facial bones in relation to the cranium, and positive halo sign, what further fracture classification is most likely to represent his signs and symptoms?

2.12/**5.** What if anything would you as the evaluating clinician have done differently in Figure 2.12.2?

2.12/**6.** Formulate a plan to further analyze any other associated conditions that could affect the outcome of this case, including possible signs and symptoms.

CASE

2.13

A 44-year-old female athlete, McKinley, presented to Kim, the certified athletic trainer at a local sports medicine clinic. McKinley had a CC of jaw soreness and constant headaches. McKinley was escorted to an examination room by Kim where she asked her to complete a medical history and pain profile. Once all the paper work was completed, Kim began the physical examination.

HISTORY

Kim begins her evaluation by reviewing McKinley's medical history and pain profiles (Figure 2.13.1). She also asks McKinley if she remembers the mechanism of injury. McKinley reports that she was struck under the chin with an elbow while playing

---

FIGURE **2.13.1**   **McKinley's pain profiles.**

1. Please rate your current level of pain at rest on the following scale (circle one):

    0   1   2   ③   4   5   6   7   8   9   10

    (no pain)   *(worst imaginable pain)*

2. Please rate your level of pain when talking on the following scale (circle one):

    0   1   2   3   4   ⑤   6   7   8   9   10

    (no pain)   *(worst imaginable pain)*

3. Please rate your level of pain while eating on the following scale (circle one):

    0   1   2   3   4   5   6   7   8   ⑨   10

    (no pain)   *(worst imaginable pain)*

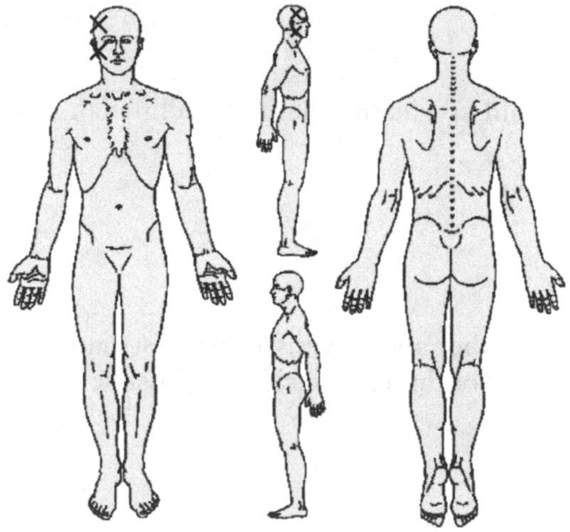

Note: General
discomfort = ✕

soccer in an over-40 women's league several weeks ago. She was not wearing her mouth-guard as she normally does, and an opposing player managed to get an elbow under the chin, striking her on the anteroinferior aspect of the mandible. Further questioning from Kim reveals that this injury occurred two weeks ago, but instead of reporting to the athletic trainer on duty during the match, McKinley ignored her symptoms. McKinley also complains of jaw pain and a clicking sensation of the jaw when talking and eating. She denies any loss of consciousness or head trauma.

PHYSICAL EXAMINATION

McKinley appears alert, cooperative, and otherwise well adjusted, but she is experiencing moderate discomfort. A minor pocket of swelling is noted along the area of the right mandibular condyle. She also has notable internal and external tenderness along the right mandibular condyle (Figure 2.13.2). She is able to open her jaw only one knuckle-width (Figure 2.13.3), and Kim notes an internal palpable click when she does this. Kim asks McKinley to smile, which demonstrates a slight malocclusion. Sensation testing about the face and neck is unremarkable. The remainder of her head, face, and neck is without sign of injury or illness.

It is decided that in order to properly manage this patient, McKinley needs to be referred to a specialist.

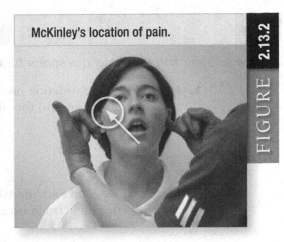

McKinley's location of pain.

FIGURE 2.13.2

Arrow and circle indicate the location of the pain and tenderness.

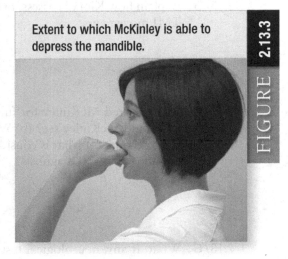

Extent to which McKinley is able to depress the mandible.

FIGURE 2.13.3

Please answer the following questions based on the above case information.

2.13/**1.** Based on the information presented in the case, determine (a) the differential diagnoses and (b) the clinical diagnosis.

2.13/**2.** Identify three to five additional history questions you would have asked as the evaluating clinician in order to properly evaluate this condition.

2.13/**3.** Explain how Kim did assess, or could have qualitatively assessed, McKinley's TMJ movements.

2.13/**4.** Kim referred McKinley for further medical care. (a) What type of specialist should McKinley see? (b) What do you believe was Kim's rationale for the referral, and what is considered to be the diagnostic gold standard for the above clinical diagnosis?

2.13/**5.** What, if any, neurological tests should an evaluating clinician perform?

T ina, a 22-year-old intercollegiate soccer goalie, was struck in the face while defending the goal (Figure 2.14.1). The school's certified athletic trainer, Dale, ran onto to the field to find Tina in obvious pain, rolling around while trying to stabilize her jaw. When Dale reached her, Tina was holding her jaw and was unable to speak or report her CC.

HISTORY

One of Tina's teammates, Rochelle, approaches the scene and informs Dale that Tina was attempting to block a shot and dove toward the goalpost to block the shot. At that moment, another player tried to kick the ball, missed, and "whacked Tina right in the side of the jaw." Dale thanks Rochelle, turning his attention to Tina. Tina has no history of facial or cervical trauma.

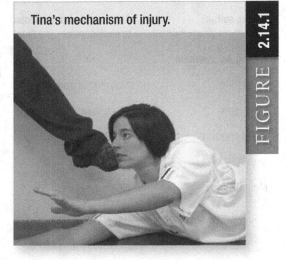

Tina's mechanism of injury.

FIGURE 2.14.1

PHYSICAL EXAMINATION

Tina is semi-alert and in severe discomfort. Dale immediately notices a marked deformity on the right side of her face near the mandibular condyle and malocclusion opposite to the deformity. Palpation over the right mandibular condyle and articular eminence is painful. Dale notes that the jaw and TMJ are beginning to swell. Tina attempts to open and close and move her jaw side-to-side at Dale's request but is unable to do so because of the intense pain. Her respirations increase from 18 at the beginning of the secondary assessment to 24 a couple of minutes later; her heart rate is also increasing (see Table 2.14.1(a) on the following page). Dale decides to stabilize the jaw and neck as a precaution and initiates the university's emergency action plan.

Once the EMTs arrive, they begin to provide care with Dale. They attempt to put a cervical collar on Tina, but it appears to be an inappropriate size for her. They remove the cervical collar and find an alternative method of stabilizing the jaw. Her vital signs en route to the hospital are located in Table 2.14.1(b).

TABLE	2.14.1	Tina's vital signs.

(a) During secondary assessment and ongoing assessment

VITAL SIGNS	FINDING
Secondary Assessment	
Pulse	122, regular and bounding
Respiration	18, normal
Blood pressure	132/86
Skin	Hot and moist
Mental status	Alert x 3 (alert and oriented to person, place, and time)
Ongoing Assessment	
Pulse	142, regular and bounding
Respiration	24, shallow and labored
Blood pressure	130/82
Skin	Hot and moist
Mental status	Alert x 3

(b) During transport

VITAL SIGNS	FINDING
Pulse	84, regular
Respiration	16, normal
Blood pressure	124/86
Skin	Warm and dry
Mental status	Alert x 3

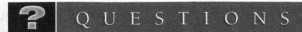

Please answer the following questions based on the above case information.

2.14/**1.** Based on the information presented in the case, determine the clinical diagnosis and the mechanism of injury.

2.14/**2.** If Tina had been wearing a mouthguard, (a) would this injury have occurred? Why, or why not? (b) If not, identify two other possible injuries that may occur.

2.14/**3.** Why is there is no mention of Dale assessing Tina's ABCs prior to initiating her physical examination?

2.14/**4.** What, if anything, did you believe Dale omitted as part of his evaluation of Tina?

2.14/**5.** During the application of the cervical collar, it was apparent the collar was the wrong size. (a) Do you believe the application of a cervical collar was appropriate given the clinical diagnosis? (b) Explain what alternative method may have been used to stabilize the jaw.

2.14/**6.** Using an algorithm, briefly outline the evaluation procedures you would take during an on-field assessment and management of the injury.

2.15

Peter, a 15-year-old high school basketball player, was struck in the mouth with an elbow as he was attempting to retrieve an offensive rebound. He immediately placed his hand over his mouth and quickly ran to the sideline. As he approached the bench, Adam, the certified athletic trainer covering the event, noticed blood dripping from the athlete's cupped hands. Adam immediately implemented the institution's blood-borne pathogen procedures and emergency action plan.

HISTORY

Once on the bench, Peter's initial CCs are of lower-lip and mandible pain. However, he also reports having some lower central incisor pain and sensitivity to the elements. He reports no loss of consciousness or difficulty breathing.

PHYSICAL EXAMINATION

Peter is alert, semi-cooperative, and in moderate discomfort. He has a through-and-through laceration of his lower lip and obvious trauma to the upper left central incisor, which has been avulsed. Once the bleeding is under control Adam is able to determine the extent of the trauma. Adam notes that the lower left lateral and central incisors appear to be elongated in an axial direction. Palpation of the left lower lateral and central incisors reveals the teeth to be mobile. Peter is able to open and close and move his jaw side to side with no pain or discomfort. He does complain of pain to the central incisor with manipulation. Normal light-touch sensation over the rest of his face is unremarkable. The remainder of his orofacial structures and head are without signs of injury and/or illness. His parents are present, and Adam suggests that Peter be transported to hospital for further evaluation.

Please answer the following questions based on the above case information.

2.15/**1.** Based on the information presented in the case, determine the clinical diagnosis and the mechanism of injury.

2.15/**2.** Identify three to five additional history questions Adam could have asked to properly evaluate this condition.

2.15/**3.** In addition to the teeth, what other bony anatomical structures or landmarks should Adam have assessed for further trauma?

2.15/**4.** Discuss the differences between a tooth's three main components: enamel, dentin, and pulp.

2.15/**5.** What are the current recommendations for handling the avulsed tooth?

2.15/**6.** Discuss how you would have handled the above situation. Would you have done anything differently?

Lauren, a 20-year-old field hockey defender, was attempting to defend her team's goal while an opposing player obstructed her play. During this brief period of obstruction, the opposing team's forward flicked the ball in Lauren's direction. Lauren did not see the ball coming at her, and the ball struck her in the left parietal area, causing her to instantly fall to the ground while grabbing her head. The referee immediately called dangerous play. Realizing Lauren was hurt, the referee stopped play. She turned to Lauren's team, calling David (the athletic trainer) and Lisa (the athletic training student) onto the field to tend to Lauren.

ON-SCENE ARRIVAL

Upon initial assessment, Lauren appeared to be alert but disoriented. Her airway, breathing, and circulation were WNL. Her vital signs were: pulse rate 108; respiration rate 22 and labored; blood pressure 132/92; skin hot and moist; and mental status alert, but disoriented. An assessment of the cervical spine and neurological screening was unremarkable. David decided it was safe to assist Lauren off the field using a two-person walking assist.

FIGURE 2.16.1

Lauren's location of palpable tenderness, within the circle.

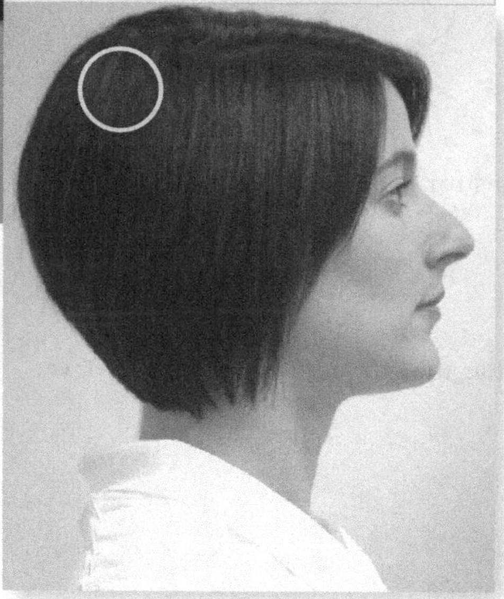

HISTORY

Once on the bench, Lauren's CCs are a headache, dizziness, tinnitus, and feeling just not quite right. She reports no loss of consciousness and is able to recall the current score; however, she does not recall the mechanism of injury. David sends Lisa over to question the referee about any loss of consciousness, which is confirmed as none.

PHYSICAL EXAMINATION

Lauren appears inattentative and denies having any problems. David notes palpable tenderness and swelling to the skull (Figure 2.16.1). Lisa returns from questioning the referee with a blank standardized assessment of con-

TABLE	2.16.1	Lauren's SAC results.	
SECTION	**FINDINGS**		**SCORE**
Orientation	Lauren is orientated to month, date, day of week, and year.		4
Immediate memory	On the first try, Lauren is able to recall the following words: (1) red, (2) balloon, (3) golf, (4) pizza, and (5) ball. She misses 1 on the second and 2 on the third attempt.		12
Concentration	Lauren is able to complete 3 reverse digit strings and repeats correctly the months of the year in reverse.		4
Neurologic	Neurological screening reveals normal distal extremity strength and dermatomes; however, a Romberg test is positive.		n/a
Exertion	Functional exertion test increases Lauren's current headache and dizziness.		n/a
Delayed recall	Lauren is able to recall 3 of the 5 previous words.		3

cussion (SAC) form. David initiates the exam (results in Table 2.16.1). A further assessment reveals normal pupil reflex and reaction.

INITIAL TREATMENT

David applies ice to Lauren's head to help control the swelling while Lisa returns to the athletic training room to retrieve Lauren's preseason SAC score. When she returns, David verifies that two months ago Lauren scored a 29. He then completes his initial graded symptoms checklist (Table 2.16.2). A reassessment of Lauren's condition 15 minutes later reveals no significant changes in her SAC or graded symptoms score. Coach Bray tries to convince Lauren to return to play. David steps in and informs the coach that, according to athletic department sports medicine policies and procedures document, Lauren is unable to return to play. Coach Bray is furious and demands that the athletic director step in. Having read and signed the policy, the director agrees with David's decision and informs the coach that Lauren will not be playing for the rest of the day.

FOLLOW-UP EXAMINATION

After the game, Lauren is escorted to the athletic training room. As David prepares her home instructions, Lisa administers the SAC and graded symptoms score again. Again, there are still no appreciable differences in the scores.

| TABLE | 2.16.2 | Lauren's graded symptoms score. |

SYMPTOMS	TIME OF INJURY	15 MIN POST-INJURY	1 HR. POST-INJURY	24 HR. POST-INJURY	48 HR. POST-INJURY
Blurred vision	0	0	0		
Dizziness	3	3	3		
Drowsiness	0	0	0		
Excess sleep	0	0	0		
Easily distracted	3	3	1		
Feel in a "fog"	3	3	5		
Feel "slowed down"	1	3	3		
Headache	3	3	3		
Inappropriate emotions	1	1	1		
Loss of consciousness	0	0	0		
Loss or orientation	3	1	1		
Memory problems	3	3	1		
Nausea	1	1	0		
Nervousness	1	0	0		
Personality change	0	0	0		
Poor balance, poor coordination	3	3	2		
Poor concentration	0	1	1		
Ringing in ears	1	1	0		
Sadness	0	0	0		
Seeing stars	3	1	1		
Sensitivity to light	0	0	0		
Sensitivity to noise	0	0	0		
Sleep disturbance	0	0	0		
Vacant stare, glassy-eyed	1	1	0		
Vomiting	0	0	0		

Please answer the following questions based on the above case information.

2.16/1. Based on the information presented in the case, determine the clinical diagnosis and the MOI.

2.16/2. According to the above case, a SAC evaluation was conducted on Lauren immediately after the injury and again at 15 minutes and 1 hour post injury. (a) What is a SAC assessment? (b) How would you have scored her initial SAC evaluation? (c) What is the clinical significance of the initial post-injury and baseline scores?

2.16/3. What is the difference between the SAC and the Sport Concussion Assessment Tool 2 (SCAT2; see Appendix B)?

2.16/4. How would you rate David's and Lisa's performances in the above evaluation? What would you have done differently in this situation, if anything?

2.16/5. What is the significance of having a concussion policies and procedures document?

2.16/6. The coach appeared more concerned with Lauren's continued participation in the game than about her health. What could David and Lisa have done to ensure that Lauren did not return to the game, if the athletic director had not intervened?

2.17

Before practice early in the collegiate women's soccer season, Coach Shelly approached Mary, the team's certified athletic trainer and 10-year veteran of the program, about one of her players. Coach Shelly explained that P.J. was having some "problems" during the team's "unofficial" practices. She further explained that earlier in the summer P.J. was joking around with her little sister and fell off a bed, striking her head on the floor. Her parents attended to her, and P.J. seemed to be fine at the time. However, during practices, P.J. appears to still be suffering from the blow and appears to be disoriented and "out of it." Mary tells Coach Shelly to have P.J. stop by around 1:30 p.m. for an evaluation.

HISTORY

P.J. arrives at the athletic training room around 2 p.m. Mary questions P.J. about her late arrival. P.J. apologizes saying, "Sorry, I lost track of time. I have been doing this often during the last couple of weeks." After accepting her apology, Mary begins questioning P.J. about what has been going on lately. P.J. states that during the summer she got knocked to the floor and struck her head on the wood floor. She reports experiencing some initial problems such as headache, confusion, occasional ringing in the ears, and other non-specific problems. Mary determines that P.J. saw her family physician and that the physician could find nothing wrong at the time of the incident. P.J. confides that since the event she has suffered from fatigue, difficulty sleeping, poor concentration, irritability, and difficulty paying attention to personal and professional conversations.

PHYSICAL EXAMINATION

P.J. is a 19-year-old female who appears restless and very anxious, and she reports sustaining a head injury one month ago, with lingering symptoms. She has no palpable skull tenderness or outward signs of trauma. Neurological testing demonstrates normal deep-tendon reflexes. Pupillary reflexes and reactions are WNL; however, some visual changes (blurred vision) are noted. Mary continues the evaluation with cognitive and neuropsychological testing. Cognitive function demonstrates slowed cognitive processing during a Serial 7's test and positive delayed memory recall. Neuropsychological testing using a Wechsler Digit Span Test and Stroop Color Word Test reveals a deficit in short-term memory, concentration, and cognitive processing speed.

While performing the neuropsychological testing, Mary observes P.J.'s level of irritability increasing. Based on this reaction, Mary decides that it would be best to conclude the evaluation. She informs P.J. that she is going to refer her to the team physician for further evaluation and possible diagnostic testing. However, in the meantime she provides P.J. with a symptoms scale to complete over the next couple of days to track her signs and symptoms.

Please answer the following questions based on the above case information.

2.17/**1.** Based on the information presented in the case determine (a) the differential diagnoses and (b) the clinical diagnosis.

2.17/**2.** (a) Do you believe Mary performed an adequate physical examination? (b) If not, what would you have done differently as the evaluating clinician?

2.17/**3.** What other history questions, if any, could Mary have asked P.J. in order to guide the evaluation?

2.17/**4.** (a) What is the relationship between the clinical diagnosis and depression? (b) Where should an athletic trainer refer an athlete who may be suffering from depression?

2.17/**5.** (a) What if any decisions need to be made regarding the disqualification of P.J. from sports? (b) When should Mary allow P.J. to resume physical activity?

CASE 2.18

It was a sunny fall afternoon, and Dennis, an athletic trainer, was covering a local club's rugby match. He was familiar with several of the players because he frequently covered this event for the group. The game had progressed without any incidents until just after the start of the second half.

HISTORY

One of the players, Paul, advances the ball and is mauled. Eventually, the referee calls for a scrum. Dennis notes that Paul is slow to get up and that he calls for a substitution. Dennis immediately goes over to assist Paul.

PHYSICAL EXAMINATION

After several minutes of evaluating Paul, Dennis diagnoses him with a grade 2 concussion using the American Academy of Neurology concussion grading scale[7] and immediately disqualifies him from further competition. Paul is referred to the local clinic for further evaluation and is provided with a set of home instructions (Figure 2.18.1). Because Dennis knows that Paul probably will not immediately see his primary-care physician, he provides Paul and also Paul's roommate with a list of conditions (Table 2.18.1) under which Paul should immediately see a doctor or go to the hospital.

FIGURE 2.18.1 Home instruction form provided to Paul.

I believe _____Paul_____ has sustained a concussion on ___November 10, 2010___. In order to ensure he/she recovers fully, please follow these recommendations. Please take him/her to the family physician after the match today for a follow-up evaluation.

1. Please review the items outlined on the enclosed Medical Referral Checklist. If any of these problems develop prior to seeing your family physican, immediately call 9-1-1. Otherwise, the patient can follow the instructions below.

2. It is ok to:
   a. Use ice packs on the head and neck as needed.
   b. Eat a light diet.
   c. Go to sleep.
   d. Rest and avoid strenuous activity.

3. There is no need to:
   a. Check pupil response.
   b. Wake up every hour.
   c. Stay in bed.

4. DO NOT:
   a. Use alcohol.
   b. Use sleeping tablets.
   c. Drive, until medically cleared.
   d. Train or play sports, until medically cleared.

TABLE 2.18.1	Medical referral checklist.[16]

PROBLEMS THE DAY OF THE INJURY	PROBLEMS THE DAY AFTER THE INJURY
1. Deterioration of neurological function*	1. Any of the findings in the day-of-injury referral category
2. Decreasing level of consciousness*	2. Increase in the number of post-concussion symptoms reported, such as headache, nausea, dizziness, drowsiness, blurry vision, feeling in a fog, personality changes, etc.
3. Decrease or irregularity in breathing*	3. Post-concussion symptoms worsen or do not improve over time
4. Decrease or irregularity in pulse*	4. Post-concussion symptoms begin to interfere with the athlete's daily activities, such as loss of orientation, memory problems, poor balance or coordination, poor concentration, etc.
5. Unequal, dilated, or unreactive pupils*	
6. Mental status changes: lethargy, difficulty maintaining arousal, confusion, or agitation*	
7. Seizure activity*	
8. Vomiting	

*These require that the athlete be transported immediately to the nearest emergency department.

Adapted from Guskiewicz, Bruce et al. 2004.

FOLLOW-UP

Two days later, Paul's roommate calls Dennis at the clinic and informs him that Paul "isn't right." Dennis asks the roommate to clarify what he means. He says: "He has had a headache that has gotten real bad over the last two days, and he doesn't always know what is going on." Dennis questions the roommate about Paul's vision, and the roommate notes that he is having problems with his vision. Dennis informs Paul's roommate to hang up the phone and call 9-1-1 immediately.

? Q U E S T I O N S   **CASE 2.18**

Please answer the following questions based on the above case information.

2.18/**1.** Based on the information presented in the case, determine (a) the differential diagnoses and (b) the clinical diagnosis.

2.18/**2.** Identify the different ways to classify the clinical diagnosis.

2.18/**3.** What is the pathophysiology of the clinical diagnosis?

2.18/**4.** What if anything would you have done differently in handling this case.

2.18/**5.** Based on the information provided in the case, what if anything did Dennis do that helped to reduce his risk of liability?

CASE

2.19

Stephanie, a 43-year-old female who was status post–anterior cruciate ligament reconstruction, was referred to the Orthopedic Sports Medicine Clinic. Stephanie was an avid tennis player recovering from surgery, and she was at the clinic to see Curtis, a certified athletic trainer, for a scheduled rehabilitation.

HISTORY

Curtis has been evaluating Stephanie's post-surgical repair and, following the surgeon's protocol, is establishing an aggressive rehabilitation program. Everything appears to be going well, and one month into her rehabilitation Stephanie's knee active range of motion (AROM) is almost within normal limits bilaterally. For this appointment, Curtis begins Stephanie's daily treatment with a leisurely stationary bike ride. While she is on the bike, Curtis is called away to answer another patient's question. An aide runs over to Curtis and yells: "Stephanie is having a seizure! She fell off the bike and hit her head on the cable column stand." Both employees run to the gym to assist Stephanie.

ON-SCENE ARRIVAL

Curtis arrives on the scene while Stephanie is still in the midst of a tonic-clonic seizure. Curtis immediately places a towel under Stephanie's head and places an intra-oral screw between her teeth.

PHYSICAL EXAMINATION

Within 30 seconds, the seizure is over, and Curtis begins a primary assessment. Stephanie appears to be unresponsive but has an adequate airway and signs of life. John, an athletic training student working with Curtis, arrives to assist and is instructed to stabilize Stephanie's cervical spine. Curtis begins a head-to-toe physical examination. He immediately detects a soft spot in the skull and notices hemorrhaging (Figure 2.19.1). He has his aide apply direct pressure to the area while he continues with the assessment. The neck, chest, abdomen, pelvis, upper extremity, and right lower extremity appear normal. The left lower extremity is angulated at the proximal tibia. Stephanie's vital signs are: pulse 92 (regular and bounding), respiration 16 (normal), and blood pressure 120/78.

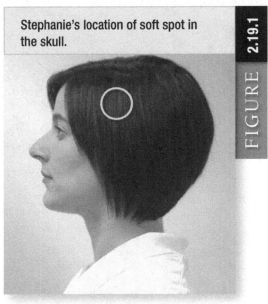

Stephanie's location of soft spot in the skull.

FIGURE 2.19.1

Circle indicates a spot soft in the skull and location of hemorrhaging.

The secretary informs Curtis that EMS has been contacted and should arrive at the clinic in 10 minutes. Once EMS arrives, Curtis and John assist in packaging Stephanie for transport. Emergency medical technicians establish an intravenous access and also administer supplemental oxygen via a non-rebreather mask at 15 L/min. Curtis informs the EMS personnel that Stephanie regained consciousness approximately 2 minutes after the trauma and appears to have a normal neurological examination.

HOSPITAL EXAMINATION

Stephanie arrives at the hospital 20 minutes after falling off the stationary bike. Upon her arrival at the hospital, the EMTs report her status and inform the on-call physician of her head trauma. During the transfer process, she begins complaining of a headache, nausea, and aphasia. Radiographs are ordered to rule out a cervical spine fracture. The ER physician's physical exam reveals the presence of anisocoria, a declining mental status, and the following changes in her vital signs: pulse rate 48 (irregular and thready), respiration rate 11, and blood pressure 142/98. Concerned, the ER physician orders a CT scan.

Please answer the following questions based on the above case information.

2.19/**1.** Based on the information presented in the case, determine the clinical diagnosis.

2.19/**2.** Explain the series of events leading to Stephanie's current condition.

2.19/**3.** If Stephanie's seizure was caused by epilepsy, how could Curtis have possibly anticipated such an outcome?

2.19/**4.** Overall, how would you rate Curtis's and John's management of the above case? What would you have done differently in this situation, if anything?

2.19/**5.** If this injury occurred during an athletic performance, describe the possible MOI for the clinical diagnosis.

CONCLUSION

Although concussions and nasal fractures top the list of acute trauma to the head and face sustained in athletics, this chapter has demonstrated that a variety of injuries to, and conditions of, the head and facial structures are possible. Unlike injuries to other joints, however, misdiagnosis or improper management of head and face injuries can have devastating effects on an athlete's career and personal life. This is because trauma to anatomical structures such as the brain, nose, and mouth all affect an athlete's ability to sustain life, making what would seem to be an inconsequential injury become life threatening and require advanced medical care.

As certified athletic trainers, we learn to handle many emergent situations on our own; however, there may come the time when local emergency medical services (EMS) need to be summoned through the activation of an emergency action plan. The EMS system assists in employing life-saving techniques to reduce morbidity and the incidence of mortality, prevent exacerbation of non-life-threatening condition(s), and facilitate the timely transfer of care of athletes and patients whose conditions are beyond the scope of the athletic trainer. Regular preparation and practice of what is learned in class, on the field, and as part of continuing professional education will prepare athletic trainers to care properly for the cases in this chapter and throughout this book.

The cases in this chapter demonstrate the variety of injuries and illness that athletic trainers will come across in their professional careers. One of the authors has personally dealt with all but three of the cases in this chapter. In fact, many of the cases presented are based on actual events. Unlike you, he did not have the chance to contemplate the seriousness of each situation, or how he would act, until he was already a certified athletic trainer. You, however, have the opportunity to learn from the authors' experiences and mistakes by going through these cases. Although you or your instructor may not agree with every decision in the chapter or text, preparation and forethought into injury management is crucial for your professional success as well as your patients' safety.

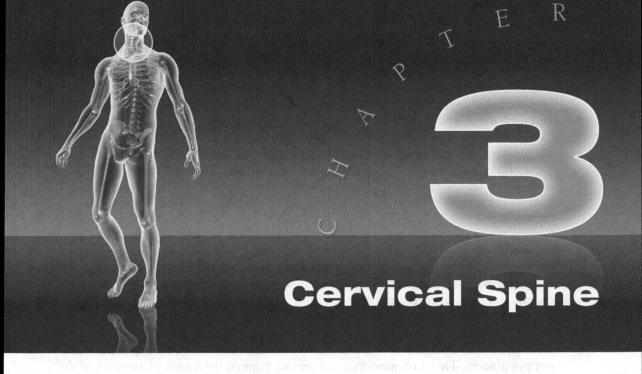

CHAPTER 3

Cervical Spine

INTRODUCTION

In this chapter we will examine the clinical evaluation and management of six cervical spine pathologies. They will be presented in a variety of settings using both on-field and off-field scenarios. The pathologies presented in this chapter include both acute and chronic pathologies. They are a good representation of injuries encountered by a certified athletic trainer. One of the cases, although considered by many to be rare in athletics, is still probable and if mismanaged is likely to have catastrophic results. Remember that some of the cases presented have been intentionally written with inappropriate actions, procedures, treatments, and general mismanagement of the case by the clinician to show that mismanagement of a cervical spine injury (CSI) could have catastrophic consequences. Additional information, such as special tests, will be discussed to help you remember previous course materials or clinical experiences. If at any time you feel that more in-depth review is needed, please refer to your favorite anatomical, assessment, and/or stress/special tests reference guides or articles.

Because the cervical spine is the most mobile of all the vertebral column sections, with its wide range of motion and its vast number of blood vessels, nerves, and spinal tissues, it is also the most vulnerable to trauma. Cervical spine injuries can range from a common "stinger" or "burner" (neurapraxia of a cervical nerve root or brachial plexus),[17] or a minor stiff neck from rotating too quickly, to a severe C5 fracture. Even worse, catastrophic injuries such as atlanto-occipital joint (AOJ) dislocation[7,12] or spinal cord syndrome[2] can result in permanent neurological injury or death.[17] Any significant trauma occurring above C3 increases the risk of death, because loss of respiratory muscle function (spinal cord damage) or damage to the hindbrain (center controlling breathing and cardiac function) can cause respiratory or cardiac arrest.

67

Acute CSI is normally the result of some type of direct blow to the neck or to an acceleration/deceleration accident that causes rapid hyperflexion or hyperextension of the spine (e.g., whiplash).[18,19] However, the major mechanism of serious cervical injuries is an axial load (combined with cervical flexion and rotation) or a large compressive force applied to the top of the head.[2,5,21] Axial loading occurs when the head and neck are flexed approximately 30°, as in head-first tackling (commonly referred to as spearing or spear tackling). In American football, axial loading is accepted as the primary cause of cervical-spine fracture and dislocation.[5]

In this position (30° of cervical flexion), the normal curve of the cervical spine disappears, removing the energy-absorbing elastic component of the region.[22] As the contact force applied to the crown of the head or helmet continues, the cervical spine experiences a compressive load from the torso.[22] Essentially, the head has stopped, but the torso keeps moving, crushing the cervical spine between the two.[5] Once the maximum vertical compression is reached, angular deformation and buckling occurs as the cervical spine fails, resulting in fracture, subluxation, or dislocation[5] and, if bony fragments or herniated disc materials encroach on the spinal cord,[2] possible concomitant spinal-cord syndrome.

Cervical spine injuries can also manifest themselves as chronic injuries and are often the result of years of repetitive microtrauma. In the workplace, musculoskeletal disorders of the neck and shoulder are frequent, and are a concern among the working population. They are more frequent among women than men.[9] Disorders of the neck and shoulder are often the result of multiple factors such as stress,[20] ergonomics (i.e., improper set-up of a computer work station or assembly line), chronic muscular fatigue[3] caused by poor cervical and thoracic posture (i.e., forward head posture), aging (changes in the chemical composition of the nucleus pulposus and annulus fibrosus that result in a progressive loss of their viscoelastic properties),[9,16] and improper lifting. A history of CSI from automobile accidents or athletic accidents may lead to the development of chronic neck pain. Years of repetitive microtrauma can also lead to degenerative changes in the vertebral disc and vertebral body. These changes can lead to spinal nerve-root irritation, affecting an individual's muscular function, ability to experience sensation, and quality of life as cervical motion is altered or lost.

FIGURE 3.1

Vertebral column.

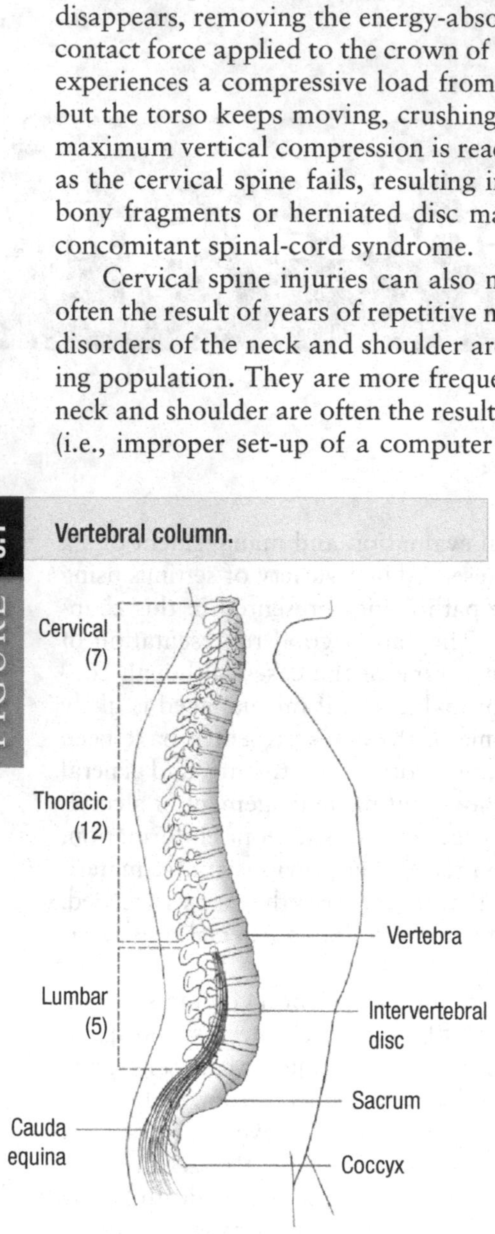

Cervical (7)

Thoracic (12)

Lumbar (5)

Cauda equina

Vertebra

Intervertebral disc

Sacrum

Coccyx

Source: NIAMS.

ANATOMICAL REVIEW

The spinal or vertebral column consists of 33 vertebrae divided into 5 regions: 7 cervical, 12 thoracic, 5 lumbar, 5 fused bones of the sacrum, and 4 fused bones of the coccyx (Figure 3.1). Our focus in this chapter is on the cervical vertebrae, which are designed more for mobility than stability[15] and consist of seven vertebrae, two of which, the atlas and axis of the craniovertebral region, are distinctly different from the other five. Each cervical vertebra is designated with a C and numbered sequentially from the atlas to the seventh vertebra—C1, C2, and so on. In general, the vertebral or spinal column is responsible for four major functions, including: (1) providing a base of support of the body in an upright posture, (2) allowing for locomotion and movement, (3) protecting the spinal cord, which resides in the spinal canal, and (4) providing shock absorption during sitting, standing, and moving via the intervertebral discs.[4,8,10,11,15]

The Atlas Vertebra

The atlas (C1) articulates superiorly with the cranium and acts as a washer between the skull and lower cervical spine, supporting the skull (Figure 3.2). The atlas has no vertebral body and supports the weight of the skull (occiput) through its articulation with the occipital condyle,[22] which functions to transmit forces from the head to the spine,[13] thereby creating the atlanto-occipital joint (AOJ). The atlas allows articulation with the axis (C2), inferiorly creating the atlanto-axial joint (AAJ).

The atlas differs from all other vertebra because it does not have a body. Rather, it consists of two lateral masses joined together by an anterior and posterior arch.[15] The transverse process of the atlas is also longer than those of the cervical vertebra, except for C7, which is the longest. The atlas transverse process is palpable between the mastoid process and mandibular angle. The length of the transverse process provides a significant leverage point and allows for a mechanical advantage when the head is rotated.[15]

The AOJ allows the cranium to move independently relative to the atlas (i.e., flexion and extension of the head on the cervical spine, known as capital flexion and extension), as when the head is nodded.[10,22] The AOJ also allows for some right and left lateral flexion and right and left rotation; however, the total amount of non-sagittal plane motion has yet to be determined.[10]

| FIGURE | **3.2** | Atlas vertebra. |

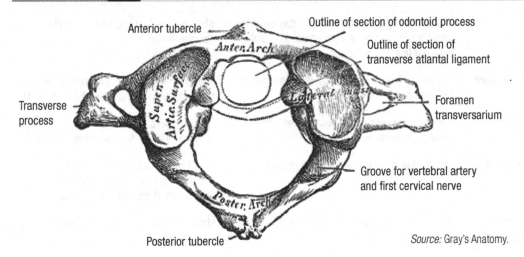

Source: Gray's Anatomy.

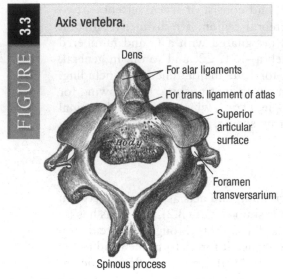

FIGURE 3.3 Axis vertebra.

Dens
For alar ligaments
For trans. ligament of atlas
Superior articular surface
Body
Foramen transversarium
Spinous process

Source: Gray's Anatomy.

The Axis Vertebra

The axis (C2), a vertical pillar of bone, projects upward from the superior surface of the axis's vertebral body and articulates with the atlas and the third cervical vertebra (Figure 3.3). The axis is unique in that it has a small body, dens or odontoid process (i.e., vertical projection from the axis body), short transverse process, and long spinous process, which provides a prominent bony landmark for palpation.[13,15] The axis lamina is thicker than any other vertebrae and provides a point of attachment for the ligamentum flava.

The superiorly directed dens also articulates with the atlas to form the atlano-odontoid joint (the median joint of the AAJ). This is where a majority of right and left cervical rotation occurs.[6,22] Rotation of the atlas around the dens is possible because of the stabilizing function of three ligaments—the transverse, alar, and apical. Together these ligaments hold the dens and make a stable structure on which the atlas can rotate.[22] The stability of the AOJ, AAJ, and atlanto-odontoid joint is provided by several ligamentous structures (Table 3.1).

TABLE 3.1 Ligaments of the upper cervical spine (C1–C2).[10,14,15]

LIGAMENT	LOCATION	FUNCTION
Nuchal ligament	Continuation of the supraspinous ligament	Serves as an area for muscle attachment and limits cervical flexion
Posterior atlano-occipital membrane	Between the posterior arch of the atlas and occiput and is a continuation of the ligamentum flavum	Stabilizes the AOJ
Tectorial membrane	A broad, strong band covering the odontoid process and is a continuation of the posterior longitudinal ligament from C2 to the occiput	Stabilizes the AOJ and AAJ and limits cervical flexion
Cruciate ligament of the dens	Divided in 3 sections and is located between the tectorial membrane and alar ligaments	Stabilizes dens, limiting anterior translation of the atlas at AAJ joint and the skull at the AOJ
Alar ligament	Two bands running on the right and left, attaching the dens to the atlas and occiput	Stabilizes dens, limiting right and left rotation of the skull at the AOJ and atlas at the AAJ
Apical odontoid ligament	Located between the dens and the occiput	Stabilizes dens by attaching it to the occiput, limiting superior and anterior translation of the head at the AOJ
Anterior longitudinal ligament	Attaches to the body of the axis, anterior tubercle of atlas, and onto the occiput	Limits extension of the cervical spine

The primary movements occurring at the AAJ are right and left rotation (e.g., saying "no"), which account for more than 50 percent of the cervical rotation in the transverse plane.[10] The AAJ also allows for limited flexion and extension and right and left lateral flexion and rotation; however, the total amount of non-sagittal plane motion has yet to be determined.

Cervical Vertebrae C3–C7

The remaining five vertebrae (C3–C7) demonstrate typical morphology with slight deviations,[10,13] and they work with the upper spine to create a lordotic curve (Figure 3.4). They function to support the axial load of the skull, maintain balance, support the reactive forces of the muscles, and provide the greatest amount of mobility in the vertebral spinal column.[10] A typical cervical vertebra is composed of a vertebral body (articulates with the intervertebral disc), vertebral arch (composed of 2 pedicles and 2 lamina), inferior and superior articular facets, and spinous and transverse processes (Figure 3.5).

The vertebral arch serves as the protective tunnel through which the spinal cord passes and narrows as it descends down the spinal column. The inferior articular facet of one vertebra (upper) and the superior articular facet of another vertebra (lower) create an apophyseal joint (facet joint), which occurs bilaterally. Facet joints contribute to overall spinal motion, decrease weight-bearing stress through the vertebral body and disc by creating two additional areas for load transmission, and create a mechanical barricade permitting certain movements and blocking others.[15] The spinous and transverse processes are points of ligament and muscular attachment. The cervical spine is unique in that the transverse processes have a transverse foramen (foramina transversaria) through which the vertebral artery passes. The vertebral artery is a branch of the subclavian artery and provides blood to the top of the spinal cord and the posterior aspect of the brain.

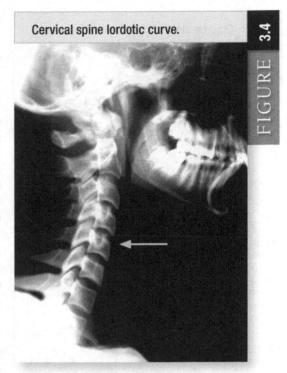

Cervical spine lordotic curve.

FIGURE 3.4

Note the normal lordosis, a normal anteriorly convex curvature of the vertebral column. When the neck is flexed 30°, the normal lordotic curve of the cervical spine disappears, removing the energy-absorbing elastic component of the region.

Source: © Ernst Daniel Scheffler/Dreamstime.com.

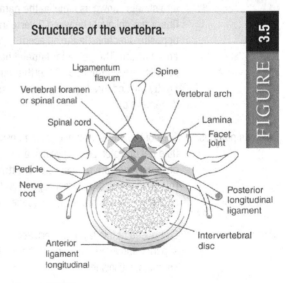

Structures of the vertebra.

FIGURE 3.5

Source: NIAMS.

FIGURE   3.6

Oblique view of the vertebral column.

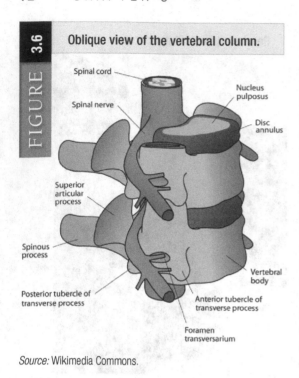

Spinal cord

Nucleus pulposus

Spinal nerve

Disc annulus

Superior articular process

Spinous process

Vertebral body

Posterior tubercle of transverse process

Anterior tubercle of transverse process

Foramen transversarium

Source: Wikimedia Commons.

Intervertebral Discs

Located between each of the vertebral bodies of C3–C7 is the intervertebral disc joint. Accounting for 25 percent of the spinal column height, each intervertebral disc acts primarily to bear the weight of the body, absorb compressive forces applied to the spine, and provide strength to the spinal column during movement.[10,14,15] The discs also act to maintain the opening between the intervertebral foramina, allowing for passage of the spinal nerve roots from the spinal cord (Figure 3.6). Composed primarily of water, each disc has an inner gelatinous portion called the nucleus pulposus, an outer fibrocartilage portion called the annulus fibrous, and two vertebral end-plates (Table 3.2). The cervical disc thickness[10,15] is approximately 3 mm and, in the cervical spine, is thicker anteriorly. The most common cause of cervical radiculopathy is a cervical disc herniation; the next most common is cervical spondylosis.[1]

TABLE 3.2	Composition and function of intervertebral discs.[4,10,14,15]

STRUCTURE	COMPOSITION	FUNCTION
Annulus fibrous	Composed of concentric rings of collagen arranged into sheets known as lamella, the parallel collagen fibers run obliquely between 2 vertebra, lying in opposite directions in the adjacent lamella to form an X pattern. The posterior lamella have a more parallel arrangement and are thinner and less tightly packed, predisposing these to trauma and degeneration.	Encapsulates the nucleus pulposus, permitting angular movement and providing stability against shear and torsion forces.
Nucleus pulpous	Core of the intervertebral disc composed of semi-fluid gel of water, proteoglycans, and collagen. The proteoglycans are responsible for attracting and retaining water. The percentage of water in the nucleus pulposus gradually decreases with aging.	Acts as shock absorber for axial forces and semi-fluid ball bearing during flexion, extension, rotation, and lateral flexion of the spinal column.
End-plate	Composed of thin layers of cartilage covering the superior and inferior surface of the vertebral body, sometimes considered part of the disc.	Acts as a growth plate, transfers nutrients from the vertebral body to the disc, and prevents the nucleus pulposus from bulging into the vertebral body.

Ligaments

Several ligaments play an important role in stabilizing the vertebral column by limiting excessive spinal motion (Figure 3.7).[10,14,15] These include the anterior and posterior longitudinal ligaments, ligamentum flava, and supraspinous and interspinous ligaments (Table 3.3).

| FIGURE 3.7 | Ligaments of the vertebral column. |

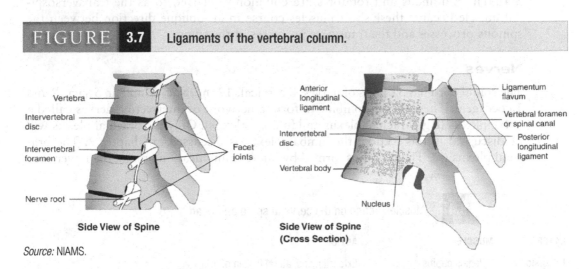

Side View of Spine

Side View of Spine
(Cross Section)

Source: NIAMS.

| TABLE 3.3 | Ligamentous stability of the vertebral column.[4,10,14,15] |

LIGAMENT	LOCATION	FUNCTION
Anterior longitudinal ligament (ALL)	Broad fibrous band, extends from the C1 and occiput to sacrum Firmly fixed to the anterior aspect of all the vertebrae bodies and discs	Maintains stability of the vertebral joints and limits extension of the spinal joints
Interspinous ligament	Short ligaments located between adjacent spinous processes of the vertebrae	Limits spinal joint flexion
Ligamentum flava	Pair of elastic ligaments located between the anterior margins of the superior and inferior vertebral lamina from C2 to sacrum Strongest in the lower thoracic region	Straightens the spinal column after it has been flexed; maintains the normal curvature of the spinal column; and limits spinal joint flexion, rotation, and lateral flexion
Ligamentum nuchae	Cervical region, occipital protuberance to C7	Limits cervical flexion
Posterior longitudinal ligament (PLL)	Narrow and weaker than ALL, extends from the C2 to sacrum Fixed to the intervertebral discs and posterior edge of the vertebral bodies in the spinal canal	Prevents hyperflexion of the spinal column and any posterior protrusion of the discs
Supraspinous	Extends along the posterior margin of the spinous processes of C7–L3/L4	Limits spinal joint flexion

Muscles

Movement of the head and cervical spine is accomplished through the coordinated movement of muscles acting on the upper and lower cervical spine. Together, the anterior, lateral, and posterior cervical musculature allows for flexion and extension of the spine and head, right and left lateral flexion, and right and left rotation (Table 3.4). The multifidus and rotatores are commonly referred to as the transversospinal muscle because these short muscles course in an oblique direction between the spinous processes and the transverse processes of the spine.

Nerves

The spinal cord has 31 pairs of nerves: 8 cervical, 12 thoracic, 5 lumbar, 5 sacral, and 1 coccygeal. These nerves combine to form a network of intersecting nerves called a nerve plexus (e.g., brachial plexus and lumbar plexus). Only the brachial plexus will be discussed in this section; the lumbar plexus is discussed in Chapter 7. The brachial plexus (see Figure 3.8) is formed by intercommunication among the lower four

TABLE 3.4   Muscles acting on the cervical spine and head.

LAYER	MUSCLE	ACTION
Intrinsic	Splenius capitis	Extension and lateral flexion of ADJ
	Splenius cervicis	Rotation of the face toward the same side, extension of cervical spine
	Iliocostalis (cervicis)	Extension and lateral flexion of vertebral column (cervical region)
	Longissimus (cervicis)	Extension and lateral flexion of vertebral column (cervical region)
	Longissimus (capitis)	Extension of the head and cervical spine, rotation of the head toward the same side
	Spinalis (cervicis)	Extension and lateral flexion of vertebral column (cervical region)
	Spinalis (capitis)	Extension and lateral flexion of the ADJ
	Semispinalis (cervicis)	Extension of the cervical and thoracic spine, rotation to the opposite side
	Semispinalis (capitis)	Extension of the ADJ, rotation to the opposite side
	Multifidus	Trunk extension, trunk side flexion, trunk rotation, spinal stabilization
	Rotatores	Trunk rotation, spinal stabilization
Extrinsic	Trapezius (upper one-third)	Extension and lateral flexion of cervical spine, rotation of cervical spine to the opposite side
	Levator scapulae	Extension of cervical spine
	Sternocleidomastoid	Flexion of cervical spine, rotation of head to the opposite side, lateral flexion of cervical spine
	Anterior scalene	Lateral flexion of cervical spine
	Middle scalene	Lateral flexion of cervical spine
	Posterior scalene	Lateral flexion of cervical spine

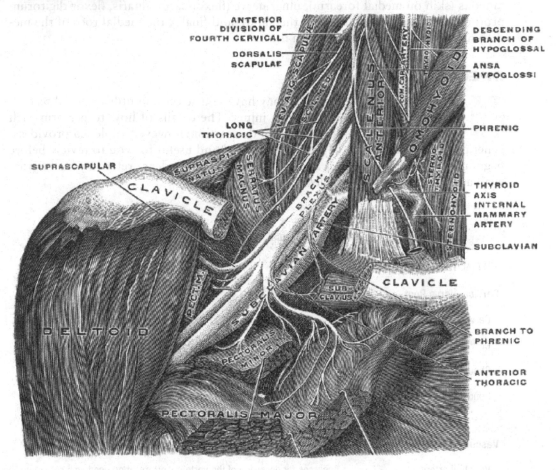

Source: Gray's Anatomy.

cervical nerves (C5–C8) and the first thoracic nerve (T1) and divides into the upper, middle, and lower trunks shortly after emerging from the intervertebral foramina. The nerve roots C5 and C6 form the upper trunk, C7 forms the middle trunk, and C8 and T1 form the lower trunk. Each trunk is further divided into anterior and posterior divisions at the clavicle region, with the anterior division innervating the upper-limb wrist and hand flexors and the posterior division innervating the wrist and hand extensors, respectively.

Continuing down the neck, the posterior division of all three of the trunks forms the posterior cord, the anterior division of the middle and upper trunks forms the lateral cord, and the anterior division of the lower trunk forms the medial cord. The posterior cord stems from the nerve roots of C5 to T1 and has five branches: upper subscapular (supplies the subscapularis), thoracodorsal (supplies latissimus dorsi), lower subscapular (teres major), axillary (deltoid, teres major), and radial nerves (triceps). The lateral cord stems from C5 to C7 and has three branches: lateral pectoral (pectoralis major), musculocutaneous (coracobrachialis, biceps brachii, brachialis), and the lateral root of the median nerve (forearm flexors). The medial cord stems from C8 to T1 and has five branches: medial pectoral (pectoralis minor and major), medial brachial cutaneous (skin on medial side of the arm), medial antebrachial cutaneous (skin on medial forearm), ulnar nerve (flexor carpi ulnaris, flexor digitorum profundus, and smaller muscles of the hand), and finally, the medial root of the median nerve that supplies the forearm flexors.

SPECIAL TESTS

The case studies in this chapter may have you select and utilize special tests in order to adequately evaluate the injury. The details of how to perform each special test are beyond the scope of this section; however, Table 3.5 provides a general list of special tests that may be required and useful for you to review before beginning the case studies. For a more thorough review, please refer to your favorite evaluation text or journal article(s).

TABLE **3.5** Special tests of the cervical spine.

SPECIAL TEST	FUNCTION
Cervical Nerve Root	
Cervical compression	Duplicates pain by increasing pressure on the cervical nerve root(s)
Cervical distraction	Assesses for nerve root compression by relieving the patient's symptoms
Shoulder abduction	Assessing for herniated disc(s) and nerve root compression
Spurling's	Assesses nerve root compression, which can be correlated by the distribution of pain along the dermatome pattern
Vascular	
Vertebral artery	Assesses for occlusion of the vertebral artery, often used as a screening technique
Herniated Disc	
Valsalva	Assesses for increased pain due to increased intrathecal pressure, which may be secondary to a space-occupying lesion, herniated disc, tumor, or osteophyte (a bony outgrowth or protuberance) in the spinal canal
Brachial Plexus	
Brachial plexus stretch	Assesses for irritation of the brachial plexus
Tinel's sign	Assesses nerve pathology to the brachial plexus and peripheral nerves

REFERENCES

1. Abbed KM, Coumans JCE. Cervical radiculopathy: pathophysiology, presentation, and clinical evaluation. *Neurosurgery*. 2007;60(Suppl 1):S-28–S-34.

2. Bailes JE, Petschauer M, Guskiewicz KM, Marano G. Management of cervical spine injuries in athletes. *J Athl Train*. 2007;42(1):126–134.

3. Buckle PW, Devereux J. The nature of work-related neck and upper limb musculoskeletal disorders. *Appl Ergon*. 2002;33(3):207–217.

4. Ebraheim NA, Hassan A, Lee M, Xu R. Functional anatomy of the lumbar spine. Seminars in *Pain Med*. 2004;2(3):131–137.

5. Heck JF, Clarke KS, Peterson TR, Torg JS, Weis M. National Athletic Trainers' Association Position Statement: head-down contact and spearing in tackle football. *J Athl Train*. 2004;39(1):101–111.

6. Hoppenfeld S. *Physical Examination of the Spine and Extremities*. Norwalk, CT: Appleton-Century-Croft; 1976.

7. Houle P, McDonnell DE, Vender J. Traumatic atlanto-occipital dislocation in children. *Pediatr Neurosurg*. 2001;34:193–197.

8. Humphreys SC, Eck JC. Clinical evaluation and treatment options for herniated lumbar disc. *Am Fam Physician*. 1999;59(3):575–582.

9. Larsson B, Søgaard K, Rosendal L. Work related neck-shoulder pain: a review on magnitude, risk factors, biochemical characteristics, clinical picture and preventive interventions. *Best Pract Res Clin Rheumatol*. 2007;21(3):447–463.

10. Levangie PK, Norkin CC. *Joint Structure and Function: A Comprehensive Analysis*. Philadelphia, PA: F. A. Davis; 2001.

11. McGill S. Functional anatomy of the lumbar spine. In: *Low Back Disorders: Evidence-Based Prevention and Rehabilitation*. Champaign, IL: Human Kinetics; 2002:45–86.

12. McKenna DA, Roche CJ, Lee WK, Torreggiani WC, Duddalwar VA. Atlanto-occipital dislocation: case report and discussion. *Can J Emerg Med*. 2006;8(1):50–53.

13. Mercer SR. Structure and function of the bones and joints of the cervical spine In: Oatis CA (Ed.), *Kinesiology: The Mechanics and Pathomechanics of Human Movement*. Baltimore, MD: Lippincott, Williams & Wilkins; 2004:451–469.

14. Moore K, Dalley A. *Clinically Oriented Anatomy* (5th ed.). Baltimore, MD: Lippincott, Williams & Wilkins; 2005.

15. Oliver J, Middleditch A. *Functional Anatomy of the Spine*. Oxford: Butterworth-Heinemann Ltd.; 1991.

16. Rao R. Neck pain, cervical radiculopathy, and cervical myelopathy. *J Bone Joint Surg Am*. 2002a;84-A(10):1872.

17. Rihn JA, Anderson DT, Lamb K, et al. Cervical spine injuries in American football. *Sports Med*. 2009;39(9):697–708.

18. Rosenfeld M, Gunnarsson R, Borenstein P. Early intervention in whiplash-associated disorders: a comparison of two treatment protocols. *Spine*. 2000;25(5):1782–1787.

19. Rosenfeld M, Seferiadis A, Carlsson J, Gunnarsson R. Active intervention in patients with whiplash-associated disorders improves long-term prognosis: a randomized controlled clinical trial. *Spine*. 2003;22:2491–2498.

20. Sjaastad O, Wang H, Bakketeig LS. Neck pain and associated head pain: persistent neck complaint with subsequent, transient, posterior headache. *Acta Neurol Scand*. 2006;114(6):392–399.

21. Swartz EE, Boden BP, Courson RW, et al. National Athletic Trainers' Association position statement: acute management of the cervical spine–injured athlete. *J Athl Train*. 2009;44(3):306–311.

22. Swartz EE, Floyd RT, Cendoma M. Cervical spine functional anatomy and the biomechanics of injury due to compressive loading. *J Athl Train*. 2005;40(3):155–161.

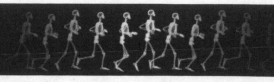

Hector, a 24-year-old United States Marine recruit, was rappelling during basic training when his safety harness detached, and he fell 20 feet to the ground. Seth was the certified athletic trainer attached to the 301st Medical Battalion, the unit responsible for the health and welfare of Hector's unit. He observed Hector falling from the wall. He immediately rushed to Hector, who lay supine and unconscious. A medic also arrived on scene within 5 seconds of Seth's arrival. Within another few seconds Hector began to regain consciousness.

HISTORY

It appears to Seth that Hector landed on the top of his head with a flexed neck. While gathering a SAMPLE history (symptoms, allergies, medications, past pertinent history, last oral intake, event leading to the situation), Seth is informed that Hector is unable to move any of his extremities and complains of neck discomfort.

PHYSICAL EXAMINATION

Hector was unconscious for 30 seconds. He is alert now but is disoriented as to his current location, date, and details of his fall. His Glasgow Coma Scale is 12 (eye opening 4, verbal 4, motor 4). Hector is tender between the spinous processes of C5 and C7. Upper and lower deep tendon reflexes are absent bilaterally. Dull and sharp sensory testing demonstrates anesthesia from the acromioclavicular joint (ACJ) into the thorax and down through the palmar aspect of the feet bilaterally. He demonstrates no other immediate signs of secondary trauma except for numerous abrasions to his face and neck. His pupils are equal, round, and reactive to light, with the remaining vital signs in Table 3.1.1a.

Seth and the two other medics apply a Stifneck cervical collar and secure Hector onto a spine board. Once the ambulance arrives, a head-immobilizing device is applied to further support the spine. Hector is transported to a stretcher for transit to the base hospital for further evaluation. His vital signs en route to the hospital are in Table 3.1.1b.

TABLE   3.1.1   Hector's vital signs.

3.1.1a Secondary Assessment

VITAL SIGNS	FINDING
Pulse	92, regular, and bounding
Respiration	18 and labored
Blood pressure	138/84
Skin	Hot and moist
Mental status	Alert, but disoriented

3.1.1b Transport

VITAL SIGNS	FINDING
Pulse	78 and regular
Respiration	15 and normal
Blood pressure	128/82
Skin	Warm and dry
Mental status	Alert, but disoriented

Please answer the following questions based on the above case information.

3.1 / **1.** Based on the information presented in the case, determine (a) the differential diagnoses and (b) the clinical diagnosis.

3.1 / **2.** Once Seth arrived at Hector's side and determined that the scene was safe, Seth should have immediately begun to assess what?

3.1 / **3.** Based on the case, once a medic arrived on scene, she should have been responsible for performing what?

3.1 / **4.** Discuss the difference between the AVPU (alert, verbal, painful, unconscious) scale and the Glasgow Coma Scale (GCS). If you were in this situation, which scale would you prefer to use and why?

3.1 / **5.** Discuss how you would have managed this situation from scene survey to packaging and transport of Hector.

T om, a 22-year-old football player, came running off the football field shaking his right arm after making a spectacular tackle. Lisa, the certified athletic trainer covering the game, jogged over to tend to Tom. During her trip over she noticed that Tom's right arm was dangling by his side (Figure 3.2.1) and that he was rubbing his arm and fingers.

FIGURE 3.2.1

Tom's arm position coming off the football field.

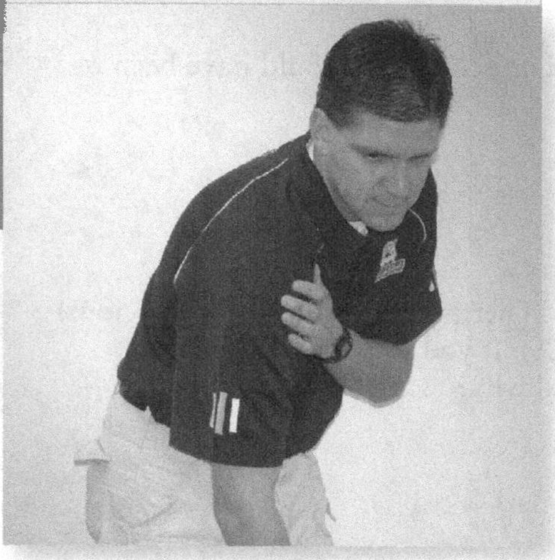

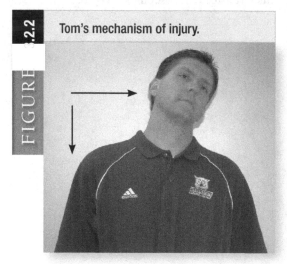

FIGURE 3.2.2

Tom's mechanism of injury.

Tom's head was forced to his left with a downward force to the right shoulder.

HISTORY

Tom explains that while he was making a tackle "my head and neck were forced to the side." Lisa continues to question Tom and determines that his head was forced laterally to the left side (i.e., left ear to left shoulder) while making the tackle (Figure 3.2.2). His immediate CCs on the sideline include the inability to raise his right arm and a "burning" sensation radiating down the right arm. After about 6 minutes, the burning sensation begins to decrease, and Tom regains minimal movement of his right arm.

PHYSICAL EXAMINATION

Upon physical examination, Tom is A&O and in moderate discomfort. There is no observable deformity of the cervical spine, shoulder girdle, and/or thorax. Tom has palpable muscle spasms along the scalene(s) (anterior and middle). Lisa instructs Tom to raise both arms overhead. He is unable, however, to abduct or flex his right arm greater than 15° and 10°, respectively. His right hand grip strength is also diminished by comparison with the uninvolved side. Cervical ROM is painful and limited into left lateral flexion, and there is bilateral rotational pain. All other motions are WNL. Cervical compression and distraction tests are negative. A neurological exam reveals paresthesia over the middle deltoid and upper medial aspect of the humeral area. There is decreased sensitivity over the lateral patch. Lisa informs the coach that Tom will be unable to return to the game until a further evaluation is completed. Lisa calls in the team's internal medicine physician for a further evaluation.

Please answer the following questions based on the above case information.

3.2 / 1. Based on the information presented in the case, determine (a) the differential diagnoses and (b) the clinical diagnosis.

3.2 / 2. Lisa asked several specific history questions to guide the physical examination. Based on the clinical diagnosis above, identify three to five additional history questions you may have asked as the evaluating clinician.

3.2 / 3. If this injury was to persist during the athletic season, what type of physician would be best suited to manage Tom's case and why?

3.2 / 4. Based on the results of functional and neurological exams presented in this case, which nerve roots and peripheral nerves are most likely to be involved?

3.2 / 5. Considering Tom's clinical diagnosis, identify the criteria Lisa should use in order to make a return-to-play decision.

3.2 / 6. (a) What other special tests, if any, should Lisa perform to confirm her clinical diagnosis? (b) Identify how to perform these tests.

Nancy, a certified athletic trainer working for Peak Physical Therapy, received a referral from Dr. Adams to evaluate and treat Tim, a 35-year-old recreational tennis player, who just left his office complaining of left-sided neck pain with paresthesia.

HISTORY

As Nancy begins her history, she notes Tim's guarding and stiffness of the cervical spine. Tim explains to Nancy that during his tennis match last week he went to serve and during his follow-through he felt a sharp, piercing pain in his neck. He reports that he kept playing for the next half hour, but by the next morning he was experiencing ". . . pinching sensations that radiate down the outside of my arm into my thumb and index finger." Further questioning from Nancy reveals that Tim was a collegiate football player who played semi-professional football for two years. Nancy also learns that Tim has a sedentary job involving 8 hours of repetitive computer work and an additional 2 hours of computer programming at home per evening.

PHYSICAL EXAMINATION

Tim presents with cervical spine-guarding and moderate discomfort (7/10). An assessment of AROM finds that Tim's pain is worsened by forward flexion (0°–30°) and right lateral flexion (0°–31°). In fact, right lateral flexion increases Tim's radi-

TABLE 3.3.1	Tim's manual muscle testing results.	
MOTION	**RIGHT**	**LEFT**
Shoulder flexion	5/5	4/5
Shoulder abduction	5/5	3+/5
Shoulder internal rotation and external rotation	5/5	4/5
Elbow flexion	5/5	3/5
Elbow extension	5/5	4/5
Pronation	5/5	4/5
Supination	5/5	3/5
Wrist flexion	5/5	4/5
Wrist extension	5/5	3+/5

ating pain. Muscle testing reveals the results shown in Table 3.3.1. During the physical examination, Nancy finds Tim's grip strength in his left hand is only 50 percent of his right-hand grip, which is the dominant hand. Right grip strength is 80 lbs. of force and left grip strength is 40 lbs. of force. Upper-extremity range of motion bilaterally are within functional limits passively. The special test in Figure 3.3.1 causes an increase in Tim's radicular symptoms, but a cervical distraction test relieves his discomfort.

Nancy believes she has enough information to make her clinical diagnosis. She explains her findings to Tim, and together they design a course of action that will include cervical traction, electrical stimulation for pain control, and ergonomic training.

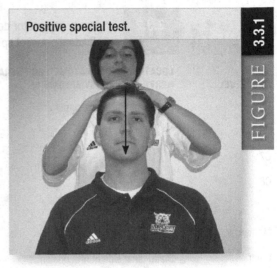

Positive special test.

FIGURE 3.3.1

Arrow indicates direction of force applied to crown of Tim's head.

❓ QUESTIONS   CASE 3.3

Please answer the following questions based on the above case information.

3.3 / 1. Based on the information presented in the case, determine (a) the differential diagnoses and (b) the clinical diagnosis.

3.3 / 2. Overall, do you believe Nancy adequately evaluated Tim's condition? If not, what would you have done differently as the evaluating clinician and why?

3.3 / 3. Which nerve root or roots are involved in this condition and how and why did you come to this conclusion?

3.3 / 4. Complete Table 3.3.2 below, which lists the location of sensory and motor deficits associated with nerve root involvement at each of the cervical spine levels and upper extremity peripheral nerves.

TABLE 3.3.2	Sensory and motor deficits in association with nerve root involvement at individual cervical spine levels and upper extremity peripheral nerves.	
DISC LEVEL	**LOCATION OF DERMATOME/PERIPHERAL NERVE SENSORY SYMPTOMS**	**MOTOR DEFICIT**
C5	Deltoid patch, lateral upper arm	
C6		
C7		Elbow extension (triceps), wrist flexion
C8		
T1	Medial elbow, arm	
Median		
Ulnar	Distal ulnar side of fifth phalange	
Radial		Wrist extension and thumb extension

3.3 / **5.** An individual's sensory perception arises from a variety of afferent receptors located within the skin that relay information to the CNS. Given the findings from the case, how and what should be assessed in order to measure Tim's sensory perception?

3.3 / **6.** During the assessment it is determined that the grip strength is decreased by 50 percent. (a) Why is grip strength assessed? (b) Should the non-dominant hand equal the dominant hand? (c) What is the reliability of dynamometers for measuring grip strength?

3.3 / **7.** What, if any, other special tests could Nancy have performed to assist in determining the clinical diagnosis?

J oel, a 25-year-veteran head athletic trainer at the University of Zion, was covering a football practice when his senior athletic training student, Rachel, suddenly began calling his name. Joel immediately rushed over to Rachel's location, realizing that Pat, one of the defensive backs, was lying on the ground. As he reached Pat, he assessed his level of consciousness (LOC) and determined that Pat was unresponsive.

PHYSICAL EXAMINATION

Joel immediately initiates the university's emergency action plan, which requires immediate stabilization of the cervical spine. The rest of the athletic training students, including Rachel, gather the emergency equipment, including an AED, a bag-valve mask, adjunct airways, and supplemental oxygen. Rachel also places a call to 9-1-1. The primary assessment using a head-tilt/chin-lift reveals adequate airway, breathing, and circulation. The lateral loop straps on Pat's helmet are removed, and the face mask is swung upward. While waiting for EMS, Sean, another certified athletic trainer, arrives and completes a head-to-toe physical exam and assesses Pat's blood pressure and pulse, which appear to be stable. Upon arrival of the EMS, the athletic training staff works with the EMTs to package the student-athlete. En route to the hospital, Pat goes into respiratory arrest, requiring intubation and positive-pressure ventilation by the EMTs.

HOSPITAL EXAMINATION

Joel sends Sean with the EMTs to the hospital to assist in appropriately removing the football equipment. Upon arrival at the hospital, the athlete's GCS is 7, with no spontaneous respirations. Removal of the football equipment is delayed until radiographs could confirm the presence of cervical trauma.

DIAGNOSTIC IMAGINING

A lateral cervical spine radiograph revealed soft tissue widening, a malalignment between the cranium and cervical spine, and widening of the atlanto-occipital greater than 7 mm.

Please answer the following questions based on the above case information.

3.4 / **1.** Based on the information presented in the case, (a) what is the likely clinical diagnosis? (b) What is the typical MOI?

3.4 / **2.** The athlete in this case went into respiratory arrest. Given the information provided in the case, why did this occur?

3.4 / **3.** (a) Pat was unconscious; so how did Joel gather any history information? (b) Had the athlete been conscious, identify three to four history questions you, as the evaluating clinician, would have asked to guide the physical examination.

3.4 / **4.** Overall, do you believe Joel appropriately managed the current situation? If not, what would you have done differently as the evaluating clinician, and why?

3.4 / **5.** Based on the clinical presentation, the football equipment was not removed until Pat's arrival at the emergency department. If you were in Sean's place, discuss how you would have removed the football equipment in the emergency room.

CASE 3.5

On a Thursday afternoon, Josh, the athletic trainer working at Sports South Health Clinic, was getting ready for his next patient. Kyla, a 23-year-old female, complained of neck pain and was referred by the local emergency room (ER) to Dr. Knight and then to Josh. A brief note in her chart read: "The patient sought medical attention after being in a golf cart accident."

HISTORY

Josh begins the evaluation by asking Kyla what happened. She explains that after making par on the fourth hole, she and her girlfriends were horsing around with the golf cart when they were rear-ended by another golf cart. She continues, stating, "This happened five days ago at a local country club. My head snapped backwards and forward, and the pain was so bad that my friends took me to the ER where they took some X-rays of my neck, which were negative for fractures. The ER doctor told me to take some anti-inflammatory medication, and they gave me a soft collar to help with the pain. From there I was referred to Dr. Knight, my family doctor, who prescribed some more anti-inflammatory medication and therapy."

Josh asks a series of questions related to Kyla's current status. Her CCs are presented in Table 3.5.1. She denies any paresthesia and any noticeable weakness of the upper extremities. Josh learns that she is an active individual and enjoys golfing, jogging, lifting, and swimming. She is unable to participate in any of these activities because of increased pain.

PHYSICAL EXAMINATION

Observation of the patient reveals Kyla is no longer wearing her soft collar. Josh notices Kyla is moving her neck very deliberately and does not appear comfortable. Josh's observation of Kyla's head posture is noted in Figure 3.5.1. The AROM of her cervical spine is limited and is painful in all directions. Flexion is 20°, extension is 20°, bilateral rotation is 20°, and bilateral lateral flexion is 25° in

TABLE 3.5.1

Kyla's CCs upon physical examination.

- Diffuse neck pain with no specific area worse than another
- Pain is better with rest, specifically when lying down
- States she has some difficulty sleeping
- Pain worse when sitting for prolonged period of time either at computer or while in class
- Complains of increased discomfort of cervical spine with movement of any kind and reports having increased headaches since accident

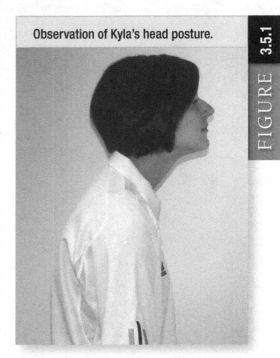

FIGURE 3.5.1

Observation of Kyla's head posture.

FIGURE 3.5.2

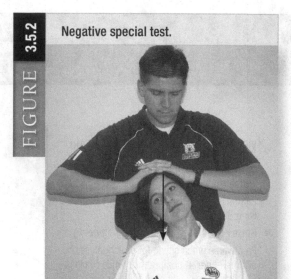

Negative special test.

Arrow indicates direction of force applied to Kyla's head.

the sitting position. Kyla's PROM is WNL throughout in the supine position, and she reports less pain. Scapular/shoulder elevation is painful, with a muscle grade of 4/5 bilaterally. Shoulder abduction causes pain of the cervical spine with resistance, while active motion is not painful. Elbow flexion reveals a full grade of 5/5 bilaterally. Elbow extension, wrist extension, wrist flexion, and finger abduction are all graded 5/5.

Kyla has difficulty performing cervical retraction in the seated position and is unable to flatten out the lordosis of the cervical spine. Protraction of the cervical spine is painful in the sitting position. When Kyla is supine, active cervical retraction motion improves; however, protraction continues to be painful in the supine position. When Josh asks Kyla to lift her head off the table, she is unable to do so because of increased pain. Sternocleidomaistoid muscle strength is 2/5 bilaterally. Cervical extension strength is 3/5. In addition, Kyla presents with tenderness of the bilateral scalenes and along the sternocleidomastoid muscles bilaterally. Light-touch sensation is intact throughout all upper extremity dermatomes. A vertebral artery test and another special test (shown in Figure 3.5.2) are negative. Josh observes the way Kyla comes to a sitting position from supine and notes that she moves into a side-lying position and helps herself up with the use of her arms.

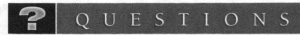

Please answer the following questions based on the above case information.

3.5 / 1. Based on the information presented in the case, determine (a) the differential diagnoses and (b) the clinical diagnosis.

3.5 / 2. Based on the results of the physical examination in this case scenario, why would AROM be limited, but PROM be within functional limits?

3.5 / 3. Overall, do you believe Josh adequately evaluated Kyla's condition given the provided information? If not, what would you have done differently as the evaluating clinician and why?

3.5 / 4. (a) What other anatomical structures, if any, should Josh have palpated to help determine the clinical diagnosis? (b) When Josh noted cervical extension strength to be a 3/5, which structures were specifically being assessed? (c) Which structure(s) were specifically involved in the clinical diagnosis, and which other structures could have been traumatized?

3.5 / 5. Based on the clinical diagnosis presented in this case, describe the MOI and provide other examples of how the injury may occur.

3.5 / 6. After completing the physical examination, Josh documented his findings electronically for Kyla's file. Using your athletic training room's computer tracking software, document your findings electronically as if you were the treating clinician. If the case did not provide information you believe is pertinent to the clinical diagnosis, please add this to your documentation. If you do not have access to injury-tracking software, consider downloading a trial version from CSMI Solutions (Sportsware) by going to www.csmi solutions.com/cmt/publish/service_software_dl.shtml and following the on-screen directions.

During a high school football game, Jared, a wide receiver, jumped up in an attempt to catch a ball that was thrown high. While in the air, he was hit in the back from behind upon catching the ball.

HISTORY

When Jared is hit unexpectedly, his head snaps forward and backwards. Once on the ground Jared is slow to get up and leaves the field holding the back of his neck in pain. As Jared walks off the field, Tyler, the athletic trainer, walks over to tend to him and begin his assessment.

PHYSICAL EXAMINATION

Jared is A&O, with no observable deformity or swelling noted; however, Jared appears to be guarding as a result of scalene and upper trapezium spasms. Upon physical examination, Jared presents with point tenderness in and around the musculature and other anatomical structures (Figure 3.6.1). Tyler performs a full neurological exam, which is unremarkable. After a few minutes, Jared tells Tyler "I want to go back into the game." Before Tyler allows Jared to return to play he re-evaluates his ROM. Active cervical ROM is specifically painful in flexion and rotation. Tyler places Jared in a supine position and begins to assess PROM; however, Jared stops Tyler from moving into flexion because of increased pain along the cervical spine (refer back to Fig. 3.7, p. 73). Because of the lack of proper PROM and the pain, Tyler decides it is best to take away Jared's helmet and remove him from play. Tyler treats him conservatively and provides some at-home instructions for the weekend. He informs Jared that he wants to see him on Monday afternoon.

FIGURE 3.6.1

Observation of Jared's point tenderness.

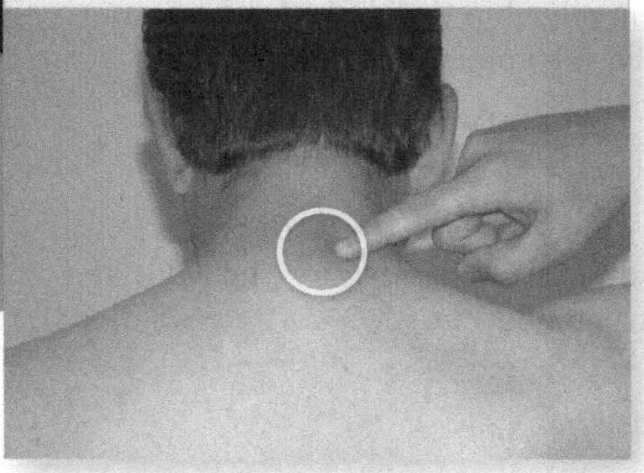

Area of tenderness and pain is located within the circle.

FOLLOW-UP PHYSICAL EXAMINATION

Jared reports to the athletic training room on Monday complaining of extreme pain in the posterior cervical spine area and spasm of the surrounding musculature. His AROM is limited severely in all directions, and PROM is painful into flexion and rotation. Muscle testing is deferred because of pain. Tyler treats him accordingly and refers him to the team physician, who is stopping by later in the day.

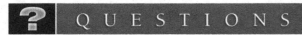

Please answer the following questions based on the above case information.

3.6 / 1. Based on the information presented in the case, determine (a) the differential diagnoses and (b) the clinical diagnosis.

3.6 / 2. Overall do you believe Jared handled the situation correctly? Would you have handled it the same way?

3.6 / 3. Given the information presented in the case, there are two very possible clinical diagnoses that are very similar and present nearly identically. What are the diagnoses, and what would lead you to determine one clinical diagnosis over the other?

3.6 / 4. According to the case study, Tyler did not appear to perform any stress or special tests. (a) Why? (b) How can a clinician adequately assess and establish the clinical diagnosis?

3.6 / 5. (a) How would you manage the injury? (b) What instructions would you have given the athlete for weekend management?

3.5 / 6. If Jared's signs and symptoms progressed to the point where Tyler needed to initiate cervical spine mobilization techniques to treat the injury, (a) which screening test should Tyler employ to rule out any contraindicating pathologies, and (b) is this test really necessary?

CONCLUSION

Cervical spine pathologies share many similar signs and symptoms and can be manifested in different locations within the body (e.g., radicular pain), making them difficult to evaluate and treat. This is why a systematic approach is often warranted. Compounding the problem is the proximity of the vital neurovascular and neurological structures that regulate a variety of biological functions. A missed diagnosis can result in just as catastrophic an outcome as a trauma of significant magnitude (e.g., spearing) if an athletic trainer is not prepared. Athletic trainers need to understand the mechanisms of injury and how to correct body mechanics and behaviors that may cause injury. Remaining up to date with the current emergency assessment and management procedures, and establishing and practicing an organized emergency action plan, are both crucial in reducing catastrophic injuries. The more often an athletic trainer practices and coordinates with the local EMS, the more likely an actual emergency event will be addressed efficiently. Finally, education is vital when dealing with either competitive or recreational athletes. The more that athletic trainers can educate their patients and athletes about proper tackling techniques in football, or about ergonomic design while working on a computer, the greater the likelihood that they can reduce the risk of acute and chronic cervical spine injuries.

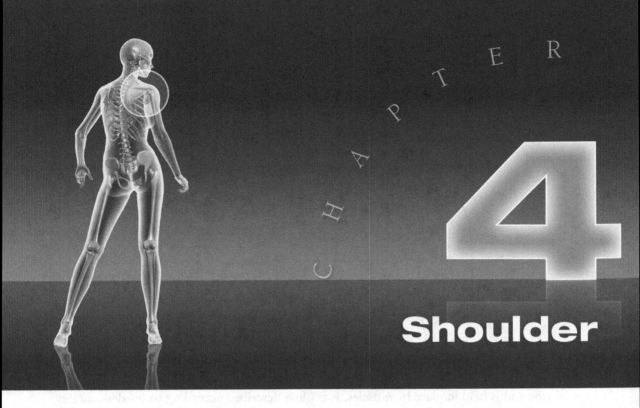

Shoulder

INTRODUCTION

I n this chapter, we will examine the clinical management of 14 shoulder pathologies, based on scenarios that depict a variety of settings with a diverse patient population, to broaden your critical-thinking skills. As with all cases presented in this text, the scenarios are either actual pathologies or modifications of injuries presented in literature. Some scenarios may intentionally contain wrong actions taken by the clinician. Each scenario provides information in order to adequately answer the questions presented; however, in some scenarios, information may be missing or extraneous information may be presented that may affect the way you decipher the scenarios. Therefore, the purpose of providing these scenarios is to facilitate your awareness of different types of acute and chronic conditions, some of which are common, and some not so common. Scapulothoracic motions and mechanics of throwing will not be covered, but a review of these concepts is deemed important for several of the case studies.

ANATOMICAL REVIEW

T he shoulder is often described as two separate anatomical structures—one called the shoulder girdle and the other called the shoulder joint. The shoulder girdle is comprised of the clavicle and scapula bones, whereas the shoulder joint is comprised of the articulation between the scapula and the humerus (Figure 4.1).[2,3]

The clavicle is S-shaped, with the medial end projecting outward and the lateral end projecting inward. The clavicle articulates between the sternum at the medial end (sternal end) and the scapula at the acromion process at the lateral end (acromial end). The clavicle is the sole attachment of the upper extremity to the trunk at the sternal end.

FIGURE   4.1   Clavicle and scapula.

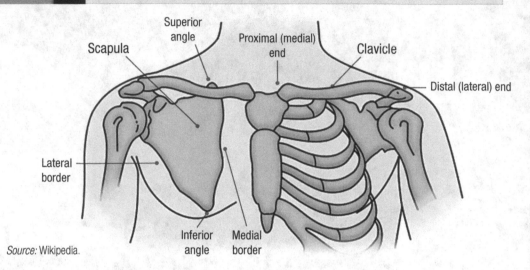

Source: Wikipedia.

The scapula is a triangular-shaped bone that lies over the posterior section of the ribs and is held in place by muscles. It is often described according to borders, angles, and articulations with the humerus and includes: a superior border, lateral border, and medial border; superior and inferior angles; and the articulation of the glenoid fossa with the head of the humerus. Two special projections arise from the scapula—one called the acromion process from the spine of the scapula that articulates with the lateral end of the clavicle and another called the coracoid process that runs anteriorly, just medial to the glenoid cavity (Figure 4.2). The coracoid process serves as a site for muscle attachment. Finally, at the lateral end, the glenoid fossa is the concave articula-

FIGURE   4.2   Anatomy of the shoulder.

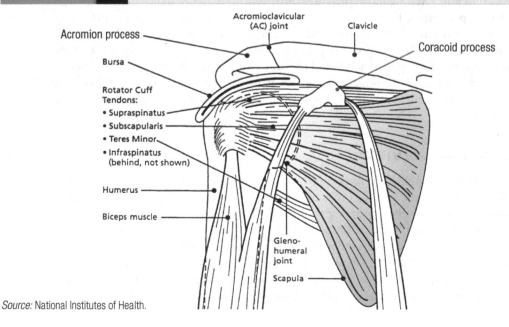

Source: National Institutes of Health.

tion that supports the head of the humerus to create a ball and socket joint (glenohumeral joint). The glenoid fossa has an outer cartilaginous lip called the glenoid labrum.

The humerus is a long bone with a superior portion that articulates with the scapula and a distal portion that articulates with the elbow (Figures 4.3, 4.4). The head of the humerus articulates with the glenoid fossa and is surrounded by a strong capsule and several ligaments. Just below the head of the humerus, and after the anatomical neck, are two bony projections called the greater and lesser tuberosities (serving as muscle attachments) and a bicipital groove located between the two tuberosity structures that houses the long head of the biceps brachii. The surgical neck is just below the tuberosities and continues inferiorly to the shaft. On the shaft, approximately halfway down, is a small bony projection called the deltoid tuberosity, which serves as the attachment site for the deltoid muscle. At the distal end of the humerus, the shaft angles outward and the ridges formed are called the medial and lateral supracondylar ridges. The capitulum is the articulation of the humerus with the radius, and the trochlea is the depression that articulates with the olecranon process of the ulna. On the anterior surface of the distal humerus is the coronoid fossa, which articulates with the coronoid process of the ulna.

Shoulder Joints and Ligaments

The shoulder has several articulating joints and ligaments (Table 4.1). The first shoulder joint is the acromioclavicular joint (ACJ). The AC joint is located at the distal end of the clavicle and the acromion process of the scapula (Figure 4.5). It is classified as a diarthrodial joint, with primarily gliding motions in all three planes of movement. Attaching the joint together is the acromioclavicular ligament (superior and inferior portions) and a thin joint capsule. In addition to the acromioclavicular ligament, the coracoacromial ligament attaches to the acromion and the coracoid process of the scapula. The joint capsule that surrounds the AC joint is weak and must be reinforced by the ligaments of this region.

FIGURE 4.3

Proximal and distal humeral articulations.

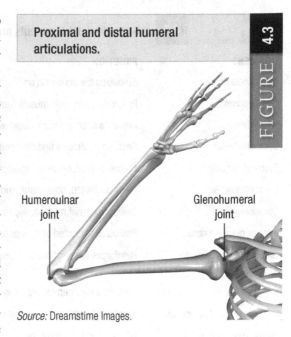

Source: Dreamstime Images.

Humeroulnar joint

Glenohumeral joint

FIGURE 4.4

Anatomical landmarks of the humerus.

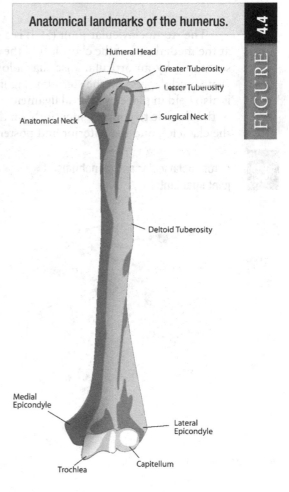

Humeral Head
Greater Tuberosity
Lesser Tuberosity
Anatomical Neck
Surgical Neck
Deltoid Tuberosity
Medial Epicondyle
Lateral Epicondyle
Trochlea
Capitellum

TABLE 4.1	Shoulder joint ligaments and major functions.[7]
LIGAMENT	**FUNCTION**
Acromioclavicular	Stabilizes the acromion on the clavicle, resists upward translation
Coracoacromial	Protects rotator cuff muscle from acromion bone
Interclavicular	Prevents depression and downward glide of the clavicle
Costoclavicular	Secures clavicle to first rib, prevents clavicular elevation
Sternoclavicular	Stabilizes joint, prevents anterior and posterior movements of the clavicle on the sternum
Coracoclavicular	Resists upward, downward, and anteroposterior movement of the clavicle on the scapula
Coracohumeral	Resists external rotation, supports limb against gravity
Inferior glenohumeral	Stabilizes abducted arm, supports inferior capsule and prevents internal rotation
Glenohumeral (superior, middle, inferior)	Reinforces the joint capsule, prevents external rotation
Superior transverse scapular	Creates a foramen for the suprascapular nerve
Inferior transverse scapular	Creates a tunnel for passage of the suprascapular nerve to innervate the infraspinatus muscle
Transverse humeral	Holds the long head of the biceps brachii in the bicipital groove

The sternoclavicular joint (SCJ) is a saddle-shaped synovial joint, with articulation at the medial end of the clavicle and the superior portion of the sternum (manubrium), separated by an articular disc that allows the clavicle to rotate, protract, retract, elevate, and depress on the sternum (Figure 4.6). A joint capsule surrounds the joint and is also held in place by several ligaments: the interclavicular (runs between the two ends of the clavicle to connect superiorly on the manubrium), the costoclavicular (first rib to the clavicle), and the anterior and posterior sternoclavicular ligaments.

FIGURE 4.5

Acromioclavicular and glenohumeral joint ligaments.

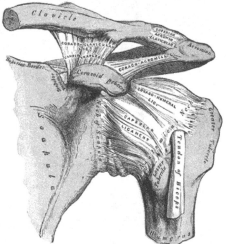

Source: Gray's Anatomy.

The coracoclavicular joint (CCJ) is the articulation between the coracoid process of the scapula and the clavicle. It is joined together by the coracoclavicular ligament (CCL). The CCL has two distinct bands, the conoid and the trapezoid. The conoid band is located more medially than the trapezoid, and both help to resist upward, downward, and anteroposterior clavicular movement. Tearing of these fibers permits the clavicle to rise up, a condition often seen in shoulder separation.

The glenohumeral joint (GHJ) is a ball-and-socket joint, and it has the fullest range of motion of any joint in the body. The stability of the joint is less than that of the ball-and-socket hip joint, because the humeral head is larger than the glenoid fossa and the glenoid is quite shallow when compared with the acetabulum at the hip. The joint is supported by the glenoid labrum, making it larger for better

FIGURE	**4.6**	Sternoclavicular joint ligaments.

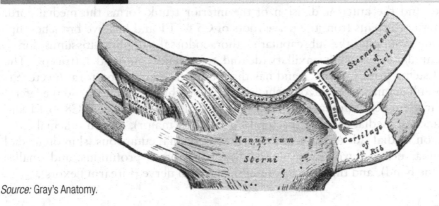

Source: Gray's Anatomy.

congruency, and it is surrounded by a joint capsule. The glenohumeral (GH) ligament (with superior, middle, and inferior bands) arises from the outer rim of the glenoid to the head of the humerus, providing necessary support on the anterior side of the joint. The coracohumeral ligament, found between the coracoid process of the scapula and the head of the humerus, provides support against superior GH dislocations. An inferior GH ligament functions to support and strengthen the inferior portion of the joint capsule and also functions as a stabilizer for the arm in the abducted position.

Other ligaments include the superior and inferior transverse scapular ligaments, found at the scapular and great scapular notches, and the transverse humeral ligament, which crosses between the intertubercular (bicipital) groove.

Nerves

The shoulder has a complex nervous system, with the brachial plexus innervating the muscles and skin in the shoulder, arm, forearm, wrist, and hand (Table 4.2). The brachial plexus arises from the nerve roots ranging from C5 to T1 and divides into upper, middle, and lower trunks as it enters the neck. The nerve roots C5 and C6 form the upper (superior) trunk, C7 forms the middle trunk, and C8 and T1 form the lower (inferior) trunk. The trunks are further divided into anterior and posterior divisions at the clavicle region, with the anterior divisions innervating the upper-limb flexors and the posterior divisions innervating the wrist and hand extensors, respectively.

TABLE	**4.2**	Myotomes and dermatomes of the upper extremity region.

NERVE ROOT	MYOTOME	DERMATOME
C4	Resisted scapula elevation	Back of neck, neck to clavicle to acromion
C5	Resisted shoulder abduction	Deltoid patch, lateral upper arm
C6	Resisted elbow flexion and wrist extension	Lateral forearm, radial side of hand, first and second phalanges
C7	Resisted elbow extension and wrist flexion	Posterior lateral arm and forearm, third phalange
C8	Resisted thumb extension and ulnar deviation	Medial forearm, ulnar border of hand, fourth and fifth phalanges
T1	Resisted finger abduction/adduction	Medial elbow, arm

Continuing down the neck, the posterior divisions of all three of the trunks form the posterior cord, the anterior divisions of the middle and superior trunks form the lateral cord, and the anterior division of the inferior trunk forms the medial cord. The posterior cord stems from the nerve roots of C5 to T1 and has five branches: upper subscapular (supplies the subscapularis), thoracodorsal (supplies latissimus dorsi), lower subscapular (teres major), axillary (deltoid, teres major), and radial (triceps). The lateral cord stems from C5 to C7 and has three branches: lateral pectoral (pectoralis major), musculocutaneous (coracobrachialis, biceps brachii, brachialis), and the lateral root of the median nerve (forearm flexors). The medial cord stems from C8 to T1 and has five branches: medial pectoral (pectoralis minor and major), medial brachial cutaneous (skin on medial side of the arm), medial antebrachial cutaneous (skin on medial forearm), ulnar nerve (flexor carpi ulnaris, flexor digitorum profundus, and smaller muscles of the hand), and the medial root of the median nerve (forearm flexors).

Muscles

The muscles of the shoulder can be grouped according to location or function: (1) flexion, (2) extension, (3) abduction, (4) adduction, (5) external (lateral) rotation, and (6) internal (medial) rotation. The major muscles and their actions are listed in Table 4.3. The muscles surrounding the joint region are used for controlling the head

TABLE 4.3	Shoulder region muscles and main functions.[4,6]
MUSCLE	**ACTIONS**
Subscapularis	Medially rotates and adducts arm and stabilizes humeral head
Pectoralis major	Adducts and medially rotates arm
Pectoralis minor	Tilts scapula anteriorly, with a fixed scapula raises the third to fifth ribs during forced inspiration
Serratus anterior	Abducts, depresses, elevates scapula
Levator scapulae	Elevates and medially rotates scapula
Latissumus dorsi	Extends, adducts, medially rotates arm
Trapezius	Elevates, retracts, rotates, depresses scapula
Rhomboid major/minor	Retracts and medially rotates scapula
Deltoid	Flexes and medially rotates arm, abducts arm, extends arm
Supraspinatus	Externally rotates and abducts arm and stabilizes humeral head
Infraspinatus	Externally rotates arm, stabilizes humeral head
Teres minor	Externally rotates arm, stabilizes humeral head
Teres major	Adducts and medially rotates arm
Biceps brachii	Supinates/flexes forearm, palm up (i.e., supination)
Brachialis	Flexes forearm, palm down (i.e., pronation)
Coracobrachialis	Flexes and adducts arm
Triceps brachii	Extends forearm, extends arm

of the humerus within the socket and for movements of the upper extremity, upper back, and chest regions.

LIGAMENTOUS AND SPECIAL TESTS

T he case scenarios in this section will require that you select and use various special tests in order to determine the pathology. A detailed explanation of how to perform these special tests is beyond the scope of this section; however, Table 4.4 will provide a list of special tests that may be required and will be useful for you to review before beginning the case studies. For a more thorough review, please refer to your favorite evaluation text or journal article(s).

TABLE 4.4	Ligamentous and special tests for the shoulder.[1,5]
SPECIAL TEST	**FUNCTION**
Apprehension	Tests for anterior dislocation and glenohumeral instability
Anterior drawer	Tests for labrum tear/glenohumeral joint integrity
Posterior drawer	Tests for posterior labrum tear/glenohumeral joint integrity
Clunk	Tests for glenohumeral labrum tear
Jobe relocation	Tests for relief of pain with an apprehensive test
Sulcus sign	Tests for inferior glenohumeral instability
O'Brien's	Tests for labrum/SLAP lesions
Speed's	Tests long head of biceps in bicipital groove, bicipital tendonitis
Yergason's	Tests for integrity of transverse humeral ligament to hold long head of biceps tendon
Empty can	Tests for supraspinatus injury/pathology
Hawkins and Kennedy impingement	Tests for shoulder joint impingement (supra spinatus or long head of biceps brachii)
Neer impingement	Tests for supraspinatus pathology
Drop-arm	Tests for rotator cuff pathology; tear
Lift-off sign	Tests for subscapularis pathology
Adson's	Tests for thoracic outlet syndrome secondary to compression of the subclavian artery by the scalene muscles
Costoclavicular syndrome (Military brace)	Tests for thoracic outlet syndrome secondary to compression of the subclavian artery as it travels under the clavicle and first rib
Allen	Tests for thoracic outlet syndrome secondary to compression by the pectoralis minor
AC joint compression	Tests for horizontal stability of AC joint
AC joint distraction/traction	Tests for coracoclavicular ligament integrity

REFERENCES

1. Anderson MK, Hall SJ, Martin M. *Foundation of Athletic Training: Prevention, Assessment, and Management*. Philadelphia, PA: Lippincott Williams & Wilkins; 2005.

2. Behnke RS. *Kinetic Anatomy*. Champaign, IL: Human Kinetics; 2001.

3. Clemente CD. *Anatomy: A Regional Atlas of the Human Body* (4th ed.). Baltimore, MD: Williams & Wilkins; 1997.

4. Kendall FP, McCreary EK. *Muscles Testing and Function* (3rd ed.). Baltimore, MD: Williams & Wilkins; 1983.

5. Magee DJ. *Orthopedic Physical Assessment* (5th ed.). Philadelphia, PA: Saunders; 2007.

6. Moore KL, Agur AMR. *Essential Clinical Anatomy* (3rd ed.). Baltimore, MD: Lippincott Williams & Wilkins; 2006.

7. Norkin CC, Levangie PK. *Joint Structure and Function: A Comprehensive Analysis*. Philadelphia, PA: FA Davis; 1992.

CASE 4.1

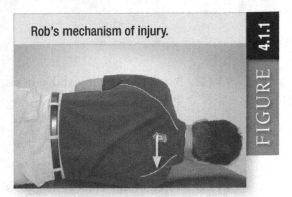

Rob's mechanism of injury.

FIGURE 4.1.1

T ony, a recent college graduate, is working as an athletic trainer at a high school wrestling match. During the first period, the visiting wrestler slams Rob, one of the student-athletes, onto the mat with all of his force. Rob falls directly onto his right shoulder with his arm against his side (Figure 4.1.1). Rob clutches his shoulder, and a medical time-out is called by the referee.

PHYSICAL EXAMINATION

Tony approaches Rob, who is lying on the mat. Tony is able to quickly determine that Rob is conscious and is breathing and con-

Arrow indicates the direction of force applied to the shoulder.

firms that Rob landed on the tip of his right shoulder. After sitting Rob up, Tony notices slight redness about the AC joint and a slight bump approximately 3 to 4 cm from the outside of Rob's deltoid. Palpation for fractures reveals slight crepitus over the lateral edge of the clavicle, and pain is elicited at the same region with a "springy" sensation. Rob has significant difficulty moving his arm and must use his left arm for support. Because of this, he is forced to forfeit the match.

FOLLOW-UP PHYSICAL EXAMINATION

In the locker room, Tony initiates a more thorough examination. The shoulder is beginning to swell. Manual muscle testing (MMT) reveals the following weaknesses: deltoids (1/5), biceps brachii (3/5), and triceps (3/5). Dermatomes of the upper extremity and deep tendon reflexes of the biceps, triceps, and brachioradialis are unremarkable. Tony instructs Rob in the correct use of cryotherapy, places him in a sling for the weekend, and asks him to return on Monday morning for further assessment.

? QUESTIONS   CASE 4.1

Please answer the following questions based on the above case information.

4.1 / **1.** Based on the information presented in the case, determine (a) the differential diagnoses and (b) the clinical diagnosis.

4.1 / **2.** Based on the clinical diagnosis, describe the common grading scale used to quantify this injury.

4.1 / **3.** Based on the clinical diagnosis, identify the ligaments that may be affected and their location.

4.1 / **4.** What would be the appropriate short-term management plan for treating this type of injury?

4.1 / **5.** Overall, do you believe Tony adequately evaluated Rob's condition given the information presented in the case? If not, what would you have done differently as the evaluating clinician?

4.1 / **6.** Based on the clinical diagnosis, what are some potential complications (short or long term) as a result of the injury?

CASE **4.2**

Brian is the athletic trainer for a local high school. The football team was playing their cross-town rivals on a warm Friday night. In the fourth quarter, while Brian was attending to another athlete, he noticed one of the other players walking off the field. As the player was exiting the field, Brian noticed him holding his arm over his chest (Figure 4.2.1).

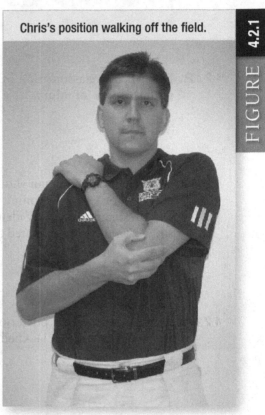

Chris's position walking off the field.

FIGURE 4.2.1

HISTORY

Chris is a 16-year-old high school football player who is tackled while his left arm is outstretched. He reports his arm was forced behind him while his body hit the ground. He complains of pain in the middle of his chest and slight difficulty breathing because of the localized pain. Chris' pain is rated as 8/10, and he complains of being unable to raise his left arm.

PHYSICAL EXAMINATION

Brian palpates under Chris' shoulder pads and cannot determine any abnormalities at this time. Brian believes it is safe to assist Chris in removing his jersey and shoulder pads, which is done with difficulty because the affected arm must be moved. Upon closer inspection, Brian notices a slight rise at the tip of the sternum and proximal clavicle. Palpation over the clavicle at the sternal end reveals a slight anterior deformity not present on the unaffected side. The athlete reports never having noticed any lumps at his sternum before, but he cannot be sure it didn't already exist prior to the incident. During AROM testing, Chris has difficulty with shoulder flexion and extension as well as scapular elevation, protraction, and retraction. All neurological tests are unremarkable. MMT reveals weakness during scapular elevation and shoulder adduction, abduction, and flexion. Biceps, triceps, and forearm strength are equal bilaterally, and his head is slightly titled to the affected side.

Please answer the following questions based on the above case information.

4.2 / 1. Based on the information presented in the case, determine (a) the differential diagnoses and (b) the clinical diagnosis.

4.2 / 2. Describe the classification of ligamentous injuries commonly associated with this type of injury.

4.2 / 3. The evaluating clinician should palpate several bony and soft tissue landmarks in order to determine the correct clinical diagnosis. Based on the clinical diagnosis above, identify the bony and soft tissue landmarks you should/would have palpated to guide the physical examination.

4.2 / 4. If this injury were a posterior dislocation as opposed to an anterior one, the injury would be classified as a potential medical emergency. Why?

4.2 / 5. As the evaluating clinician, describe how you would initially manage this injury.

CASE 4.3

A s an athletic trainer for the water sport teams at a Division III institution, Kari has been providing treatment for various injuries and conditions throughout the year. One particular water polo athlete, 19-year-old Jillian, has been complaining of shoulder pain that seems to be getting worse. Despite the pain, she has never sought treatment or evaluation and has been playing through the pain and discomfort. Finally, after her coach questioned why her performance had changed, Jillian confessed to having a problem, particularly with increased pain upon exertion, and the coach decided she needed to seek medical services.

HISTORY

Kari begins by asking Jillian history questions such as: "When did the injury become noticeable?" "What type of pain are you experiencing?" and "What activities exacerbate and/or relieve the pain and discomfort?" Jillian says that the problem has been progressively getting worse. She states: "Over the summer I fell water skiing and sprained my shoulder. I thought I could just work through it, but about two months ago I noticed more popping of the joint, almost like it is sliding in and out of place." Kari also asked about arm dominance, history of injury to the shoulder, neck, and elbow, and about past rehabilitation and current employment status (Jillian is a restaurant server). Jillian's pain profile information is presented in Figure 4.3.1.

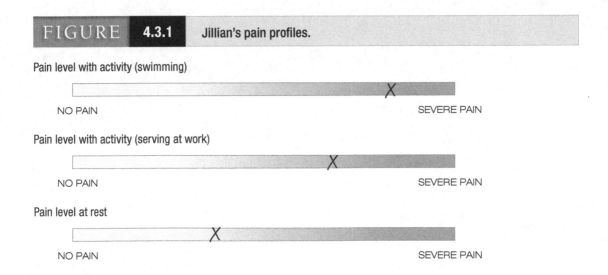

FIGURE **4.3.1** Jillian's pain profiles.

Pain level with activity (swimming)

NO PAIN   SEVERE PAIN

Pain level with activity (serving at work)

NO PAIN   SEVERE PAIN

Pain level at rest

NO PAIN   SEVERE PAIN

FIGURE 4.3.2

Positive ligamentous test.

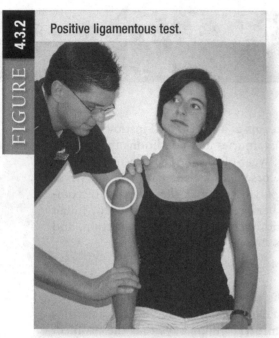

Test revealed a puckering of the skin around the circle.

PHYSICAL EXAMINATION

Jillian is alert, oriented, and in minimal discomfort as Kari begins her evaluation. A general observation of the shoulder reveals joint stiffness, apparent rotator cuff weakness, pain when reaching backwards overhead, and forward slumping of the shoulder. Jillian also complains of slight burning/tingling in her hand and numbness in her deltoid. There is no apparent swelling or discoloration. During ROM testing, Kari notices that external rotation at 90° of abduction is limited and painful. She also notices that Jillian has more external than internal rotation flexibility. Kari performs a special ligamentous test that is positive (Figure 4.3.2). A positive load and shift test reveals more laxity in the involved arm than the non-involved arm. An anterior apprehension test is also positive. Kari does notice some clunking sensation during these tests.

Please answer the following questions based on the above case information.

4.3 / **1.** Based on the information presented in the case, determine (a) the differential diagnoses and (b) the clinical diagnosis.

4.3 / **2.** Identify any other possible pathologies occurring secondary to this kind of injury.

4.3 / **3.** Figure 4.3.2 demonstrates a positive ligamentous stress test. What is the name of this test, and what important step is necessary to ensure a proper clinical decision?

4.3 / **4.** What other special tests could be used to make the clinical diagnosis?

4.3 / **5.** What management options would you use to treat this condition?

4.3 / **6.** After completing the physical examination, Kari documented her findings and sent a copy of the report over to the athletic administration office. Please document your findings as if you were the treating clinician. If the case did not provide information you believe is pertinent to the clinical diagnosis please feel free to add this information to your documentation.

anuel, a 21-year-old recreational water polo player, was performing a lat pull-down during early season conditioning, when he felt pain in his shoulder. His pain did not subside after waiting a couple of days, so he decided to seek medical attention. Manuel went to the local sports medicine clinic, where Julie, a certified athletic trainer, proceeded to evaluate his condition after having him complete several documents, including Figure 4.4.1.

HISTORY

Julie begins her evaluation by reviewing the paperwork completed by Manuel, noting that the injury occurred two days earlier. Nothing in the completed paperwork stands out as a red flag. Manuel said he was attempting to perform a set of six reps at 90 percent of his 5 ROM. He completed only two reps because he felt some pain and discomfort in his right shoulder. Manuel stated, "When I began pulling down on the lat bar, I felt my shoulder area become tight on the first rep. When I started the second rep, I began experiencing some pain and decided to quit the set before I hurt myself anymore. Although the pain was mild to moderate, I thought I just 'tweaked' something in my shoulder and stretching would help." He says he continued to perform his other conditioning drills and had only slight pain with activities involving his shoulder. His rated his pain as 3/10 at rest and 6/10 with arm movements over the head.

| FIGURE | 4.4.1 | Manuel's pain chart. |

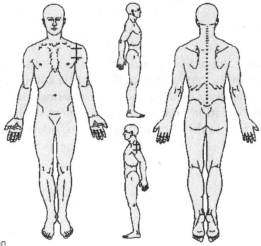

Note: Crosses equal location of general pain.

PHYSICAL EXAMINATION

Manuel is alert and in minor to moderate discomfort (5/10) with no obvious guarding or joint splinting. Upon inspection, Julie does not note any swelling or deformation. Manuel has full ROM in all shoulder and arm movements bilaterally, with some notable discomfort at the end range of shoulder flexion and external rotation. Resisted ROM testing reveals slight discomfort and weakness in shoulder flexion (4–/5) and bicep curls with the palm up (4–/5). Impingement and instability tests cause relatively minor discomfort. The Yergason's test and the special test in Figure 4.4.2 elicit pain. All other physical examination findings, such as reflexes and dermatomes, are normal.

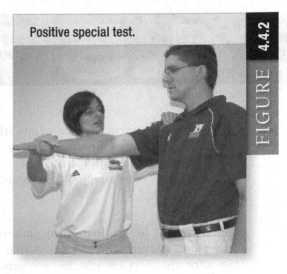
Positive special test.

FIGURE 4.4.2

| ? | QUESTIONS | CASE 4.4 |

Please answer the following questions based on the above case information.

4.4 / 1. Based on the information presented in the case, determine (a) the differential diagnoses and (b) the clinical diagnosis.

4.4 / 2. What anatomical structures provide support for the long head of the biceps in the bicipital groove?

4.4 / 3. Figure 4.4.2 demonstrates a positive special test performed on Manuel. (a) What is the name of this test, and (b) did it appear to be performed correctly?

4.4 / 4. (a) What is the purpose of the Yergason's test? (b) Why is the hand of the examiner placed over the bicipital groove?

4.4 / 5. Why would performing a lat pull down cause this type of injury?

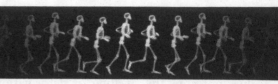

Alexis is working as a part-time athletic trainer for a tennis facility while attending graduate school. She works mostly with younger athletes. One afternoon, while sitting in the athletic training room, a 15-year-old female tennis player approaches her complaining of right shoulder pain.

HISTORY

Alexis begins her evaluation by gathering some general information about Doreen, the tennis player. Doreen reports that she has been having deep anterior shoulder pain for about six months, but it is getting progressively worse, especially while serving. A thorough questioning of her playing habits reveals that she has been playing tennis competitively for five years. She practices or has matches about four to five times a week, lasting anywhere from one to four hours. Alexis inspects her tennis racquet to determine if its size and weight are appropriate for Doreen. Doreen reports using the same type and brand racquet for the past three years. Doreen denies any significant injury to the shoulder.

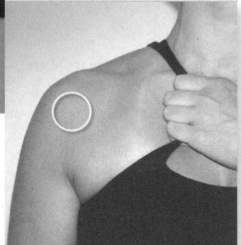

FIGURE 4.5.1

Doreen's location of swelling and pain.

PHYSICAL EXAMINATION

Doreen is alert and in minor discomfort (3/10 on a numerical pain scale). Under general observation, Doreen's right shoulder appears normal (Figure 4.5.1). Alexis palpates the shoulder area, including the humeral head, acromion, clavicle, and all associated musculature in the region. All palpation feels normal (no crepitation), and she has no remarkable deficits. However, Doreen does report discomfort when palpating around the bicipital groove area. MMT of the shoulder and upper arm reveals weakness and discomfort with shoulder flexion and abduction. Doreen's ROM testing results can be found in Table 4.5.1. Neurological tests are unremarkable.

Alexis discusses her findings with Doreen and informs her that she needs to speak with Doreen's mother in order to determine the next course of action.

TABLE	4.5.1	Doreen's range of motion results.		
			FINDINGS	
MOTION	**JOINT**		**RIGHT**	**LEFT**
AROM	Shoulder flexion*		170°	180°
	Shoulder extension		52°	60°
	Abduction		175°	180°
	Horizontal adduction		130°	135°
RROM	Shoulder flexion		3+/5 with pain	
	Shoulder extension		4+/5	
	Abduction		4/5	
	Horizontal adduction		4/5 with pain	

* Pain increases to 7/10 with active flexion and passive extension.

Please answer the following questions based on the above case information.

4.5 / **1.** Based on the information presented in the case, determine (a) the differential diagnoses and (b) the clinical diagnosis.

4.5 / **2.** Based on the physical examination, Alexis clearly forgot to perform ligamentous or special shoulder tests. List and describe at least three special tests you as the evaluating clinician may have performed in order to guide the physical examination. Explain why each test will assist in making the clinical diagnosis.

4.5 / **3.** Besides forgetting the ligamentous and special tests to the shoulder, do you feel that Alexis assessed the injury adequately enough? If you were the evaluating clinician, what if anything would you add to the evaluation? What might you expect to find clinically?

4.5 / **4.** Why does Alexis need to speak with Doreen's mother?

4.5 / **5.** If you were the evaluating clinician, how would you rehabilitate this injury during the next month?

A 38-year-old female, Erin, has been referred to Juan's orthopedic physical therapy clinic by her orthopedic surgeon for immediate evaluation and treatment. When Erin arrives, Juan finds that the prescription from the physician is illegible, and he can decipher only that Erin has some type of shoulder pathology. He attempts to contact the physician, but the answering service says they are "out of the office for lunch." Juan decides to evaluate Erin and then call the physician later in the afternoon for further clarification and to thank him for the referral.

HISTORY

Erin begins by stating that she has had left shoulder pain sporadically for the past several years with no complete resolution of the problem. She vaguely remembers that the previous diagnosis had something to do with shoulder impingement with throwing, but she is not sure. She continues by stating that: "Over the last couple of months my shoulder pain has progressively worsened, so much so that I am having difficulty lifting my left arm over my head." She also claims she has difficulty sleeping at night, which is affecting her job performance.

PHYSICAL EXAMINATION

Erin has minor-to-moderate discomfort (4/10 on a numerical pain scale). A pain diagram (Figure 4.6.1) below describes Erin's pain pattern. An observation of Erin's

| FIGURE | 4.6.1 | Erin's pain chart. |

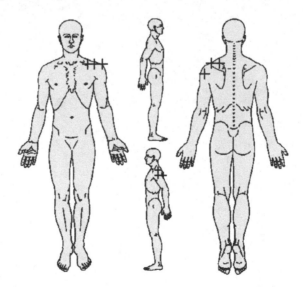

Note: Crosses equal location of general pain.

shoulder reveals noticeable atrophy around the suprascapular fossa. A posterior postural examination reveals a winging scapula. Erin's AROM produces pain in the arc of motion from about 60° to 120° of abduction and forward flexion, with substitution movements of the shoulder. Muscle testing identifies weakness during scaption (2+/5) and shoulder flexion (3/5). Capsular testing reveals increased humeral head translation in the anteroinferior direction. The Hawkins-Kennedy test and empty can test are positive on the left side. Neurological and circulatory tests are unremarkable.

DIAGNOSTIC IMAGING

Plain film radiographs confirmation from the radiologist identifies a type III shaped acromion and a decreased subacromial space.

? QUESTIONS   CASE 4.6

Please answer the following questions based on the above case information.

4.6 / 1. Based on the information presented in the case, determine (a) the differential diagnoses and (b) the clinical diagnosis.

4.6 / 2. Identify three to four additional history questions you may have asked in order to differentiate between the above condition and other shoulder pathologies.

4.6 / 3. Answer the following questions about the palpation portion of the physical examination: (a) What are the bony and soft tissue structures that should have been palpated as part of the physical examination? (b) Based on the clinical diagnosis, where would one expect the patient to be point tender? (c) When should the palpation portion of the physical examination be conducted?

4.6 / 4. What type of functional active ROM testing could a clinician perform to determine an overall sense of the patient's shoulder function? Describe the test and what motions the test assesses.

4.6 / 5. Identify a second special test other than the commonly used empty can test that a clinician may use to identify the specific rotator cuff pathology in this case. What makes this test useful for clinicians?

4.6 / 6. When trauma occurs to the involved structure, as in this case, it may result in two types of tears: partial thickness and full thickness. (a) Identify the difference between the two types. (b) Compare and contrast the signs and symptoms using an evidenced-based approach that allows a clinician to discriminate between the two conditions during a clinical evaluation.

CASE 4.7

During a lacrosse match, Jeremy, a 24-year-old, was hit by his own player while going for a loose ball. After falling to the ground, Jeremy walks over to Kyla, the athletic trainer covering the game, with his arm held to the side and holding it with his unaffected arm (Figure 4.7.1). Kyla notes that the arm appears to be in slight external rotation as he walks over to the sideline.

FIGURE 4.7.1

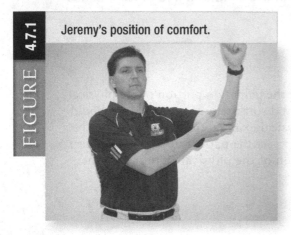

Jeremy's position of comfort.

FIGURE 4.7.2

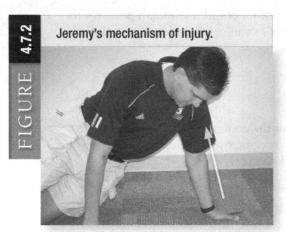

Jeremy's mechanism of injury.

Arrow indicates the direction of force transmitted through the limb.

HISTORY

Kyla supports Jeremy's left arm while trying to determine what happened. Jeremy reports that another team player hit him by accident, knocking him to the ground (Figure 4.7.2). He states: "When I hit the ground it felt like my arm popped." His CCs are discomfort and lack of movement. He reports that he thought he heard a popping sound at the time of the injury but is not certain.

PHYSICAL EXAMINATION

Kyla asks Jeremy to sit on the bench while she begins her physical examination. Jeremy is alert and in moderate-to-severe discomfort (7/10). As Kyla palpates the shoulder bilaterally under Jeremy's lacrosse pads she notices an irregularity at the shoulder joint that is not consistent with the unaffected side. She notes a flattened deltoid muscle and a slight lump in the anterior deltoid/pectoralis space. Once she is able to remove the shirt and pads with caution she notices a more prominent acromion. Kyla assesses the distal pulse, which is evident and appears normal. Jeremy denies any other neurological problems. Jeremy cannot move his shoulder in any direction without physical discomfort. Kyla believes the best course of action would be RICE and referral to the emergency room immediately for further evaluation.

| ? | Q U E S T I O N S | CASE 4.7 |

Please answer the following questions based on the above case information.

4.7 / 1. Based on the information presented in the case, determine (a) the differential diagnoses and (b) the clinical diagnosis.

4.7 / 2. The injury in this case scenario can occur in several directions. (a) Identify the most common directions for the clinical diagnosis, and (b) identify which anatomical structures are compromised.

4.7 / 3. What is the proper short-term management of this injury?

4.7 / 4. Explain why the structural integrity of the joint predisposes athletes to this injury.

4.7 / 5. Kyla provided basic first-aid care on the field. What are some basic rehabilitation strategies or techniques a clinician may use for this injury?

4.7 / 6. If you were the evaluating clinician in this case, how would you determine if the athlete is ready to return to competition?

4.8

Jon, a certified athletic trainer, was covering men's gymnastics practice at a Division I university. He was assisting another athlete when he heard a thump, immediately followed by an athlete screaming in pain. It appeared that a gymnast slipped and fell during exercises on the pummel horse. Jon immediately ran to the event apparatus and found Paul lying on the ground.

FIGURE 4.8.1

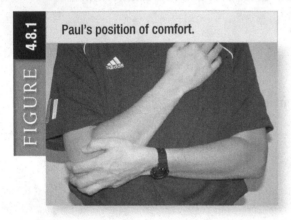

Paul's position of comfort.

TABLE 4.8.1

Paul's vital signs.

VITAL SIGNS	FINDING
Pulse	88 and regular
Respiration	13 and normal
Blood pressure	124/78
Mental status	Alert and oriented

HISTORY

Jon immediately calms Paul down while Paul supports his right arm (Figure 4.8.1). When Jon asked what happened, Paul states: "I was performing a double back twist on the horse, and when I landed I lost my balance and fell to the floor, landing on my right shoulder." Paul continues to grimace in pain. He describes his pain as intense and sharp and states it is 9/10.

PHYSICAL EXAMINATION

While Paul is talking, Jon inspects the injured shoulder. Jon notes that Paul's right shoulder appears abnormal compared with his left shoulder, with noticeable deformity anteriorly near the lateral end of his clavicle where it articulates with the acromion.

Jon calls over to Mary, an athletic training student, and asks her to bring over the splint bag. While waiting for the splint bag, Jon assesses Paul's vital signs, shown in Table 4.8.1.

Please answer the following questions based on the above case information.

4.8 / **1.** Based on the information presented in the case, determine (a) the differential diagnoses and (b) the clinical diagnosis.

4.8 / **2.** Based on the information presented in the case, what should Jon do next?

4.8 / **3.** Jon asked a couple of history questions to guide his physical examination. Based on the clinical diagnosis above, identify three to five additional history questions you may have asked as the evaluating clinician.

4.8 / **4.** Jon identified several signs and symptoms related to the injury. If you were the evaluating clinician what other signs and symptoms associated with the injury would you be looking to identify?

4.8 / **5.** Overall, do you believe Jon adequately evaluated Paul's condition, considering the information provided? If not, what would you have done differently as the evaluating clinician?

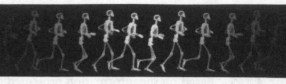

CASE 4.9

Bernardo, a 20-year-old college football player, felt posterior shoulder pain after he sustained a direct trauma to the back of his right shoulder when he was blocked onto his back. He was able to continue playing but later pulled himself from the game. The next day the pain worsened. Bernardo sought out the assistance from Laurel, one of the first-year graduate student–certified athletic trainers assigned to football.

HISTORY

Laurel begins her assessment by asking Bernardo what happened. He tells her about the block to his back during the game the day before and explains that the pain had gotten worse and that he had difficulty sleeping the previous night because he could not find a comfortable position. He states that he is experiencing pain at his upper back with arm movement. Laurel also determines that he is a defensive back and never experienced previous shoulder pain or injury to this area.

PHYSICAL EXAMINATION

Bernardo is alert, oriented, and in moderate discomfort at this time. As Laurel begins her observation, Bernardo is holding his right arm flexed 90° at the elbow, with his forearm adducted and supported close to his body. There is no obvious deformity of the shoulder. She notes that his pain is localized (Figure 4.9.1), with diffuse palpable tenderness around the supraspinatus and infraspinatus. The AROM of the shoulder is full in all directions but very painful. Resisted ROM is weak in abduction, particularly in the early stages of the range and in external rotation. Laurel also notes that Bernardo has poor scapulothoracic rhythm with active movement. Ligamentous and special tests are unremarkable. Neurologically Bernardo appears intact.

Laurel is a little stumped. She believes she has an idea of the clinical diagnosis, but she knows she probably needs radiographs to confirm the diagnosis. She refers Bernardo to the team physician.

FIGURE 4.9.1

Bernardo's location of pain.

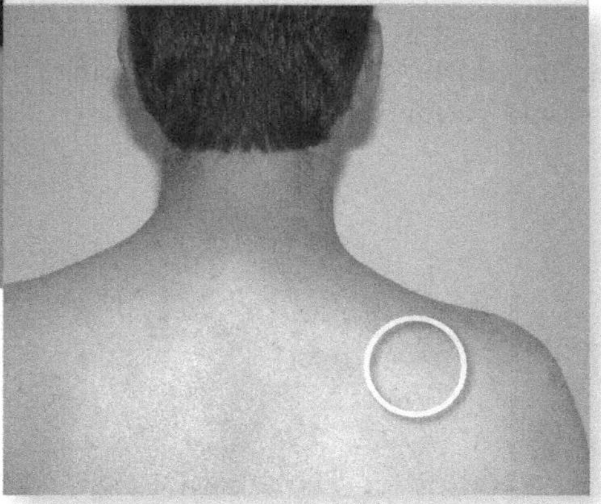

Area of pain is within the circle.

Please answer the following questions based on the above case information.

4.9 / **1.** Based on the information presented in the case, determine (a) the differential diagnoses and (b) the clinical diagnosis.

4.9 / **2.** If you were the evaluating clinician, what would lead you to the clinical diagnosis?

4.9 / **3.** After reviewing the X-ray with the team physician, the clinical diagnosis is clear. What are the common types/locations and the mechanisms of injury associated with this injury?

4.9 / **4.** What is/are the treatment options for the clinical diagnosis?

4.9 / **5.** Given the clinical diagnosis, when can the athlete return to play?

During a high school women's field hockey practice, Sadie noticed a collision between two opposing players. The collision occurred while both players were going for the ball. The defensive player careened into the offensive player's right shoulder and flank. Both players fell to the ground but immediately got up and continued playing.

HISTORY

During a break, Sadie approaches both players. The defensive player, Samantha, reports no associated injury, pain, or discomfort. However, the offensive player, Caitlin, age 16, reports some unusual numbness on her right side (Figure 4.10.1). This is the first time she has experienced such a problem, and she says she has never had any injuries up to this time.

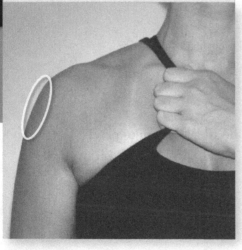

FIGURE 4.10.1

Caitlin's location of numbness.

Area of numbness is along the lateral humerus within the circle.

PHYSICAL EXAMINATION

After conducting the history, Sadie begins to examine Caitlin's shoulder. Because they are on the sidelines, Sadie asks Caitlin to walk over to the grandstand. Sadie wants to give Caitlin privacy, because observation of the shoulder would be easier without a shirt and Caitlin says she is wearing a sports bra. Upon visual inspection, both shoulders appear to look normal with no apparent deformity or unusual markings. Palpation of both shoulders reveals similar findings. Caitlin's ROM testing results are shown in Table 4.10.1. Ligamentous testing is WNL.

After completing the physical examination, Sadie pulls Samantha from the practice and discusses her findings with Samantha's mom. She recommends that Samantha follow up with a neurologist.

TABLE	4.10.1	Caitlin's ROM results.

MOTION	JOINT	FINDINGS		
			RIGHT	LEFT
AROM	Shoulder flexion		170°	180°
	Shoulder extension		52°	60°
	Abduction		30°	180°
	Adduction		130°	135°
	Internal rotation		70°	70°
	External rotation		65°	90°
RROM	Shoulder flexion	5/5		
	Shoulder extension	5/5		
	Abduction	4/5		
	Adduction	2+/5		
	Internal rotation	4/5		
	External rotation	4/5		

? Q U E S T I O N S   **CASE 4.10**

Please answer the following questions based on the above case information.

4.10 / **1.** Based on the information presented in the case, determine (a) the differential diagnoses and (b) the clinical diagnosis.

4.10 / **2.** How does a blunt trauma cause this type of injury? Is there another MOI that a clinician should be aware of?

4.10 / **3.** Describe the anatomical landmarks as the structure associated with the clinical diagnosis traverses through the shoulder area.

4.10 / **4.** Based on the findings of the physical examination, ligamentous testing was WNL. What other special or neurological tests may be used to help differentiate this condition?

4.10 / **5.** If Sadie had been a male, would anything need to change in the clinical evaluation?

J ordan is the athletic trainer for a women's Division III collegiate volleyball team. The season has been unremarkable for acute and/or major injuries. However, a blocker has been having some shoulder and muscle weakness of her right arm. Jordan has been notified that the player has been affected by these symptoms for approximately two weeks. Although the player has these symptoms, she has not asked for or sought any treatment.

HISTORY

The player, Teresa, finally approaches Jordan after practice with complaints of her condition worsening approximately 10 weeks into the season. She reports that her serve is not as powerful and that she has had some pain and discomfort about the left shoulder, neck, and scapula areas.

PHYSICAL EXAMINATION

During the inspection, Jordan notices that Teresa has rounded shoulders and forward head posture. Jordan also notices a slight protuberance of the left scapula as compared with the right (elevation of the medial border). She has decreased AROM for shoulder extension and horizontal abduction, tight latissimus dorsi and upper trapezius and rhomboids. Bilateral shoulder movement reveals inconsistencies in the scapulohumeral rhythm of her affected side. MMT shows that she has weak forward flexion and elevation movements. Dermatome testing is inconclusive.

? | Q U E S T I O N S | CASE 4.11

Please answer the following questions based on the above case information.

4.11 / **1.** Based on the information presented in the case, determine (a) the differential diagnoses and (b) the clinical diagnosis.

4.11 / **2.** How does the injury in this case occur with repetitive use?

4.11 / **3.** What other sports or activities may predispose the athlete to this injury?

4.11 / **4.** Describe the anatomical landmarks associated with the clinical diagnosis as the structure traverses through the shoulder region.

4.11 / **5.** Identify the myotomes an athletic trainer should assess to accurately determine the clinical diagnosis.

4.11 / **6.** Identify the dermatomes an athletic trainer should assess to accurately determine the clinical diagnosis.

4.11 / **7.** What are some special tests available to an athletic trainer to help with the differential diagnoses?

Marge, an athletic trainer with three years of experience, was checking in on the tennis team. While she was talking with the coach about the university's drug testing policy, Rosa, a 19-year-old female player from Italy, approached Marge. Rosa waited until Marge and the coach were finished talking before striking up a conversation with Marge.

HISTORY

After some small talk, Marge asks Rosa if anything is going on. Rosa states, "I will tell you, but promise not to tell coach?" Marge thinks for a second and agrees. Rosa begins explaining that she has been experiencing shoulder pain for the past several weeks. She describes her pain as intense while serving and achy during most overhead shots and any other movement and notes pain at night. She reports that the pain developed several weeks ago and that it had been getting progressively worse and now is affecting her serve velocity.

PHYSICAL EXAMINATION

Marge's initial observation is unremarkable. She did note palpable point tenderness near the greater tuberosity (Figure 4.12.1). Results of Rosa's ROM results are in Table 4.12.1. During MMT of Rosa's biceps, deltoids, triceps, internal and external rotators, and elbow flexors and extensors, Marge observes weakness and also notices that Rosa resists abducting the shoulder (3/5) and external rotation at 0° (3/5) as compared with the unaffected arm. The scapular stabilizers on the affected side also appear weak, and these movements cause discomfort for Rosa. Ligamentous testing about the shoulder is unremarkable. Marge performs the following special tests: Neer, Hawkins-Kennedy, empty can, and Yergason's.

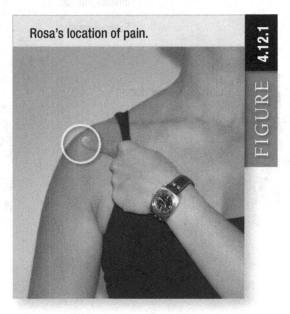

Rosa's location of pain.

FIGURE 4.12.1

Area of pain is located under the finger and within the circle.

TABLE	4.12.1	Rosa's ROM results.		

MOTION	JOINT	FINDINGS	
		RIGHT	**LEFT**
AROM	Shoulder flexion	168°	180°
	Shoulder extension	55°	60°
	Abduction	135°	180°
	Adduction	135°	135°
	Internal rotation	60°	70°
	External rotation	75°	90°
PROM	Shoulder flexion	Minimal-to-no discomfort	
	Shoulder extension	Increased pain end range motion	
	Abduction	Minimal-to-no discomfort	
	Adduction	Minimal-to-no discomfort	
	Internal rotation	Increased pain end range motion	
	External rotation	Minimal-to-no discomfort	

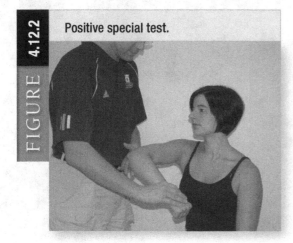

FIGURE 4.12.2   Positive special test.

Only the special test shown in Figure 4.12.2 is positive. Dermatomes and deep tendon reflexes are WNL.

Marge discusses the results of her physical examination with Rosa. Marge suggests that Rosa take a couple of days off to allow the shoulder to calm down. Rosa, however, gets upset because that would require telling the coach. She confides further in Marge that the coach stated that if she missed any games or practices she would lose her chance of All-American status. Marge is unsure what to do.

Please answer the following questions based on the above case information.

4.12 / **1.** Based on the information presented in the case, determine (a) the differential diagnoses and (b) the clinical diagnosis.

4.12 / **2.** Figure 4.12.2 demonstrates a positive special test. What is the name of this test? Why did only this test reveal discomfort and not the Neer test?

4.12 / **3.** As the evaluating clinician, what other concerns or issues should you be concerned about? Identify some of the main causes of this injury.

4.12 / **4.** Describe the stages of Neer's classification system used in the clinical diagnosis.

4.12 / **5.** What rehabilitation techniques are indicated for Rosa?

4.12 / **6.** Clearly, Marge has placed herself in a difficult position by initially agreeing not to share the results of her physical examination with the coach. If you were the evaluating clinician, how would you have handled this situation? Would you have agreed to keep the information quiet?

4.13

Brian is an athletic trainer for several high schools in the local school district. Because the schools cannot afford to have an athletic trainer on staff at each individual school, Brian travels to each school to meet with and treat athletes. Today he is greeted by Ricky, a 17-year-old right-handed baseball pitcher, who presents with right shoulder pain.

HISTORY

Ricky explains that his pain is worse with activity, especially with throwing and overhead activity. He has not tried to throw any new pitches. However, his team is in the playoffs, and he has been on a more frequent rotation. The pain came on gradually over the last two weeks. The pain tends to be worse at night, now making it difficult for him to sleep. Ricky prefers to hold his right arm at his side. He has not experienced shoulder pain before.

PHYSICAL EXAMINATION

The pain is localized over the point of the shoulder, over and below the acromion. There is no obvious deformity of the shoulder. Pain is increased with flexion and abduction above 90°, but AROM is maintained. There is no weakness of the rotator cuff with the elbow at the side. Impingement signs are mildly positive, but the drop-arm test is negative. There is no hypermobility of either shoulder. Tests of the right shoulder for SLAP (superior labral from anterior to posterior) tears are negative. Neck ROM is WNL.

? | Q U E S T I O N S   CASE 4.13

Please answer the following questions based on the above case information.

4.13 / 1. Based on the information presented in the physical examination, determine (a) the differential diagnoses and (b) the clinical diagnosis.

4.13 / 2. How did you arrive at the clinical diagnosis?

4.13 / 3. Impingement syndrome can lead to many of the same shoulder pain symptoms as the clinical diagnosis. How can you, as a practicing clinician working in conjunction with a physician, make an accurate diagnosis?

4.13 / 4. Why is treatment in the form of rest, oral medication, therapeutic modalities, and possibly even a shoulder injection so important?

A 42-year-old active female, Jean, developed acute left neck and arm pain while swimming. At the time, she experienced pain shooting down her left arm. The pain had gotten somewhat better with rest, but it never completely resolved. Three months later, Jean still experiences numbness down her left arm with over-head activity (both athletic and activities of daily living). She has been unable to return to swimming because of the continued pain, numbness, and heaviness.

HISTORY

In her initial examination with Alex, PT/ATC, Jean reports a past history of a motor vehicle accident in which she sustained a significant cervical strain (whiplash injury). The symptoms related to this have completely resolved.

PHYSICAL EXAMINATION

Jean is alert and in minor-to-moderate discomfort (4/10 at rest and 6/10 with activity). Alex's general observation of Jean's neck and shoulder reveals no neck deformity, though the left shoulder appears slightly elevated as compared to the right. There is no palpable deformity of the neck or shoulder. Numbness is reproduced upon examination and affects the ulnar and radial sides of the hand and wrist. Alex assesses neck AROM, which is limited slightly in extension and left lateral bending. Strength and AROM of the neck are otherwise normal. Both of Jean's shoulders are stable in all directions. Apprehension and Jobe Relocation tests are negative. Impingement signs are negative. Alex positions the arm above the head and reproduces the arm symptoms. Positioning the arm as in Figure 4.14.1 also reproduces Jean's symptoms, especially the heaviness. The radial pulse does change in the above arm positioning. The arms show no edema. Other than generalized decreased sensation in the hand and wrist, the upper extremity neurological examination is unremarkable. Spurling's test of the neck demonstrates localized neck pain but no radiation of arm symptoms.

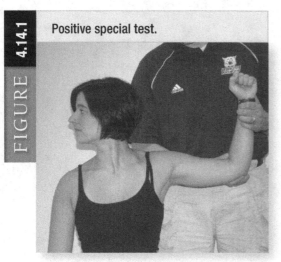

FIGURE 4.14.1

Positive special test.

Please answer the following questions based on the above case information.

4.14 / **1.** Based on the information presented in the case, determine (a) the differential diagnoses and (b) the clinical diagnosis.

4.14 / **2.** Based on the information presented in the case, explain how you determined the clinical diagnosis.

4.14 / **3.** Explain at least three different physical examination maneuvers that may help an evaluating clinician determine the clinical diagnosis.

4.14 / **4.** What are the treatment options for this condition?

4.14 / **5.** Given her condition, when can Jean begin swimming again?

CONLCUSION

T he majority of the case scenarios presented in this chapter are typical injuries seen by athletic trainers. The goal of this chapter was to recreate scenarios that are typically seen in the athletic training setting, but some of the scenarios presented may be rare. Nonetheless, each scenario should have resulted in the athletic trainer reviewing shoulder anatomy, evaluation, and rehabilitation skills. In addition, many of the scenarios or answers to the scenarios omit information or reveal tests/evaluation procedures that are questionable in certain circumstances. With assistance from your instructor, physician, clinical instructor, or other experienced allied health professional, discuss what could/should be performed if necessary. Questions regarding outcomes, such as when to have the athlete "return to play," or about other similar or related conditions that can mimic the injury presented, are necessary for development and refinement of the skills of an athletic trainer. The more practice one has, the better the chance of becoming a knowledgeable and competent clinician.

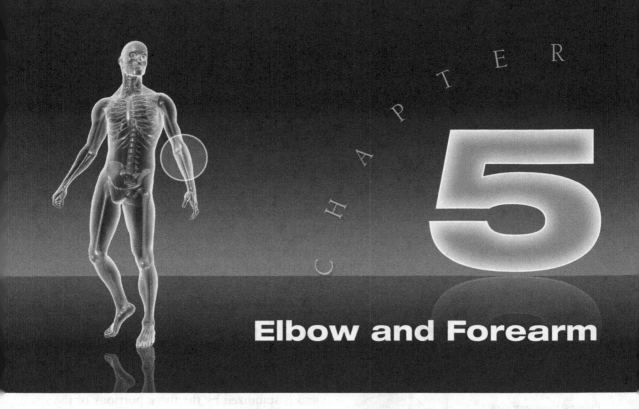

5

Elbow and Forearm

INTRODUCTION

In this chapter we will examine the clinical evaluation and management of 16 elbow pathologies, using a combination of on-field and off-field scenarios presented in a variety of settings with a diverse patient population. The elbow pathologies presented are a mixture of acute and chronic conditions. Although we have tried to identify many of the common conditions frequently seen by athletic training students, we also believe in exposing students to rare and/or unusual cases they may run across during their careers. Finally, some of the cases presented have intentionally been written with inappropriate actions, procedures, treatments, or general mismanagement of the case by the clinician. It is our hope that by critically analyzing these cases you will be able to identify the inappropriate decision(s) and provide the appropriate gold-standard treatment.

ANATOMICAL REVIEW

The elbow and forearm, which together serve as a link between the upper arm and shoulder and the wrist and hand, are composed of the distal humerus, radius, and ulna. Together these structures form four separate joint articulations, three at the elbow complex (humeroulnar, humeroradial, and proximal radioulnar joints) and one at the wrist (distal radioulnar joint) (Figure 5.1). Functionally, the elbow complex is a stable joint, supported by a single joint capsule and medial and lateral ligament restraints, which help reinforce the joint capsule.[10] Combined with its bony configuration and medial and lateral supports, the elbow complex can withstand substantial forces,[17] particularly when in extension. The elbow complex is used in almost all athletic activities, such as throwing, pushing and pulling, and activities of daily living. Activities

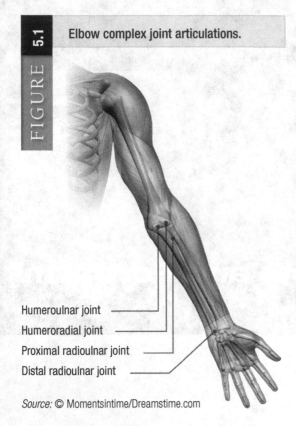

FIGURE 5.1 Elbow complex joint articulations.

Humeroulnar joint
Humeroradial joint
Proximal radioulnar joint
Distal radioulnar joint

Source: © Momentsintime/Dreamstime.com

of daily living normally require from 30° to 130° of elbow flexion and 50° to 55° of forearm pronation and supination, respectively.[10] Certain athletic sports, such as gymnastics, in which terminal elbow extension is necessary to perform certain activities, may require an even greater degree of motion.

Humeroulnar Joint

The humeroulnar joint, a hinge joint, is formed by the articulation between the hourglass-shaped trochlea of the distal humerus and the trochlea notch of the ulna, allowing the joint 1° of freedom. Flexion and extension are the primary movements, with extension limited by the bony configuration between the olecranon fossa of the humerus and the olecranon process of the ulna. This joint is most stable when placed in extension and is stabilized by the three portions of the ulnar (medial) collateral ligament (UCL of the elbow), the anterior and posterior bundles, and the transverse ligament (Table 5.1). The anterior bundle is functionally the most significant, is easily distinguishable from the

TABLE 5.1 Ligamentous stability of the humeroulnar joint.[5,6,10,12]

LIGAMENT	LOCATION	FUNCTION
Anterior bundle of medial collateral ligament	Originates on the anterior aspect, tip and medial edge of the medial epicondyle passing anterior to the axis of rotation, to insert onto the medial aspect of the ulnar's coronoid process	Primary restraint against a valgus force at the elbow
		Anterior band of anterior bundle, taut in full extension and in full flexion, primary restraint at 30°, 60°, 90° of elbow flexion and co-primary restraint at 120°
		Posterior band of anterior bundle, primarily taut beyond 55° of flexion, is co-primary restraint at 120° and secondary restraint at 30° and 90° of elbow flexion
Posterior bundle of medial collateral ligament	Originates on the posterior aspect of the medial epicondyle to insert onto the medial edge of the olecranon process	Secondary restraint against a valgus force at the elbow
		Taut with the elbow flexed beyond 55°–90°
Transverse ligament	Originates on the medial olecranon process, spanning the medial aspect of the trochlea notch, to insert onto the inferior medial coronoid process	Offers no medial support because the origin and insertion both arise from the ulna

joint capsule, is the strongest and stiffest,[14] and is the primary restraint against a valgus force.[4,9,14,18] The posterior bundle, a fan-shaped thickening of the joint capsule, becomes taut somewhere between 55° and 90° of elbow flexion and plays a less significant role in resisting a valgus force.[5,7,14] The transverse ligament offers no valgus stability due to its origin and insertion on the same bone.[6]

Humeroradial Joint

The humeroradial joint, a gliding joint, is formed by the articulation between the spherically shaped capitulum of the humerus and the proximal radial head. Unlike the humeroulnar joint, where there is constant contact between the articulating surfaces of the humerus and ulna during flexion and extension,[14] the humeroradial joint has no contact between the articulating surfaces during full extension. This joint is most stable when placed in 90° of elbow flexion with the forearm supinated 5°. Stabilized by four separate ligaments, each with a varying degree of lateral elbow support, the humeroradial joint is rarely stressed, and injury to the lateral support is not associated with any specific activity.[6] However, the risk of injury to the lateral support structures does increase, especially with significant traumas such as elbow dislocations and/or fracture-dislocations.[11] The four components of the lateral elbow support are the radial collateral ligament, the lateral ulnar collateral ligament, the annular ligament, and the accessory lateral collateral ligament[12] (Table 5.2). The radial (lateral) collateral ligament (anterior, middle, and posterior band), a fan-shaped thickening of the joint capsule, which is poorly localized, is primary restraint against a varus force because it is taut throughout flexion.[13,14]

TABLE	5.2	Ligamentous stability of the humeroradial joint.[6,10,12,14]

LIGAMENT	LOCATION	FUNCTION
Radial collateral ligament	Originates on the lateral epicondyle and inserts on the annular ligament	Primary restraint against a varus force at the elbow Anterior band taut in extension Middle band taut throughout flexion and extension Posterior band taut in flexion
Lateral ulnar collateral ligament	Originates on the middle of the lateral epicondyle and inserts onto the supinator crest of the ulna	Secondary restraint against a varus force at the elbow Taut in extreme range of elbow flexion and during the application of a varus stress Prevents medial and lateral rotatory instability of the humeroulnar joint
Annular ligament	Encircles the radial head, attaching to the anterior and posterior edges of the radial notch on the ulna	Binds the radius to the ulna, allowing for forearm pronation and supination Anterior fibers taut during end-range supination Posterior fibers during end-range pronation Prevents proximal radioulnar joint dislocations and subluxations
Accessory lateral collateral ligament	Originates on the inferior aspect of the annular ligament and inserts onto the supinator crest of the ulna	Assists annular and radial collateral ligament in preventing displacement of the radius when a varus force is applied to the elbow

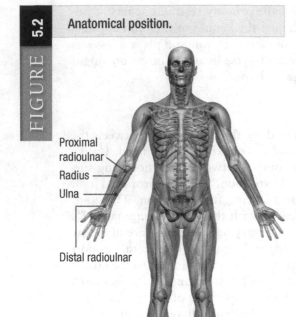

Source: © Momentsintime/
Dreamstime.com

FIGURE 5.2 **Anatomical position.**

Proximal
radioulnar
Radius
Ulna

Distal radioulnar

Radioulnar Joint

The proximal radioulnar joint of the elbow complex works in conjunction with the distal radioulnar joint, forming what is commonly referred to as the forearm. Classified as a pivot joint, the radioulnar joint allows for forearm pronation and supination. It therefore allows for 1° of motion as the radial head articulates with and rotates within the radial notch of the ulna (proximal) and as the ulnar notch of the radius moves around the head of the ulna (distal). When supinated in the anatomical position (palm up) the ulna and radius lie parallel to each other (Figure 5.2). During pronation the radius is allowed to roll and cross over the ulna, with joint motion eventually limited by contact of the radius on the ulna or by soft tissue tension. Three ligaments provide stability to the proximal radioulnar joint: the annular ligament, the quadrate ligament, and the oblique cord. The distal portion is stabilized by the triangular fibrocartilage complex (TFCC) (Table 5.3). The TFCC is formed by the dorsal and

TABLE 5.3 **Ligamentous stability of the radioulnar joints.**[10]

LIGAMENT	LOCATION	FUNCTION
Proximal annular ligament	Encircles the radial head, attaching to the anterior and posterior edges of the radial notch on the ulna.	Binds the radius to the ulna allowing for forearm pronation and supination.
quadrate ligament	Originates on the inferior edge of the ulna's radial notch and inserts onto the neck of the radius.	Reinforces the inferior joint capsule and limits radial head rotation during pronation and supination.
oblique cord	Flat facial band originating on the tuberosity of the ulna running distally to insert just distal to the radial bicipital tuberosity.	Function is unclear, believed to assist in preventing separation of the radius and ulnar.
Distal dorsal radioulnar ligament*	Originates on the dorsal aspect of the ulnar notch of the radius and inserts onto the ulnar fovea and ulnar styloid process.	Provides support to the distal radioulnar joint.
palmar radioulnar ligament*	Originates on the palmar aspect of the ulnar notch of the radius and inserts onto the ulnar fovea and ulnar styloid process.	Provides support to the distal radioulnar joint.
triangular fibrocartilage	Runs from the distal radius to the distal ulna, blending into the capsular and ligamentous structures of the distal radioulnar joint	Stabilizes the distal radioulnar joint by binding the radius and ulna together.

*The exact motion limited by these ligaments is unclear.

palmar radiocarpal ligaments, triangular fibrocartilage (articular disc), and the ulnar collateral ligament complex. The ulnar collateral ligament complex and TFCC will be discussed in Chapter 6, because its prime function is to support the wrist joint. The interosseous membrane, a dense band of fibrous tissue, assists in transmitting impact forces applied to the radius, to the ulna, and up through the humerus to the shoulder complex, stabilizing both the proximal and distal segments and is a site of attachment for the forearm muscle.

Muscles

Dynamically, the elbow is also stabilized by muscles crossing the joint which provide a compressive force to the irregular but congruent joint surfaces.[15] There are nine muscles crossing the anterior elbow, and only three of these (biceps brachii, brachioradialis, brachialis) (Figure 5.3) have a primary function (flexion) at the elbow.[10,12] However, five of the remaining six muscles (pronator teres, flexor digitorum superficialis, flexor carpi ulnaris, and the flexor carpi radialis long and brevis)—all of which have a primary function at the wrist—are believed to supply the medial elbow complex with a varus moment, thus resisting valgus forces imparted on the medial elbow.[1] The palmaris longus, the remaining muscle, crosses anterior to the elbow. Together, the remaining six muscles also act as weak elbow flexors because they arise from a common tendon of the elbow's medial epicondyle.[10]

The muscles crossing the anterior surface, depending on their bulk, are also believed to assist in reducing hyperextension injuries.[15,16] Posteriorly, the triceps (Figure 5.4) and anconeus have a primary function at the elbow of allowing for elbow extension. Laterally, several muscles originating from the lateral epicondyle have a primary function at the wrist. Together the extensor digitorum comminus, the extensor carpi radialis brevis and longus, the anconeus, and the extensor carpi ulnaris are believed to stabilize the lateral elbow by producing a valgus moment, thereby resisting a varus force.[12]

Neurovascular Structures

There are three major nerves and one major vascular structure crossing the elbow complex that can be injured as a result of acute trauma or repetitive stress: the brachial artery, the ulnar nerve, the median nerve, and the radial nerve. The brachial artery crosses anterior to

FIGURE 5.3

Muscle crossing the anterior elbow complex.

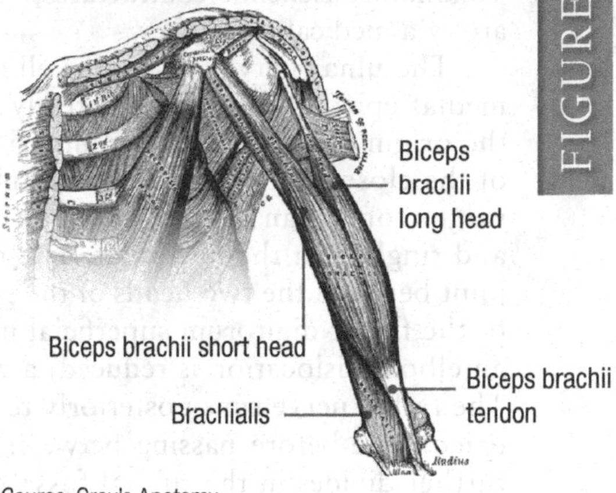

Biceps brachii long head

Biceps brachii short head

Brachialis

Biceps brachii tendon

Source: Gray's Anatomy.

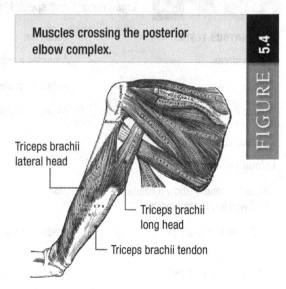

FIGURE 5.4

Muscles crossing the posterior elbow complex.

Triceps brachii lateral head

Triceps brachii long head

Triceps brachii tendon

Source: Gray's Anatomy.

the cubital fossa and passes between the biceps tendon and the median nerve before splitting into the radial and ulnar arteries. Lack of blood flow from trauma, such as an elbow dislocation or fractures,[3,8] increases the risk of compartment syndrome and Volkmann's ischemic contractures,[19] making any compromise to the radial or ulnar artery a medical emergency.

The ulnar nerve crosses the elbow's joint line medially and posteriorly to the medial epicondyle and is relatively superficial passing between the two heads of the origin of the flexor carpi ulnaris muscle before entering the forearm. Because of the close relationship between the ulnar nerve and the medial elbow, excessive valgus forces can cause a traction force on the ulnar nerve, resulting in numbness and tingling in the fifth digit. The median nerve crosses over the anterior elbow joint between the two heads of the pronator teres, running down the forearm deep to the flexor digitorum superficial muscle. When compressed or entrapped (when an elbow dislocation is reduced) a patient may develop pronator teres syndrome. The radial nerve runs posteriorly to the humerus, where it crosses over the lateral epicondyle before passing between the brachialis and brachioradialis muscle. It further divides in the cubital fossa to form the posterior interosseous and the superficial radial nerve.

LIGAMENTOUS AND SPECIAL TESTS

The case scenarios in this chapter may require you to select and use different types of ligamentous and special tests in order to evaluate the injuries adequately. The details of how to perform each special test are beyond the scope of this section; however, Table 5.4 provides a general list of special tests that may be required and useful for you to review before beginning the case studies. For a more thorough review and to determine the sensitivity of and specificity of each test, please refer to your favorite evaluation text or journal article(s).

TABLE 5.4	Ligamentous and special tests of the elbow and forearm.
LIGAMENTOUS TESTS	**FUNCTION**
Varus stress	Assesses integrity of radial (lateral) collateral ligament
Valgus stress	Assesses integrity of ulnar (medial) collateral ligament
Radioulnar joint stress	Assesses integrity of the radioulnar joint (i.e., annular ligament)
SPECIAL TESTS	
Lateral Epicondylitis	
Resistive tennis-elbow (Cozen's) (active lateral epicondylitis)	Assesses for lateral epicondylitis
Resistive tennis-elbow	Assesses for lateral epicondylitis, isolating the extensor carpi radialis brevis
Passive tennis-elbow	Assesses for lateral epicondylitis

(continued)

TABLE 5.4	Continued.

Medial Epicondylitis

| Resistive or active medial epicondylitis | Assesses for medial epicondylitis |
| Passive medial epicondylitis | Assesses for medial epicondylitis |

Nerve Compromise

Tinel's sign	Assesses ulnar nerve pathology
Elbow flexion	Assesses ulnar nerve compression or entrapment in the cubital tunnel
Pronator teres	Assesses median nerve compression caused by muscle hypertrophy of the pronator teres
Pinch grip	Assesses anterior interosseous nerve pathology between the 2 heads of the pronator muscle

REFERENCES

1. An KN, Hui FC, Morrey BF, Linscheid RL, Chao EY. Muscles across the elbow joint: a biomechanical analysis. *J Biomech.* 1981;14:659–669.

2. An KN, Kaufman KR, Chao EY. Physiological considerations of muscle force through the elbow joint. *J Biomech.* 1989;22:1249–1256.

3. Berg EE. Elbow dislocation with arterial injury. *Orthop Nurs.* 2001;20(6):57–59.

4. Cain EL, Dugas JR, Wolf RS, Andrews JR. Elbow injuries in throwing athletes: a current concepts review. *Am J Sports Med* [electronic version]. 2003; 31:621–635. Available from: http://ajs.sagepub.com/cgi/content/abstract/31/4/621. Accessed July 7, 2007.

5. Callaway GH, Field LD, Deng XH, Torzilli PA, O'Brien SJ, Altchek DW, et al. Biomechanical evaluation of the medial collateral ligament of the elbow. *J Bone Joint Surg Am.* 1997;79-A(8):1223–1231.

6. Cohen MS, Bruno RJ. The collateral ligaments of the elbow: anatomy and clinical correlation. *Clin Orthop Relat Res.* 2001;(383):123–130.

7. Fuss FK. The ulnar collateral ligament of the human elbow joint: anatomy, function and biomechanics. *Am J Anat.* 1991;175:203–212.

8. Kaminski TW, Power ME, Buckley B. Differential assessment of elbow injuries. *Athl Ther Today.* 2000;5(3):6–11.

9. Langer P, Fadale P, Hulstyn M. Evolution of the treatment options of ulnar collateral ligament injuries of the elbow, *Br J Sports Med* [electronic version]. 2006;40:499–506. Accessed July 31, 2007.

10. Levangie PK, Norkin CC. *Joint Structure and Function: A Comprehensive Analysis.* Philadelphia, PA: F.A. Davis; 2001.

11. McKee MD, Schemitsch EH, Sala MJ, O'Driscoll SW. The pathoanatomy of lateral ligament disruption in complex elbow in stability. *J Shoulder Elbow Surg.* 2003;12:391–396.

12. Moore K, Dalley A. *Clinically Oriented Anatomy* (5th ed.). Baltimore, MD: Lippincott Williams & Wilkins; 2005.

13. Olsen BS, Sojbjerg JO, Dalstra M, Sneppen O. Kinematics of the lateral ligamentous constraints of the elbow joint. *J Shoulder Elbow Surg.* 1996;5(5):333–341.

14. Regan WD, Korinek SL, Morrey BF, An KN. Biomechanical study of ligaments around the elbow joint. *Clin Orthop Relat Res.* 1991;271:170–179.

15. Safran MR, Baillargeon D. Soft-tissue stabilizers of the elbow. *J Shoulder Elbow Surg.* 2005;14:179S–185S.

16. Safran MR, Bradley JP. Elbow injuries. In: Fu FH, Stone DA eds. *Sports Injuries: Mechanisms, Prevention, Treatment* (2nd ed.). Philadelphia, PA: Lippincott Williams & Wilkins; 2001:1049–1084.

17. Schultz SJ, Houglum PA, Perrin DH. *Examination of Musculoskeletal Injuries* (2nd ed.). Champaign, IL: Human Kinetics; 2005.

18. Sojbjerg JO, Ovesen J, Nielsen S. Experimental elbow instability after transection of the medial collateral ligament. *Clin Orthop Relat Res.* 1987;(218):186–190.

19. Wu J, Perron AD, Miller MD, Powell SM, Brady WJ. Orthopedic pitfalls in the ED: pediatric supracondylar humerus fractures. *Am J Emerg Med.* 2002;(6):544–550.

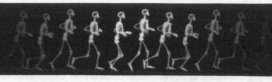

5.1

I t is Friday morning, early in the baseball season, and Sean, an athletic trainer, is working with the Ogden Falcons. The minor league baseball team is getting ready for practice. Jack, a 23-year-old pitcher, walks into the athletic training complex complaining of elbow pain. Jack has been with the team for the past two years, and Sean has treated him in the past for medial epicondylitis.

HISTORY

Sean begins the evaluation by taking a detailed history. Jack explains that during the last couple of weeks his right medial elbow has been getting progressively worse. However, Jack cannot pinpoint a specific date or event that may have caused the initial pain, saying, "it just keeps getting worse since I started throwing this season." Jack explained that most of the pain occurs "during the late cocking and acceleration phase of my pitch." Sean further questions Jack and determines that after throwing 25 to 30 pitches he begins feeling "pins and needles" radiating down the inside of his elbow to his ring and little finger. Jack is very concerned because he has had medial elbow problems in the past, particularly several episodes of medial epicondylitis, but says that those episodes went away with rest.

Sean reassures Jack and excuses himself for a few minutes to review some of Jack's pitching videos. When he returns, Sean informs Jack that there appear to be some changes in his mechanics from last season. In particular, Jack's trunk rotation appears to be off slightly, in that he is not squaring his body and his elbow appears to be dropping during the late cocking and early acceleration phase, rather than being in line with his shoulder.

PHYSICAL EXAMINATION

Sean begins the physical examination by asking Jack to remove his shirt. An observation of Jack's posture reveals obvious signs of structural changes. Observation of the elbow itself reveals an increased carrying angle greater than 15° on the involved side. Jack also appears to be carrying the elbow at 70° of flexion for comfort. Pain with palpation over the flexor-pronator muscle mass and ulnar nerve is noted. Sean places Jack's elbow into 70° flexion and notes pain with palpation from the inferior aspect of the medial epicondyle to the medial aspect of the coronoid process diagonally (Figure 5.1.1). The AROM of the cervical spine is WNL; however, Jack's shoulder AROM for external rotation is less than the uninvolved side and increased for shoulder abduction. Elbow flexion and extension AROM are also decreased because of pain. Wrist flexion and

FIGURE   5.1.1

Palpation of medial elbow at 70° of flexion.

Circle indicates general location of palpable tenderness. Arrow indicates specific location of the palpable tenderness.

extension ROM appears to be WNL. Ligamentous testing with the elbow at 25° flexion demonstrates increased pain and laxity over the medial epicondyle. An increase in neurological symptoms down the medial side of the right elbow into the fourth and fifth fingers is also noted. A moving valgus stress and Tinel's sign are positive. A golfer's elbow test is negative.

? QUESTIONS   CASE 5.1

Please answer the following questions based on the above case information.

5.1 / **1.** Based on the information presented in the case, determine (a) the differential diagnoses and (b) the clinical diagnosis.

5.1 / **2.** Sean asked several history questions to guide the physical examination. Based on the information presented in the case, (a) do you believe Sean took an adequate history? If not, (b) what questions would you have asked as the evaluating clinician?

5.1 / **3.** The injury in this case presents as a chronic condition with an insidious onset. What piece of information obtained as part of the history could have led Sean to believe that the injury was acute in nature?

5.1 / **4.** (a) Identify the dynamic and static stabilizers of the medial elbow joint. (b) Identify the location of the static stabilizers. (c) Which structures were specifically involved in the injury and why?

5.1 / **5.** During the assessment, Sean performed several stress and special tests. If the athlete asked you to explain why the elbow is flexed to 25°, (a) what would your response be? (b) What is the purpose of the Tinel's sign in this case?

5.1 / **6.** (a) What is a moving valgus stress test, and how is it performed? (b) If you were the evaluating clinician, would you have performed this test and why? (c) If not, what other tests might you have performed?

CASE

5.2

atsuko, a 28-year-old female recreational racquetball player, has been referred to a sports medicine clinic by her internist. The prescription states: "lateral elbow pain, evaluate and treat." Don, the certified athletic trainer who will be evaluating her, assumes she is suffering from lateral epicondylitis and prepares a generic home exercise program before she arrives. When she arrives, she has an interpreter with her.

HISTORY

Don initiates the evaluation by asking Natsuko several questions through her interpreter. He is able to determine that she was backpedaling and lost her balance while playing racquetball. As she fell backward, she tried to brace herself, and when she landed, she immediately began experiencing pain along the outside of the elbow. Her CCs include lateral elbow pain, recurrent snapping with activity, and pain with supination-pronation.

PHYSICAL EXAMINATION

Natsuko is alert, oriented, and in moderate discomfort (5/10 on a numerical pain scale). The diagram in Figure 5.2.1 describes Natsuko's pain pattern. An observation of Natsuko's elbow reveals noticeable swelling on the lateral side of the left elbow. Active elbow flexion and extension ROM is 0° to 135° (R) and 4° to 120° (L). Left elbow active supination and pronation demonstrates a 10° deficit in both directions. Muscle testing identifies pain and weakness during supination and pronation

| FIGURE | 5.2.1 | Natsuko's pain chart. |

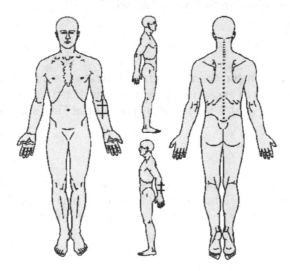

Crosses equal location of general pain.

(3/5) and elbow flexion (3+/5). Wrist flexion and extension muscle testing is WNL. Don performs a valgus stress test and posteromedial rotatory instability test, both of which are negative. Neurological and circulatory tests are unremarkable. Don's immediate reaction is that Natsuko sustained a hyperextended elbow. He sets her up with cryotherapy and High TENS electrical stimulation to help with her pain. At the end of the treatment, he fits her with a compression sleeve and instructs her in home exercises. He also instructs her to use ice 45 to 60 minutes 3 to 4 times a day.

? QUESTIONS   CASE 5.2

Please answer the following questions based on the above case information.

5.2 / **1.** Based on the information presented in the case, (a) what is the likely clinical diagnosis? (b) What makes this clinical diagnosis unique?

5.2 / **2.** Don asked several specific history questions to guide the physical examination. However, there was one question that may have assisted in narrowing down the clinical diagnosis, which he either did not ask or which may not have been answered appropriately because of a translation error. Can you identify this question?

5.2 / **3.** If Natsuko presented with the same clinical findings from the case but also had weakness with wrist extension, (a) would your clinical diagnosis possibly change? (b) What would cause you to make this change?

5.2 / **4.** Do you believe Don adequately evaluated Natsuko's condition? If not, what would you have done differently as the evaluating clinician?

5.2 / **5.** In this case, a language barrier existed. Fortunately, a translator was able to assist Don during the physical examination. If you were placed in a situation in which you were unable to communicate with a patient because of a language barrier, how would you handle the situation?

Monica is a certified athletic trainer and manager of an industrial physical medicine clinic for a large manufacturing company. She was working on her daily reports and follow-up employee evaluations when the phone rang. The head nurse over in the acute care center wanted to know if Monica could evaluate one of the employees who reported to the clinic about two hours earlier. She informed Monica that Dr. Smith had made the request and said, "He trusts your clinical skills and will follow up with the employee and you later." Dr. Smith had already ordered radiographs but was called away for an emergency before he could evaluate the employee. Monica agreed to see the employee and informed the nurse to send him over immediately.

HISTORY

Eugene, the employee, arrives at the physical medicine clinic with his arm in a sling. Monica begins her physical exam by gathering some general information. She then proceeds by asking, "So tell me what happened?" Eugene replies, "I was working on the line yesterday when I stepped to the left and tripped over a block of metal. I lost my balance and fell. I tried to save the piece I was working on and ended up landing on my left arm." After some further questioning, Monica determines the MOI to be a fall on the outstretched hand with the elbow in mid-flexion as Eugene tried to brace himself when he hit the ground. Eugene described feeling a slight "popping" sensation at the back of the elbow. He complained of pain with active elbow extension and flexion. His pain was rated as 6/10. He has a history of diabetes mellitus (type II) and denies any previous history of elbow trauma.

PHYSICAL EXAMINATION

Eugene is alert and oriented. He presents with an elastic wrap, which Monica removes. He has moderate swelling about the elbow and forearm. Palpable tenderness and what appears to be a slight palpable defect at the insertion of the triceps are noted. The forearm is non-tender and demonstrates no signs of muscle tension. Eugene's ROM results are presented in Table 5.3.1. Muscle testing reveals moderate-to-significant weakness while trying to actively extend the elbow against gravity. Monica completes a neurovascular physical exam, which is unremarkable. She then accesses the radiographs ordered by Dr. Smith electronically.

TABLE 5.3.1 Eugene's humeroulnar ROM measurements.

MOTION	RIGHT	LEFT
AROM	0°–130°	45°–90°
Passive	1–0°–135°	20°–110°

DIAGNOSTIC IMAGING

The lateral-view radiographs reveal what appears to be a small piece of bone separated from the olecranon process. Monica treats Eugene accordingly, documents her findings for the Workmen's Compensation Insurance, and then dictates a note for his chart and Dr. Smith's records.

? QUESTIONS   CASE 5.3

Please answer the following questions based on the above case information.

5.3 / **1.** Based on the information presented in the case, determine (a) the differential diagnoses and (b) the clinical diagnosis.

5.3 / **2.** The MOI in this case study was a fall on the outstretched hand with the elbow in mid-flexion. During Eugene's fall, what specific action was being performed by the tissue involved in the injury?

5.3 / **3.** If you were the evaluating clinician, what "general information" would you have gathered at the beginning of the history?

5.3 / **4.** In addition to the clinical observations presented in the case, what other signs or symptoms may be presented depending on how old the injury is?

5.3 / **5.** If you were in Monica's position, (a) discuss how you would have assessed Eugene's muscular strength against gravity. (b) Why was he still able to extend the elbow?

5.4

During a collegiate conference track meet, Tabatha, the top junior javelin thrower, was warming up for her event when she began to experience medial elbow pain. Coach Quinn was concerned about Tabatha's current pain, especially considering a previous history of elbow problems, and immediately sought out McKinley, the team's certified athletic trainer. When Coach Quinn found McKinley, she was talking with the team's internist, Dr. Martinez, who was the physician on call for the home meet.

HISTORY

As McKinley begins gathering her history, she notes that Tabatha is supporting and rubbing her right elbow. Tabatha explains to McKinley that during warm-ups she misstepped and lost her balance as she approached the line, causing her to forcefully snap the wrist as she was releasing the javelin. Tabatha said, "As I released the javelin, I felt a pull on the inside and top of my right arm. I wanted to try to throw again, but the pain was really bad when I was just trying to hold the javelin." Tabatha denies any popping or unusual sounds. Her pain is 4/10 when not throwing and 7/10 to 8/10 when throwing.

PHYSICAL EXAMINATION

Tabatha is alert, oriented, and anxious to get back to competition. McKinley identifies palpable tenderness over the medial epicondyle, medial forearm, and pronator teres. Active ROM with wrist flexion and pronation produces moderate pain. MMT reveals weakness in the right wrist flexors (3+/5) and pronator teres (3+/5) when compared with the left. Grip strength testing and a neurovascular exam are unremarkable. Dr. Martinez, who is watching the examination, sends her over to health services for a set of radiographs (AP, lateral, and 110° oblique radiographic views) because of the medial epicondyle tenderness. These are unremarkable.

McKinley decides it is best to remove Tabatha from competition. Coach Quinn has a different opinion. He begins pressing McKinley to allow Tabatha to compete. When McKinley does not agree, Coach Quinn seeks out Dr. Martinez. After a lengthy conversation behind closed doors, Dr. Martinez emerges, draws up 60 mg of ketorolac tromethamine, injects Tabatha's elbow, and allows her to return to the meet.

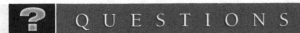

Please answer the following questions based on the above case information.

5.4 / **1.** Based on the information presented in the case, determine (a) the differential diagnoses and (b) the clinical diagnosis.

5.4 / **2.** McKinley asked several history questions to guide the physical examination. Based on the information presented in the case, do you believe she took an adequate history? If not, what questions would you have asked as the evaluating clinician?

5.4 / **3.** McKinley assessed AROM and muscle strength but failed to assess PROM. If you were the evaluating clinician, how would you assess PROM, and what would you expect to find?

5.4 / **4.** (a) What is ketorolac tromethamine? (b) Is this an appropriate course of action?

5.4 / **5.** If you were the evaluating clinician, what if anything would you do regarding the coach's actions?

Paul, a 42-year-old weightlifter and avid water skier, arrived at Sam's rehabilitation clinic one day after suffering a water-skiing accident. He was out for a day of fun with his family when he hit a wake while water skiing. When Paul arrived at the clinic, his right shoulder was in a homemade sling (his elbow was being held at a 45° angle), and he appeared to be in moderate discomfort.

HISTORY

Paul reports crossing back over his wake, causing him to lose his balance. As he tried to regain his balance, Paul experienced a forceful, unanticipated extension of his arms as his elbows were actively flexed. Unfortunately, he was unsuccessful at keeping his balance. He reports experiencing immediate pain and felt a popping sensation "in the front part of my right elbow near the crease." Paul also reports difficulty swimming back to the boat. He states, "It felt as though I had no strength or ability to move my elbow."

PHYSICAL EXAMINATION

One day post injury, Paul presents with moderate discomfort (5/10–6/10 on the numeric pain scale [NPS]). An observation of Paul's cubital fossa reveals moderate swelling and ecchymosis. A closer observation reveals some minor swelling into the right forearm and hand. Active ROM is slightly decreased (5°–10°) during elbow flexion and forearm pronation. Forearm supination ROM is decreased by 50 to 60 percent. Paul's AROM of the shoulder in flexion is slightly decreased; all other active motions of the shoulder and PROM are WNL. Capsular and ligamentous testing are not performed, because of increased swelling and pain. Special tests are positive. Tests for fractures are unremarkable. Neurologically, Paul is intact.

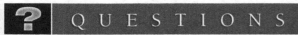

Please answer the following questions based on the above case information.

5.5 / **1.** Based on the information presented.in the case, determine (a) the differential diagnoses and (b) the clinical diagnosis.

5.5 / **2.** What, if any, other signs should Sam have observed during the physical examination that may have helped to guide his clinical diagnosis?

5.5 / **3.** Based on the clinical diagnosis, (a) what component of the physical examination did Sam forget? (b) What is the clinical significance of omitting this part of the physical examination?

5.5 / **4.** According to the case report, the special tests were positive. Based on your clinical diagnosis, (a) name at least one test that you feel could have been positive. (b) Describe how to perform the test.

5.5 / **5.** Would radiographic studies be useful in this case? Why, or why not?

CASE 5.6

J eff was the head athletic trainer covering a high school state wrestling meet along with four other certified athletic trainers and six athletic training students. The day had been relatively calm with only minor injuries. As he was walking by the center mat, Jeff stopped to watch the 185-pound weight class where one of his school's wrestlers was competing. Adam was in control for several seconds until his opponent escaped. Once the opponent escaped and regained his composure, he performed a single leg tackle. Adam was not prepared for this attack, and as he fell to the mat, he tied to brace himself. As soon as he landed, Adam began screaming, and the referee called injury time. Jeff and Sue, an athletic training student, ran onto the mat.

HISTORY

Jeff immediately calms Adam down while Sue begins to stabilize the left elbow. Because Jeff had witnessed the incident, he already knew that Adam had tried to brace himself with his elbow extended and supinated. Adam states, "When I hit the mat my elbow popped, and now I can't move it."

FIGURE 5.6.1

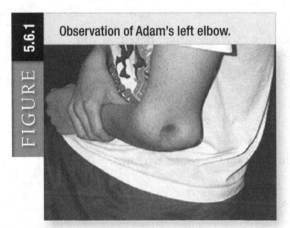

Observation of Adam's left elbow.

TABLE 5.6.1

Adam's vital signs.

VITAL SIGNS	FINDING
Pulse	90, regular
Respiration	15, normal
Blood pressure	136/82
Mental status	Alert

PHYSICAL EXAMINATION

Adam is alert, oriented, and in severe discomfort. He has observable joint deformity at the elbow, with the elbow held in a fixed position around 90° (Figure 5.6.1). The joint and forearm are beginning to swell. Jeff believes the ulna has moved posterolateral to the humerus, but he is not completely sure. Adam has palpable tenderness around the posterior and anterior elbow. Muscle and ROM testing are deferred because of pain. Jeff asks Sue to bring over the splint bag. While they wait for the splint bag, Jeff takes Adam's vital signs, shown in Table 5.6.1.

Sue stabilizes the elbow while Jeff splints the injury using a SAM SPLINT and an elastic wrap. Jeff notices that the hand is beginning to look pale and feels cooler than the noninvolved hand. Once stabilized, the elbow is put into a commercial sling. Adam's parents arrive, and Jeff and Sue explain what just occurred. They inform them that Adam needs to be seen in the ER as quickly as possible. His parents decide to drive Adam to the hospital themselves rather than wait for an ambulance.

? QUESTIONS   CASE 5.6

Please answer the following questions based on the above case information.

5.6 / **1.** Based on the information presented in the case, determine (a) the differential diagnoses and (b) the clinical diagnosis.

5.6 / **2.** Based on the clinical diagnosis above, identify three to five additional history questions you may have asked as the evaluating clinician.

5.6 / **3.** Do you believe Jeff and Sue adequately evaluated Adam's condition? If not, what would you have done differently as the evaluating clinician?

5.6 / **4.** Given the clinical diagnosis, describe the exact MOI and which, if any, other structures may have been injured.

5.6 / **5.** If you were the athletic trainer in this case, would you have provided the same type of immediate care? Why, or why not? Describe the steps you would have used.

S asha, a certified athletic trainer for a Division II women's ice hockey team, was at the rink Monday afternoon preparing for ice hockey practice and was working with one of the athletic training students on clinical proficiencies. The coach called the office asking if she could come over and talk for a few minutes about a player. Sasha left the office to talk to the coach. While Sasha was gone, Raquel, the team captain and starting center, arrived at the athletic training room. The only person available was Al, the athletic training student. He informed Raquel that Sasha was talking with the coach and would be back in a few minutes. They began to chat and Raquel asked if Al could look at her elbow. Al replied, "Why don't we wait till Sasha gets back?" Sasha arrived 10 minutes later to find Raquel and Al sitting there.

HISTORY

After some discussion of the game on Saturday, Sasha asks why Raquel is here. Raquel says, "Do you remember when I got tripped and fell on the ice? I put out my right hand to catch myself and felt pain in my elbow. It didn't really bother me then, but over the weekend my elbow swelled and it hurt to move." Sasha asks, "Did you land with your arm in front of you or behind you?" Raquel replies, "In front." Further questioning reveals some loss of elbow function. Pain is rated as 6/10.

PHYSICAL EXAMINATION

Raquel is alert and oriented. Her elbow is currently wrapped with an elastic wrap; however, ecchymosis is noted on the dorsal aspect of the hand. Sasha unwraps the elbow, noting moderate swelling around the elbow (Table 5.7.1). Raquel is also holding the elbow in a fixed position around 45° of flexion. Palpable tenderness is noted along the proximal radius, particularly with supination and pronation. An elbow-extension test is positive, and ROM is decreased in all planes. Ligamentous testing reveals gapping of the right UCL when compared with the left. Sasha completes a neurovascular physical exam, which is unremarkable. The results of the findings, particularly the elbow-extension test, concern Sasha, so she decides it would be best to refer Raquel to the team's orthopedic surgeon for further evaluation. However, the surgeon cannot see Raquel until Tuesday afternoon.

TABLE 5.7.1	Raquel's elbow girth measurements.		
POSITION	**RIGHT**	**LEFT**
Epicondyles	12.5"	11"
3" below	11"	10"
6" below	9"	7.5"

? Q U E S T I O N S CASE 5.7

Please answer the following questions based on the above case information.

5.7 / **1.** Based on the information presented in the case, determine (a) the differential diagnoses and (b) the clinical diagnosis.

5.7 / **2.** (a) Explain why Raquel presented with palpable tenderness with supination and pronation. (b) Would you suspect the pain to be worse with the elbow in flexion or extension?

5.7 / **3.** Given the MOI presented in this case, why did Sasha find increased laxity over the UCL?

5.7 / **4.** Overall, do you believe Sasha adequately evaluated Raquel's condition given the provided information? If not, what would you have done differently as the evaluating clinician? Why did Sasha seem so concerned about the elbow-extension test?

5.7 / **5.** If you were the athletic trainer and your athlete could not get in to see the orthopedic surgeon until the next day, what type of immediate care would you have provided? Describe the steps you would have used.

5.8

Justin, a 35-year-old recreational athlete and college professor, was participating in an intramural lacrosse league. During the game, an opposing player struck Justin in the right arm with his stick as Justin was trying to block his face (Figure 5.8.1). The opposing player was given a penalty for slashing Justin. Justin immediately grabbed his arm in pain, and he pulled himself out of the game to get an ice pack. After 20 minutes of ice, his pain was still pretty intense. The referee suggested that Justin seek out the athletic trainer, Shane, who is responsible for caring for intramural and club sports athletes.

FIGURE   5.8.1

Position of forearm during impact with a lacrosse stick.

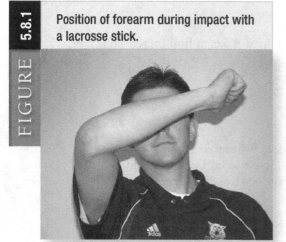

HISTORY

Justin recounts the hit to Shane. His CCs are severe pain and decreased ROM about the elbow. Justin reports no past history of elbow or forearm trauma.

PHYSICAL EXAMINATION

Justin is alert, cooperative, and in moderate discomfort. His right arm appears swollen around the mid-forearm. No visible deforming is observable. Palpable tenderness is noted along the medial mid-forearm only. Elbow flexion and extension and forearm supination and pronation ROM are decreased as compared with the left. Shane makes his clinical diagnosis and immobilizes Justin's arm as a precaution. After some discussion Justin agrees to call his wife and heads over to the urgent care center to be seen by the on-call physician. Once Justin leaves, Shane completes the necessary paperwork to document the care he provided.

❓ QUESTIONS   CASE 5.8

Please answer the following questions based on the above case information.

5.8 / 1. Based on the information presented in the case, determine the clinical diagnosis.

5.8 / 2. What is the colloquial term for this clinical diagnosis?

5.8 / 3. Shane asked a couple of history questions to guide his physical examination. Based on the clinical diagnosis above, identify three to five additional history questions you may have asked as the evaluating clinician.

5.8 / 4. Do you believe Shane adequately evaluated Justin's condition? If not, what would you have done differently as the evaluating clinician?

5.8 / 5. Discuss how you as the evaluating clinician would have managed this situation once the physical examination has been completed.

5.8 / 6. After completing the physical examination, Shane documented his findings and sent a copy of the report to the administration office. Please document your findings as if you were the treating clinician. If the case did not provide information you believe is pertinent to the clinical diagnosis, please feel free to add this information to your documentation.

5.9

S herrie, a mother of three boys (ages 6, 8, 13) and a certified athletic trainer by profession, was attending her six-year-old son's T-ball game. During the fourth inning, Jeremy, another six-year-old, was knocked down while defending home plate. He instantly began to cry out in pain and was rolling around on the ground. Sherrie quickly got up from her chair in order to attend to Jeremy. When she arrived, she quickly explained to Jeremy what she was going to do. As Sherrie was palpating Jeremy's elbow, his mother arrived.

HISTORY

After calming Jeremy down, Sherrie determines that Jeremy landed on an outstretched arm in an extended position. Jeremy complains of "really bad pain on the outside of my arm." He also states, "I can't move my arm, and it feels funny." Sherrie questions Jeremy's mother about any past elbow history, which she denies.

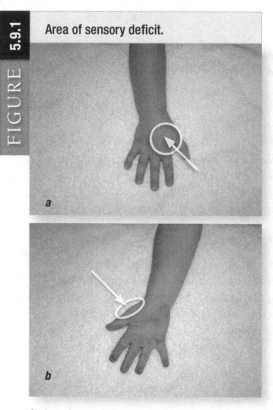

FIGURE 5.9.1

Area of sensory deficit.

a

b

Circle and arrow indicate area of sensory deficit.

PHYSICAL EXAMINATION

Jeremy is in obvious pain, and this has made his mother very anxious. Sherrie begins the physical exam by quickly palpating his lower legs and working her way up to the torso. She quickly assesses for injuries distal to the elbow, which already appears swollen. The elbow also appears to have a definite shift or angulation in the position of the humerus. He presents with palpable tenderness around the joint, particularly around the lateral supracondylar ridge. She also feels what she considers to be the olecranon prominence posterior to its normal anatomical position. Jeremy refuses to move the elbow because of the pain he is experiencing; however, Sherrie does note a deficit in grip strength and inability to extend the wrist on the involved side. A neurovascular physical examination reveals delayed capillary refill and what appears to be a sensory deficit (Figure 5.9.1) on the involved site. The results of these findings concern Sherrie. She discusses the results of her physical examination with Jeremy's mom, who appears confused by the end of the discussion.

Please answer the following questions based on the above case information.

5.9 / **1.** Based on the information presented in the case, determine the clinical diagnosis.

5.9 / **2.** Sherrie was able to determine the MOI by questioning the patient, in this case falling on an outstretched hand with the elbow extended. If you were the evaluating clinician, do you believe you would have been able to arrive to the same conclusion? Why or why not?

5.9 / **3.** (a) Identify the bony and soft tissue structure Sherrie should have palpated as part of her evaluation specific to the elbow. (b) Identify the neurological and vascular structures at greatest risk, based on the clinical diagnosis. (c) Identify the anatomical landmarks in Figures 5.9.2 and 5.9.3.

5.9 / **4.** According to the case, Sherrie notes a deficit in grip strength and the inability to extend the wrist on the involved side. What does this indicate?

5.9 / **5.** Given the age of the patient in this case, would you have handled the situation any differently? If so, why?

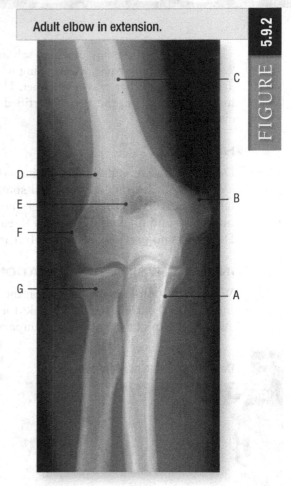

Adult elbow in extension.

FIGURE 5.9.2

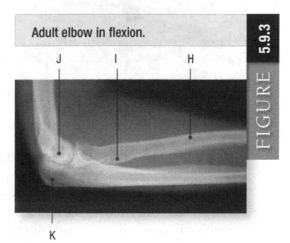

Adult elbow in flexion.

FIGURE 5.9.3

During the first play of a high school semi-final football game, Derick, a 17-year-old running back, was rushing when he abruptly and forcefully struck his right arm against another player's helmet. He immediately fell to the ground, supporting his right arm. Tim, the team's certified athletic trainer, was called onto the field to evaluate Derick.

HISTORY

Derick's CCs are mid-forearm pain and some loss of wrist function. Tim questions Derick about hearing any unusual sounds or sensations. Derick responds, "Yeah, I felt and heard a snap." Tim further questions about any abnormal sensation such as numbness and tingling in Derick's forearm. Derick responds, "No, it's just painful." Derick has no previous history of forearm trauma and is otherwise healthy.

INITIAL PHYSICAL EXAMINATION

While Tim completes his history on the field, he observes the way Derick is supporting his arm (Figure 5.10.1) and looks for DOTS (deformity, open wounds, tenderness, swelling). Tim's observations are unremarkable. He assists Derick to his feet, and they

FIGURE 5.10.1

Derick supporting his right arm.

manage to walk over to the sideline. Once on the sideline, Tim completes his evaluation, noting pain and tenderness over the mid-forearm, crepitus, swelling, guarding, and an unwillingness to move his wrist. Derick's distal pulses and sensation are intact. Tim's clinical decision is a fractured forearm. He splints the arm and applies ice to the fracture site. Tim walks over to inform the coach that Derick will not be returning to the game. As Tim returns to Derick, his parents are talking to him through the fence. Tim explains the situation to Derick's parents and recommends they take him to the ER immediately. Derick, however, wants to stay with his team and watch the game. After some discussion, Derick is allowed to stay, and his parents agree to take him to an ER right after the game is over. After 20 minutes, the ice was removed, and Derick's arm was splinted again and placed into a sling.

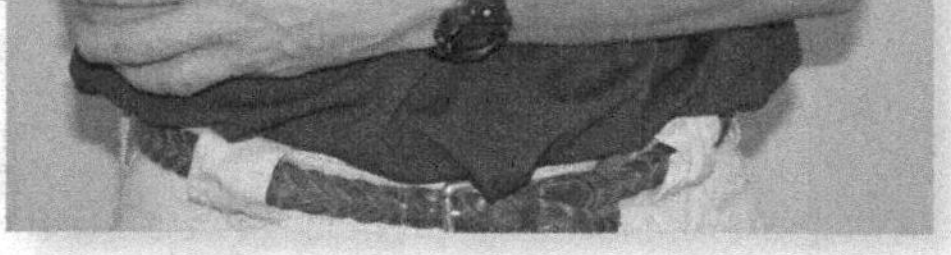

FOLLOW-UP PHYSICAL EXAMINATION

After the game was over a couple of hours later, Derick approaches Tim about his arm, saying "Tim, my arm is throbbing and my fingers are starting to go numb." Concerned, Tim removes the splint and begins re-evaluating the arm. Derick presents with numbness and increasing pain on the anterior surface of the forearm and in the wrist. The pain appears disproportionate for the injury after several hours. Another physical exam reveals increased firmness over the volar compartment of the forearm, swelling distal to the injury site, and slightly pale skin. Tim is also concerned that Derick is experiencing pain with active and passive metacarpophalangeal and interphalangeal joint motion. Tim realizes this is not a good sign and immediately informs Derick and his parents together that this is a medical emergency and to drive Derick to the ER right away. He continues to explain to the parents that this injury has a high risk of irreversible soft-tissue damage that could affect Derick's ability to play sports and have a normal life. Derick's parents are now scared they made a bad decision by letting Derick watch the rest of the game.

? **QUESTIONS**   **CASE 5.10**

Please answer the following questions based on the above case information.

5.10 / **1.** Based on the information presented in the case, determine the initial clinical diagnosis and the secondary clinical diagnosis based on the follow-up examination.

5.10 / **2.** Based on the clinical findings of the initial and secondary physical examinations, and your knowledge of the secondary clinical diagnosis, (a) what six signs and symptoms are common to the diagnosis? (b) In what order do they often present?

5.10 / **3.** Why did Tim seem so concerned about Derick experiencing pain with active and passive metacarpophalangeal and interphalangeal joint motion?

5.10 / **4.** If Derick presented with just paresthesia distal to the injury and minor throbbing over the injury site during the second assessment, how would you react? What could be occurring?

5.10 / **5.** Overall, do you believe Tim adequately handled the situation and his interaction with Derick's parents? If not, what would you have done differently as the evaluating clinician?

CASE 5.11

Harry, a 51-year-old triathlete and tennis player, was referred to an outpatient physical therapy clinic three days after seeing his family doctor for anterior elbow pain. A note was faxed from the doctor's office stating: "paresthesia and motor weakness over the thumb and second and third digits, treat accordingly." When Harry arrived, he presented his paperwork to the office staff. In the paperwork, the ICD-9 was written as 955.1. Harry then completed several forms including a *Notice of Privacy Practices,* medical history, and pain profile. Once all the paperwork was completed, Harry was escorted to a room where he would be evaluated by Ron, a certified athletic trainer.

HISTORY

Ron begins his physical examination by reviewing Harry's past medical history and gathering additional information as necessary. He then proceeds by asking, "So tell me what is going on?" Harry responded, "For several months I have been training for a triathlon that takes place in a couple of months and have begun to experience pain here (he points to the location shown in Figure 5.11.1), particularly when lifting and riding my bike for long periods of time. In fact my tennis game is also starting to be affected as well. The pain tends to be worse when I serve or am involved with a long ralley." Further questioning reveals a reduction in pain and symptoms at night and with periods of rest from activity. Harry's pain profile information is presented in Figure 5.11.2.

FIGURE 5.11.1

Harry's location of elbow pain.

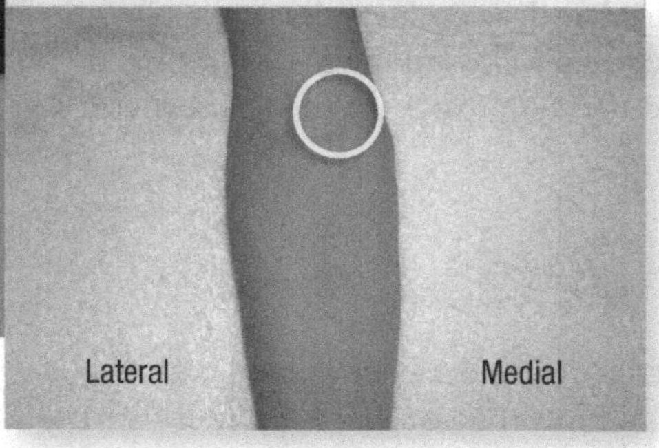

Lateral   Medial

Location of pain is within the circle.

PHYSICAL EXAMINATION

Harry is alert, oriented, and in minimal discomfort at this time. Palpable tenderness and pain are noted with forceful compression of proximal medial forearm musculature. Active elbow flexion and extension and forearm supination and pronation ROM appear normal. Resisted pronation of the involved elbow exacerbates and reproduces Harry's anterior elbow pain. Ligamentous testing is WNL. Neurological testing reveals a positive Tinel's sign over the anterior cubital fossa and sensory deficits over the palmar surface of the thumb and the second and third digits.

After completing the physical examination, Ron discusses options with Harry, including referral to another physician for a second opinion if conservative treatment fails. After Harry agrees to Ron's suggested course of treatment, Ron treats him accordingly.

FIGURE 5.11.2   Harry's pain profiles.

Pain level with activity (weight lifting, tennis)

NO PAIN   SEVERE PAIN

Pain level at rest

NO PAIN   SEVERE PAIN

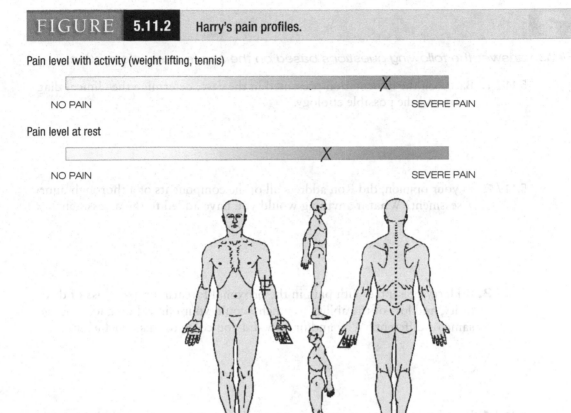

Note: Cross = general pain;
triangle = numbness and tingling

Please answer the following questions based on the above case information.

5.11 / **1.** Based on the information presented in the case, determine the clinical diagnosis and the possible etiology.

5.11 / **2.** In your opinion, did Ron address all of the components of a thorough injury assessment? What if anything would you have added to the assessment?

5.11 / **3.** If Harry presented with pain in the proximal forearm or arm, loss of dexterity, and loss of the ability to pinch, would your clinical diagnosis be the same or different? Why and/or how did you come to this conclusion?

5.11 / **4.** If you were the treating clinician, outline a conservative rehabilitation program.

5.11 / **5.** As mentioned in the case, Ron suggests referral to another physician if conservative treatment does not work. What type of physician would you consider referring Harry to, and why?

5.11 / **6.** Overall, do you believe Ron adequately evaluated Harry's condition? If not, what would you have done differently as the evaluating clinician, and why?

CASE 5.12

Recruit Jones, a 23-year-old FBI trainee, reported to the training center's medical facilities complaining of left medial elbow and forearm pain. Because the entire medical staff was in a meeting, the triage nurse sent Recruit Jones to the physical medicine department for a physical examination. Celina, the certified athletic trainer on duty, was assigned the case. Before the physical exam began, Celina brought up Recruit Jones's complete electronic medical record from the medical center's database.

HISTORY

Celina begins the assessment by reviewing Recruit Jones's medical history with him. Prior to his arrival at the training center, Recruit Jones played collegiate baseball at a local university where he was a starting pitcher. Celina questions Recruit Jones regarding his time playing baseball at the university. She learns that he has had three episodes of left medial epicondylitis. The medical records also reveal that in his sophomore year of college he sustained a second-degree ulnar collateral ligament sprain. He also fractured his left olecranon process while playing broom ball when he was 19 years old.

On this particular day, Recruit Jones is complaining of medial forearm pain and decreased motor function in his left hand and wrist, which had been progressively getting worse since he started his physical training at the center. He also states, "It has really gotten worse since we started defensive training and grappling." Further questioning from Celina reveals complaints of weak grip strength and clumsiness with training objects (e.g., holding a gun or baton). Recruit Jones recalls no specific incident that would explain his injury. He rates his pain as 4/10 at rest and 7/10 or 8/10 while training.

PHYSICAL EXAMINATION

Recruit Jones is alert, oriented, and in moderate discomfort. Celina notes minor-to-moderate swelling medially. She also notes palpable tenderness and pain over the medial epicondyle, olecranon process, and in the area of the ulnar nerve and cubital tunnel. Direct palpation of the ulnar nerve elicits pain and numbness distally from the elbow, mimicking the symptoms Recruit Jones experiences while training. Active and passive ROM (flexion) of the elbow is decreased (AROM 135° R/128° L, PROM 140° R/132° L) with pain at the end range of active motion. His wrist active and passive ROM results are shown in Table 5.12.1. Muscle testing reveals mild weakness with

TABLE 5.12.1

Recruit Jones's wrist range of motion results.

MOTION	JOINT MOTION	FINDINGS	
		RIGHT	LEFT
AROM	Flexion	80°	69°
	Extension	70°	68°
	Radial deviation	20°	16°
	Ulnar deviation	30°	20°
PROM	Flexion	WNL	
	Extension	Mild-to-moderate pain end-range motion	
	Radial deviation	Moderate-to-severe pain end range	
	Ulnar deviation	WNL	

TABLE	5.12.2	Recruit Jones's neurological results.

TEST	LOCATION	FINDINGS
Deep tendon reflex	C5	WNL
	C6	WNL
	C7	WNL
Dermatomes	C5	WNL
	C6	WNL
	C7	WNL
	C8	WNL
	T1	WNL
	T2	WNL
Myotomes	C5	WNL
	C6	WNL
	C7	WNL
	C8	WNL
	T1	WNL
Two-point discrimination to the peripheral nerves	Dorsal web space between thumb and index finger	WNL
	Lateral palm, thumb, index, middle finger, and lateral half of ring finger	WNL
	Medial palm, medial fifth finger, and medial half of ring finger	Positive

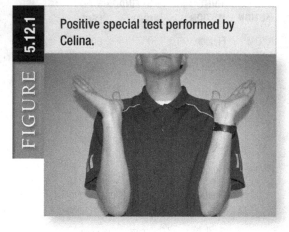

FIGURE 5.12.1

Positive special test performed by Celina.

elbow flexion and extension, moderate weakness with wrist flexion and ulnar deviation, and moderately decreased grip strength measured with a dynamometer. His neurological findings are located in Table 5.12.2. Radial collateral stress testing is negative. Ulnar collateral stress testing reveals medial elbow pain with minimal laxity on the involved elbow. Testing for cervical compression, brachial plexus nerve stretch, and thoracic outlet syndrome (TOS) is negative. A Tinel's sign and the special test shown in Figure 5.12.1 are positive.

After completing the physical examination, Celina documents her findings and sends a copy of the report to Dr. Taylor's office. Dr. Taylor calls Celina the next day to discuss her findings. Together they agree Recruit Jones warrants further diagnostic testing and immediate treatment, including the use of pharmacological agents.

? | QUESTIONS **CASE 5.12**

Please answer the following questions based on the above case information.

5.12 / **1.** Based on the information presented in the case, determine (a) the differential diagnoses and (b) the clinical diagnosis.

5.12 / **2.** Celina asked several history questions to guide her physical examination. Based on the information presented in the case, do you believe she took an adequate history? If not, what questions would you have asked as the treating clinician?

5.12 / **3.** If Recruit Jones had reported a popping or clicking sound or sensation with elbow flexion, (a) how would this have affected your clinical diagnosis? (b) Would you have altered your evaluation?

5.12 / **4.** (a) What is the elbow flexion test, and (b) how is it performed? (c) If you were the evaluating clinician, would you have performed this test? Why or why not? If not, (d) what other test might you have performed?

5.12 / **5.** After completing the physical examination, Celina documented her findings and sent a copy of the report to Dr. Taylor's office. Please document your findings as if you were the treating clinician. If the case did not provide information you believe is pertinent to the clinical diagnosis, please add this information to your documentation.

5.13

Bill, a certified athletic trainer for a Division III football team, was in the university's athletic training room getting ready for practice. This was his first job since graduating with his master's degree in athletic training. The football team had already been practicing for three weeks when Chris arrived to speak with Bill. They chatted for awhile, as Bill was trying to acquaint himself with all of the players better.

HISTORY

After talking about how Chris liked the season so far and about his job over the summer, Bill began questioning Chris regarding the purpose of his visit. Chris states, "Well, my elbow is swollen, and it hurts to bend and straighten my arm and to touch my elbow. It's like every time I get tackled I keep landing on my elbow. What can I do to stop this from happening?" Further questioning reveals no previous history of elbow trauma. Chris's pain is rated as 5/10 or 6/10 at rest and 8/10 or 9/10 when participating in athletics.

PHYSICAL EXAMINATION

Chris is alert and oriented. An observation of the elbow can be seen in Figure 5.13.1. Bill notes that Chris appears to be holding the joint around 45° of flexion. A cursory palpation of the joint (just over the swelling site) reveals pain, particularly with deep palpation, and swelling over the posterior elbow to the outer tip of the olecranon process.

FIGURE 5.13.1

Observation of the posterior elbow.

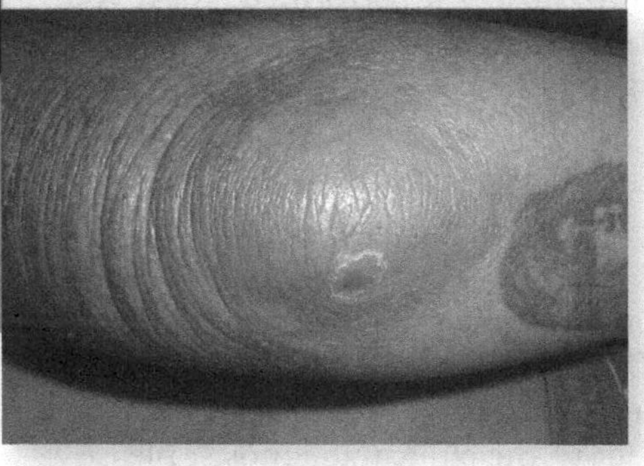

Bill notices the women's volleyball team has arrived and knows that he needs to tape them. Confident in his clinical diagnosis and not wanting to take any more time to evaluate Chris's elbow, Bill instructs Chris to ice his elbow 20 to 30 minutes every 3 to 4 hours. He fits him with a compression sleeve and sends him to the equipment room to get an elbow pad from the equipment manager.

FOLLOW-UP PHYSICAL EXAMINATION

Two days later, Chris's elbow pain has progressively gotten worse. He arrives back at the athletic training room, only this time, not only is Bill there, but the team physician Dr. Pedersen is there. After getting a medical history and observing Bill's elbow, Dr. Pedersen notes warmth and erythema around the elbow, which Chris reports having two days ago. He now also presents with a purulent discharge from the elbow. Dr. Pedersen is very upset and asks Helen, the GA covering the doctor's clinic, to prepare a 20mL syringe and a 22 gauge, 1-inch needle. Once all of the athletes are seen by Dr. Pedersen, she sits Bill down for a discussion. During this meeting, Dr. Pedersen questions Bill's clinical diagnosis. Bill denies noting the presence of any warmth and erythema around the elbow.

Please answer the following questions based on the above case information.

5.13 / 1. Based on the information presented in the case, identify what you believe was Bill's original clinical diagnosis and what the clinical diagnosis should have been.

5.13 / 2. Why do you believe Dr. Pedersen asked Helen to prepare a 20mL syringe and a 22 gauge, 1-inch needle?

5.13 / 3. (a) Overall, do you believe Bill handled the situation correctly? If not, what would you have done differently as the evaluating clinician? (b) Should Bill have had more concern for Chris's condition?

5.13 / 4. What professional standards, if any, did Bill fail to follow?

5.13 / 5. If you were Dr. Pedersen, how would you address this situation with Bill?

CASE 5.14

by Susan Stevenson, MS, ATC, CSCS, Northern Illinois University, DeKalb, IL

R ichard, a 20-year-old receiver on the Division III college football team, stopped in the athletic training room before the team's first practice to talk to Crystal, the certified athletic trainer assigned to football during the season. After a few minutes of catching up, Crystal asks Richard what really brings him into the athletic training room. Richard says that he has had an ongoing aching pain in his right elbow all summer, and he is concerned it will affect his ability to catch the football during the season. He was wondering what he could do to help it.

HISTORY

Crystal begins by asking Richard what happened over the summer to cause his elbow to hurt. He states that nothing happened; he just worked a new summer job moving furniture and, while initially all his muscles were sore, eventually the soreness in his body subsided except for the soreness in his elbow. He tried icing after work, but the pain gradually increased over the summer despite his efforts. Further questioning reveals that Richard's girlfriend taught him how to play tennis during the summer.

PHYSICAL EXAMINATION

First Crystal notes generalized swelling about the right elbow joint, with no discoloration or deformity present when compared with the uninvolved arm. When asked, Richard states his current pain is 4/10 but that it increases to 7/10 while working and 9/10 at the end of a workday. Upon palpation, Richard jumps a little when Crystal presses on the area shown in Figure 5.14.1. Passive ROM is WNL, with increased pain in the right lateral forearm with wrist flexion and pronation with the elbow extended. Active ROM is also WNL, with reproduction of pain during wrist extension. Bilateral strength is equal at 5/5, except in wrist extension where the right is 4/5. Provocative testing for soft tissue irritability includes the Cozen's and the Mill's test, both of which are positive for pain over the lateral epicondyle. After completing her evaluation Crystal discusses her findings and outlines a clinical course of action.

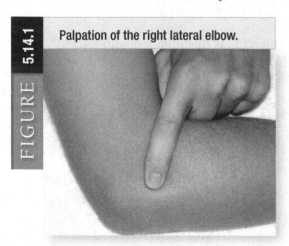

FIGURE 5.14.1

Palpation of the right lateral elbow.

Location of pain is under the index finger.

? QUESTIONS   CASE 5.14

Please answer the following questions based on the above case information.

5.14 / **1.** Based on the information presented in the case, determine (a) the differential diagnoses and (b) the clinical diagnosis.

5.14 / **2.** In addition to the information Crystal gained from the history, identify three to four additional history questions she could have asked to help guide the physical examination and to help rule out the differential diagnoses.

5.14 / **3.** Why did Richard have significant discomfort with palpation of the lateral epicondyle?

5.14 / **4.** (a) Do you believe that Crystal thoroughly evaluated Richard's condition? If not, (b) what would you have done differently as the evaluating clinician?

5.14 / **5.** If you were the athletic trainer in this case, what would your next step be, knowing that Richard is on his way out to the first practice of the season?

CASE

5.15

by Shane Stecyk, Ph.D, ATC, CSCS, University of California, Northridge

J enny is a 14-year-old pitcher on a junior league baseball team. One evening she complained to her parents that her arm had been feeling tired and that she had been experiencing pain over the medial aspect of her right elbow for the past five or six weeks. Her mother, a college professor who teaches in a nursing program, decided to speak with Anita, one of her colleagues who teaches in the athletic training education program at the nearby university. Anita, a certified athletic trainer and physical therapist, agreed to evaluate Jenny.

HISTORY

Jenny and her mom meet Anita in her office after classes. Anita begins her evaluation by gathering some general information. She determines that Jenny typically pitches four times per week: twice as a starter (70–75 pitches) and twice as a reliever (25–30 pitches). Further probing reveals the complaints of a tired arm and pain normally occurs before and after throwing and during her pre-game stretch (PROM wrist extension). More questioning also reveals that Jenny played short-stop until six weeks ago, at which time she was converted to a pitcher. In fact, she now pitches and plays short-stop on her non-pitching days (1 day per week). Jenny also states that she felt pain while arm-wrestling last weekend with her older brother to see who would have to do the dishes.

PHYSICAL EXAMINATION

Anita's initial observation is unremarkable. She does note palpable point tenderness over the medial epicondyle and insertion of the wrist flexor muscles. There is slight point tenderness on the lateral epicondyle and extensor tendons, posterior rotator cuff tendons and muscle bellies, scapular stabilizers, and the pectoralis minor. Results of Anita's ROM testing are found in Table 5.15.1. Ligamentous testing

TABLE	5.15.1	Jenny's ROM results.
MOTION	**JOINT**	**FINDINGS**
AROM	Wrist	Pain primarily with wrist flexion and pronation; some pain with extension
	Shoulder	Limited internal rotation, extension, and abduction
PROM	Wrist	Limited wrist extension and supination secondary to pain
	Elbow	Limited elbow extension secondary to pain
	Shoulder	Decreased internal rotation, extension, horizontal adduction, and abduction
RROM	Wrist	3+/5 wrist flexion secondary to pain; 4/5 pronation secondary to pain
	Elbow	4+/5 flexion; 5/5 extension
	Shoulder	4/5 abduction; 3+/5 external rotation at 90°; 3+/5 horizontal abduction; 4/5 flexion, 4+/5 extension
	Scapula	3+/5 rhomboids/middle trapezius; 3+/5 lower trapezius; 4/5 serratus anterior

around the elbow is unremarkable. Testing of the shoulder reveals some anterior laxity but no complaints of instability. Resistive wrist flexion and passive wrist extension testing are positive. An empty can test is positive. Neurovascular testing is unremarkable. Anita discusses the results of her physical examination with Jenny's mom. She agrees with Anita that Jenny needs to be seen by a specialist for further physical examination.

? QUESTIONS   CASE 5.15

Please answer the following questions based on the above case information.

5.15 / **1.** Based on the information presented in the case, determine (a) the differential diagnoses and (b) the clinical diagnosis.

5.15 / **2.** Overall, do you believe that Anita completed a thorough history? What if anything would you have done differently?

5.15 / **3.** In this case, the clinical diagnosis appears not to be an isolated injury but rather a symptom of a larger problem. Discuss what the larger problem is and how it may exist.

5.15 / **4.** What are your thoughts regarding Jenny's pitch count? Is she within the pitching limits required by USA baseball?

5.15 / **5.** Why do you believe Anita wanted to refer Jenny to a specialist? Would you have made a similar recommendation?

Barry has worked as a certified athletic trainer at a small Division III college for the last 20 years. He was covering football during a cold and snowy winter practice, and the conditions on the field made traction and maneuvers difficult for the players. During one particular drill, an offensive lineman slipped and fell to the ground, landing on his elbow region as other linemen piled on top of him. After the play cleared, the offensive lineman, Tuppu, rolled on the ground grasping his left elbow area. Barry got to Tuppu as quickly as he could and immediately verified the presence of an airway, breathing, and circulation. Tuppu was in obvious pain and discomfort.

HISTORY

Tuppu explains to Barry what happened. His CCs are severe pain (10/10) and decreased ROM about the elbow and shoulder. Tuppu reports no past history of elbow or forearm trauma.

PHYSICAL EXAMINATION

Tuppu is alert, apprehensive, and in severe discomfort. Barry inspects the left arm and immediately notices that the elbow and distal humerus do not look congruent. Barry notices that the region looks abnormal, with a medial protrusion (not through the skin) just above the elbow joint. Tuppu refuses to move the elbow and supports his lower arm with his other hand. Distal pulses and sensation at the wrist are normal.

Please answer the following questions based on the above case information.

5.16 / **1.** Based on the information presented in the case, determine (a) the differential diagnoses and (b) the clinical diagnosis.

5.16 / **2.** What is the common mechanism for this type of injury?

5.16 / **3.** If you were in Barry's situation, how would you have managed the situation?

5.16 / **4.** Suppose Barry removed the player from the field, splinted the injured area, and noticed the distal pulses were compromised. What should he then do?

5.16 / **5.** Should Barry, who is the only athletic trainer on the field, call for emergency medical services and, if necessary, go with the athlete to the hospital?

5.16 / **6.** Based on this type of injury, what are some complications that could result?

CONCLUSION

E lbow injuries, like most injuries, range from a mild case of olecranon bursitis to a severe elbow dislocation with concomitant neurovascular damage. Regardless of the severity of the injury though, all elbow injuries must be properly evaluated and managed to reduce functional limitations and disability. Injuries such as elbow dislocations or elbow sprains, even minor sprains if not properly managed, can impair or restrict an athlete's ability to participate in sport or a patient's ability to perform activities of daily living and/or work. Imagine, if you sustained a dislocated elbow, what impact it would have on your activities of daily living. How would you wash or comb your hair, eat dinner, or dress your kids or yourself? Would you be able to perform the duties of your job, such as taping, performing joint mobilizations, or even evaluate an athlete appropriately?

As athletic training students, you have been taught a conceptual framework for physical examination of musculoskeletal injuries and general medical conditions. For most of you, this framework consists of history, observation, palpation, and stress/special tests (forming the acronym "HOPS"). The cases in this chapter demonstrated all or part of this process. However, this chapter also demonstrated the necessity not only of gathering the HOPS information but also of linking this information, such as the history and the patients' symptoms, to common and not-so-common impairments and disorders, as well as being able to recognize that occasionally this information does not always coincide with what you have learned.

The cases also demonstrated the need for communication at a level appropriate to your population or situation. The case involving the translator may seem unusual to you as a student, but many professionals experience this type of challenge on a daily basis. One of the authors held a previous job in a major metropolitan city as a physical therapist, where she used translators from a variety of languages on a daily basis when treating her patients. In fact, she had to learn some basic Cantonese, because without it she would have never been able to properly diagnosis and manage her patients. Remember that a physical examination and the therapeutic interventions following it are only as good as your ability to ask and receive the correct information.

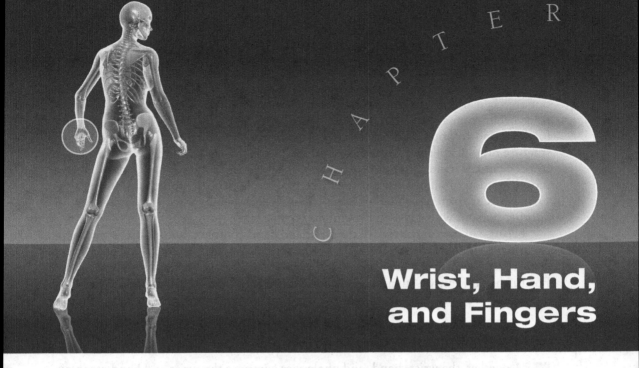

6

Wrist, Hand, and Fingers

INTRODUCTION

T his chapter will examine the clinical evaluation and management of 17 different wrist, hand, and finger pathologies, using a combination of on-field and off-field scenarios presented in a variety of settings with a diverse patient population. The traumatic and overuse injuries to the wrist and hand complex presented in this chapter are a mixture of acute and chronic pathologies as well as bony, ligamentous, and neurovascular conditions. We have attempted to identify many of the injuries frequently encountered in clinical practice by athletic trainers. As a reminder, some of the cases presented in this chapter and other chapters in this text have been intentionally written with inappropriate actions, procedures, treatments, or general mismanagement of the case by the clinician in order to allow you to critically analyze the cases, identify the inappropriate decisions, and provide the appropriate gold-standard treatment when applicable.

Injuries to the wrist are often the result of direct violent trauma, axial loading when falling on an outstretched hand, rotational force, and/or repetitive movements. Injuries to the hand and wrist account for 3 to 9 percent of all athletic injuries[25] and 1.5 to 20 percent of all emergency room visits in the general population.[8,9] Among the carpal (wrist) bones, the scaphoid is the most commonly fractured (79 percent)[1,28] and at the greatest risk for developing avascular necrosis, because of the bone's poor vascular supply.[25] The lunate is the most commonly dislocated carpal bone, becoming dislocated when an athlete falls on an outstretched hand or braces herself as the wrist is forced into hyperextension (e.g., blocking in football).[23] Trapezoid fractures are the rarest of all carpal fractures, accounting for just 2 percent of carpal fractures.[21] The increase in computer usage has also demonstrated an association between work position at the computer and musculoskeletal symptoms and disorders (MSDs) of the wrist and hand complex.[32]

Metacarpal trauma is often the result of some type of direct violent blow, such as being struck with an object (e.g., stick, ball, etc.), being stepped on, falling on an outstretched arm, or striking an opponent or object.[26] Phalange fractures and dislocations occur from a wide variety of mechanisms, including bending, direct blow, axial loading, and rotation, and these occur in a variety of types.[10] One study examining fracture rates in collegiate athletes found that, by location, fractures were most likely to occur at the hand[12] and that fractures to the fourth and fifth metacarpals are the most common of all metacarpal fractures.[2,16] Fractures of the fourth and fifth metacarpals occur from punching an immovable object, such as the ground, the wall, or another person, with a closed fist and no boxing mitt.

Because of the complexity of the wrist and hand complex, both from an anatomical and physiological perspective, the brief anatomical review will provide only a very cursory overview of the anatomical arrangement and basic functioning of the joints. For further review, we suggest reading texts and journal articles that specifically examine the structure and function of the wrist and hand complex.

ANATOMICAL REVIEW

Together, the wrist, hand, and phalanges compose the wrist and hand complex, which is made up of 27 bones (Figure 6.1) and 24 muscles—all responsible for the work, protection, and performance of athletes and patients. Located at the distal end of the upper extremity, the wrist and hand complex is responsible for carrying out the work of the upper extremity. As people instinctively place the wrist and hand in harm's way to protect the rest of the body and head, it is therefore exposed to, and at risk for, injury while working, competing, or recreating.[8,11]

The coordinated relationship between the bony and soft tissue (ligaments, muscles, tendons) arrangement of the wrist and hand complex is designed in such a way as to enable both independent and concert movement of the many bones and joints in the complex.[22] The combination of active muscular, passive ligamentous, and compressive forces in the wrist and hand complex provides a much needed base of support for positional adjustments, allowing for the development and maintenance of optimal length-tension relationships in the longer finger muscles.[14] Muscles such as the flexor digitorum superficialis and profundus depend on this constant correction and maintenance of the length-tension relationship in order to generate enough tension to permit fine adjustments of grip (power and precision handling) and motor-control performance. Without these gripping and fine and gross motor-control adjustments, an athlete or physically active individual would not be able to grip or throw a baseball, hold and swing a bat, hold the bowstring of a violin, or engage in activities requiring precise control.

FIGURE 6.1

Bones of the wrist and hand complex.

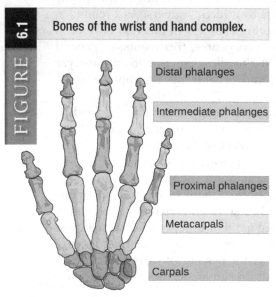

Distal phalanges

Intermediate phalanges

Proximal phalanges

Metacarpals

Carpals

Source: Wikipedia.

Wrist Complex

The wrist joint consists of two main articulations—the radiocarpal and midcarpal. These are collectively known as the wrist complex. The radiocarpal joint is situated between the distal ends of the radius and the radioulnar disc (part of the triangular fibrocartilage complex, TFCC) and the proximal row of carpal bones. The midcarpal joint is created through the individual articulations of the proximal and distal carpal rows (Table 6.1) and has its own joint capsule and synovial lining separate from the radiocarpal joint.[14,19] In addition to the radiocarpal and midcarpal joint are several smaller intercarpal joints (including the scapholunate, the scaphotriquetral, the lunotriquetral, and the capitotriquetral). These small articulations do not contribute to joint motion of the wrist and hand complex individually, but rather, they work as a group to provide the necessary joint motion required for activities of daily living. Together, the wrist complex allows 2° of freedom, flexion and extension and radial and ulna deviation ROM, depending on the position of the upper extremity as a whole.

Flexion and extension occur in a sagittal plane around a frontal axis and normally range between 0° and 80° and 0° and 70°, respectively. Because there are no direct muscular attachments to the proximal carpal row, flexion and extension occur with the proximal carpal row acting as a mechanical link between the radius and distal carpal row and metacarpals. Movement at the radiocarpal joint occurs predominantly through a gliding of the proximal carpal row on the radius and radioulnar disc. The proximal row is also the level of the wrist complex most associated with injuries.[13,15,17,25]

Radial and ulnar deviation occurs in the frontal plane around a sagittal axis and normally has a range between 0° to 20° or 0° to 30°. Radial and ulnar deviation is even more complex in its structure and function than flexion and extension and requires simultaneous flexion and extension of the proximal and distal carpal rows, depending on the movement. Radial deviation is normally greatest at the midcarpal joint, with ulnar deviation occurring equally at the radiocarpal and midcarpal joints.

TABLE	6.1	Bony configuration of the distal and proximal carpal row.

CARPAL ROW	RADIAL TO ULNAR SIDE	
Distal	Trapezium, trapezoid, capitate, and hamate	A = scaphoid B = lunate C = triquetrum D= pisiform E = trapezium F = trapezoid G = capitate H = hamate
Proximal	Scaphoid, lunate, triquetrum, pisiform*	

*The pisiform is anatomically part of the proximal carpal row, but it does not participate in the radiocarpal articulation. It functions as a sesamoid bone, floating on the triquetrum, and is believed to increase the lever arm of the flexor carpi ulnaris.

Wrist complex ligamentous structures

The ligaments of the wrist complex are categorized as extrinsic and intrinsic carpal ligaments,[5,29,30] based on whether they are on the palmar or dorsal surface. The extrinsic ligaments originate on the forearm and attach distally on the carpal bones, providing stabilization to the radiocarpal joint. Intrinsic ligaments originate and insert wholly onto the carpals, providing stabilization to the midcarpal joint. The major extrinsic ligaments are the radial and ulnar collateral and palmar and dorsal intercarpal ligaments. The intrinsic ligaments are categorized as palmar and dorsal midcarpals and the interosseous. The extrinsic and intrinsic carpal ligaments are the primary stabilizers of the wrist complex (Table 6.2), working together with the individual fibrous joint capsules of the radiocarpal and midcarpal joints and the traverse carpal ligament. Figures 6.2 and 6.3 provide a general observation of the dorsal and volar ligaments of the wrist complex. Anatomical textbooks such as Keith L. Moore's *Clinically Oriented Anatomy* and Frank H. Netter's *Netter's Clinical Anatomy* will provide more detailed information related to the wrist-hand complex ligaments and other structures that make up the complex.

TABLE 6.2	Extrinsic and intrinsic ligaments of the wrist.	
SURFACE	**LIGAMENT**	**LOCATION AND FUNCTION**
EXTRINSIC LIGAMENTS		
Palmar and radial	Radial collateral	Radial styloid process to the scaphoid and trapezium; limits ulnar deviation
Ulnar	Ulnar collateral	Ulnar styloid process to medial aspect of the triquetrum dorsally and pisiform palmarly; limits radial deviation
Dorsal	Dorsal radiocarpal	Dorsal side from the radius to the carpal bones; limits wrist flexion
Palmar	Palmar radiocarpal	
	Radioscaphocapitate	Anterior surface of the distal radius to scaphoid and capitates; limits extension
	Radiolunotriquetral	Anterior surface of the distal radius to lunate and triquetrum; limits extension
	Radioscapholunate	Anterior surface of the distal radius to scaphoid and lunate; limits extension
	Short radiolunate	Anterior surface of the distal radius to proximal surface of lunate; limits extension
	Long radiolunate	Palmar rim of the distal radius to palmar horn of the lunate; limits extension
Palmar	Palmar ulnocarpal	
	Ulnolunate	Anterior surface of the distal ulna to the lunate; limits extension
	Ulnotriquetral	Anterior surface of the distal ulna to the triquetrum; limits extension
	Ulnocapitate	Anterior surface of the distal ulna to the capitate; limits extension

TABLE 6.2	Continued.	
INTRINSIC LIGAMENTS*		
Palmar	Palmar midcarpals	
	Scaphotrapezium-trapezoid	Anterior surface of scaphoid to trapezium and trapezoid
	Scaphocapitate	Anterior surface of scaphoid to capitate
	Triquetrocapitate	Anterior surface of triquetrum to capitate
	Triquetrohamate	Anterior surface of triquetrum to hamate
Dorsal	Dorsal midcarpals	
	Dorsal scaphotriquetral	Posterior surface of scaphoid to triquetrum
	Dorsal intercarpal	Connects the scaphoid, triquetrum, and capitate
Dorsal and palmar	Interosseous	
	Scapholunate	Scaphoid to the lunate
	Lunotriquetral	Lunate to the triquetrum
	Trapezium-trapezoid	Trapezium to the trapezoid
	Trapeziocapitate	Trapezium to the capitate
	Capitohamate	Capitate to the hamate

* Intrinsic ligaments stabilize and limit motion (e.g., rotational) between the carpal bones.

FIGURE 6.2	Dorsal wrist ligaments.

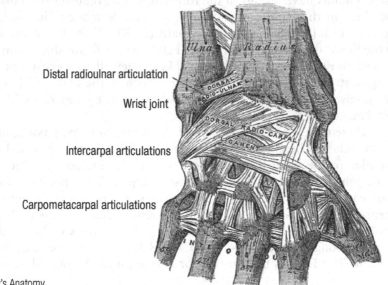

Distal radioulnar articulation

Wrist joint

Intercarpal articulations

Carpometacarpal articulations

Source: Gray's Anatomy.

FIGURE 6.3   Palmar wrist ligaments.

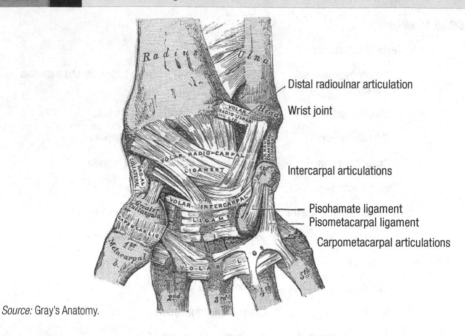

Distal radioulnar articulation

Wrist joint

Intercarpal articulations

Pisohamate ligament
Pisometacarpal ligament

Carpometacarpal articulations

Source: Gray's Anatomy.

Musculature

The musculature, or rather, the muscular tendons crossing the wrist complex are responsible for providing a broad array of activities and therefore require the ability to constantly adapt to changes in position of the upper extremity and hand complex. Muscle tendons crossing the wrist complex are classified into four groups: (1) those crossing the anterior (volar) surface, (2) those crossing the posterior surface, (3) those crossing the radial surface, and (4) those crossing the ulnar surface.

There are six muscle tendons that cross over the volar aspect of the wrist. These muscle tendons have origins in the forearm and travel distally to insert onto various locations in the hand complex. The six muscle tendons include: (1) the palmaris longus (PL), (2) the flexor carpi radialis (FCR), (3) the flexor carpi ulnaris (FCU), (4) the flexor digitorum superficialis (FDS), (5) the flexor digitorum profundus (FDP), and (6) the flexor pollicis longus (FPL). They all act as either primary or secondary agonists for wrist flexion, with some, such as the FDP and FDS, acting as primary agonist of DIPJ and PIPJ flexion, respectively, by way of their insertion onto the phalanges.

Nine muscle tendons cross the dorsum of the wrist complex, passing under the extensor retinaculum. These muscle tendons have origins in the proximal to distal forearm, similar to the wrist flexors. The nine muscles include: (1) the extensor carpi radialis longus (ECRL), (2) the extensor carpi radialis brevis (ECRB), (3) the extensor carpi ulnaris (ECU), (4) the extensor digitorum communis (EDC), (5) the extensor digiti minimi (EDM), (6) the extensor digiti indicis (EDI), (7) the extensor pollicis longus (EPL), (8) the extensor pollicis brevis (EPB), and (9) the abductor pollicis longus (APL). The ECRL, ECRB, and ECU are responsible for wrist extension. The EDC is responsible for extension of the lateral four fingers' metacarpophalange joints and also joins the extensor hood mechanism, which is comprised of the extensor tendon, sagittal bands, and conjoined tendons of the intrinsic muscles, lumbricals, and interossei.[10] The EDI and EDM are responsible for independent movements of the second and fifth fingers rather than additional strength or additional actions.[14] The EPL, EPB, and APL all act to extend or abduct the thumb. Radial deviation is controlled by the FCR, ECRL, and ECRB. Ulnar deviation is controlled by the FCU and ECU.

Hand Complex

The hand consists of three main joint articulations: the carpometacarpal joint (CMCJ), the metacarpophalangeal joint (MCPJ), and the interphalangeal joint (IPJ). These are collectively known as the hand complex (Figure 6.4).

Carpometacarpal joints

The five CMCJs are situated between the distal carpal row and five metacarpals (MC). Each metacarpal aligns with a distal row of carpals. Starting from radial to ulnar side, the first MC (thumb) articulates with the trapezium, the second MC articulates with the trapezoid, the third MC articulates with the capitate, and the fourth and fifth MCs articulate with the hamate. The first CMCJ is a saddle joint with a unique structure that allows for 2° of freedom, permitting thumb flexion and extension, abduction, and adduction (Table 6.3). Precision handling (e.g., picking up small objects such as a quarter) is accomplished through axial rotation at the thumb, known as opposition. Opposition is an accessory motion that permits the tip of the

---

FIGURE **6.4** Joint articulations of the hand complex.

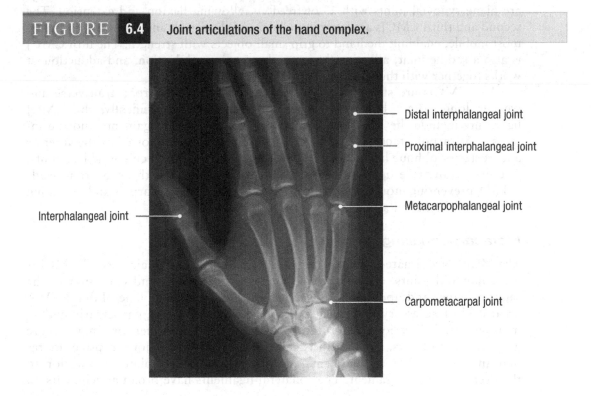

Distal interphalangeal joint

Proximal interphalangeal joint

Metacarpophalangeal joint

Interphalangeal joint

Carpometacarpal joint

TABLE 6.3	Range of motion in joints of the hand complex.			
THUMB JOINTS	**FLEXION**	**EXTENSION**	**ABDUCTION**	**ADDUCTION**
First CMCJ	0°–15°	0°–20°	0°–70°	0°–10°
MCPJ	0°–50°–60°	0°	n/a	n/a
IPJ	0°–80°	0°–20°	n/a	n/a
FINGER JOINTS				
Second CMCJ	0°–2°	0°	n/a	n/a
Third CMCJ	0°	0°	n/a	n/a
Fourth CMCJ	10°	0°	n/a	n/a
Fifth CMCJ	20°	0°	n/a	n/a
OTHER JOINTS				
MCPJ	0°–90°–110°	0°–45°	20°	20°
PIPJ	0°–100°–120°	0°	n/a	n/a
DIPJ	0°–80°–90°	0°	n/a	n/a

thumb to oppose or touch the tips of the fingers. The second through fourth CMCJs are plane synovial joints with 1° of freedom, allowing flexion and extension. The second and third CMCJs are fairly immobile, and the fourth and fifth CMCJs are the most mobile, enabling the hand to grip small objects with strength. The fifth CMCJ is also a saddle joint, allowing flexion and extension, abduction, and adduction. It works together with the thumb to permit opposition.

The CMCJs are stabilized by their joint capsules and strong transverse and weaker longitudinal ligaments volarly and dorsally.[14] Specifically, the CMCJ ligaments include the dorsal and palmar carpometacarpal ligaments and the interosseous carpometacarpal ligaments. The thumb is also supported by the anterior and posterior oblique ligaments as well as the radial and ulnar collateral ligaments. The deep transverse ligament spans the second through fourth metacarpal heads volarly, preventing more than minimal abduction of the metacarpals and providing stability to the MCPJ as well.

Metacarpophalangeal joints

The MCPJs are situated between the metacarpal bones and phalanges. The MCPJs are condyloid joints, allowing for 2° of freedom, flexion and extension in the sagittal plane, and abduction and adduction in the frontal plane (Table 6.3). A great deal of accessory movement takes place at these joints, particularly gliding motions in all directions and rotation, which enables a firmer and more secure grasp around objects. The MCPJ is stabilized by its fibrous joint capsule, its radial and ulnar collateral ligaments, and its palmar (volar) plate, in addition to the deep transverse ligament. The collateral ligaments have broad attachments on the side of the metacarpal heads, attaching proximally onto the head of the metacarpal and distally onto the base of the proximal phalanx. These collateral ligaments are responsible for the primary support of the MCPJ[18] and limit abduction and adduction beyond a neutral position, as they become taught during MCPJ flexion. The volar or palmar plate is a thick ligamentous-like disc that consists of tough fibrocartilage located from the area just proximal to the head of the MC to the base of each proximal phalange. Structurally, the volar plate prevents dorsal dislocation of the MCPJ—but only when it is in full extension.[18]

Interphalangeal joint

Nine IPJs are situated between the phalanges of the fingers, creating three separate articulations: the proximal interphalangeal joint (PIPJ), distal interphalangeal joint (DIPJ), and the interphalangeal joint. The PIPJ is located between the proximal and middle phalange bones of fingers two through five. The DIPJ is located between the middle and distal phalange bones of fingers two through five. The interphalangeal joint is located between the proximal and distal phalanges of the thumb only. The IPJs are plane synovial joints allowing for 1° of freedom, flexion, and extension in the sagittal plane (Table 6.3).

The major ligaments supporting the IPJs include the fibrous joint capsule, the PIPJ and DIPJ radial and collateral ligaments, and the palmar (volar) plate (Figure 6.5). The radial and ulnar collateral ligaments are primary restraints against a varus or valgus force[7] and attach proximally onto the head of the more proximal phalanx and distally onto the base of the distal phalanx.[14] On the volar surface, the fibrocartilaginous volar plate makes up the floor of the joint. It is ligamentous at the proximal origin and cartilaginous at the distal insertion[27] and allows the flexor tendons to glide past the joint without catching.[10] The volar plate is the primary structure preventing PIPJ extension beyond the joint's anatomical position.[6]

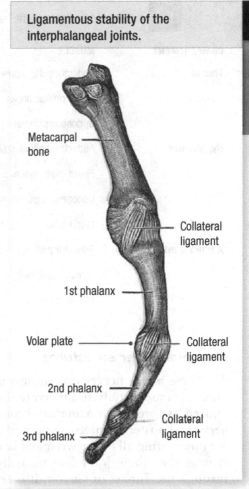

FIGURE 6.5

Ligamentous stability of the interphalangeal joints.

Metacarpal bone

Collateral ligament

1st phalanx

Volar plate

Collateral ligament

2nd phalanx

Collateral ligament

3rd phalanx

Source: Gray's Anatomy.

Musculature

Dynamically, the hand complex musculature has its origins and insertion on the carpal, metacarpals, or phalanges. These intrinsic muscles are also classified into four groups: (1) thenar eminence, (2) hypothenar eminence, (3) central, and (4) adductor interosseous compartments (Table 6.4).

TABLE	6.4	Intrinsic muscles of the hand complex.

COMPARTMENT	MUSCLE	ACTION
Thenar	Abductor pollicis brevis	Thumb abduction
	Flexor pollicis brevis	Thumb MCP flexion
	Opponens pollicis	Thumb opposition
Hypothenar	Abductor digiti minimi	Fifth finger MCP abduction
	Flexor digiti minimi brevis	Fifth finger MCP flexion
	Opponens digiti minimi	Fifth finger opposition
Central	Lumbricals	Finger MCP flexion and IP extension
Adductor interosseous	Adductor pollicis	Thumb adduction
	Palmar interossei	Finger MCP adduction
	Dorsal interossei	Finger MCP abduction

Neurovascular structures

The three major nerves (radial, median, and ulnar) that crossed the elbow complex continue distally to innervate the wrist and hand complex, and these can be injured as a result of acute or chronic injuries. The motor portion of the radial nerve and posterior interosseous nerve (a branch of the radial nerve) is responsible for innervating all of the wrist and hand extensor muscles. The ulnar nerve, which crosses the elbow joint line medially, continues down the forearm and passes through the Tunnel of Guyon. It is responsible for innervating structures such as the FCU, a portion of the FDP, the dorsal and palmar interossei, and the muscles of the hypothenar eminence. The ulnar nerve is at the greatest risk for compression, entrapment, or palsy where the nerve passes superficially through the Tunnel of Guyon. Often called "handlebar palsy" or "cycle palsy," entrapment of the ulnar nerve at the Tunnel of Guyon occurs with prolonged periods of direct pressure on the ulnar nerve from gripping bicycle handlebars.[24]

The flexor muscles, lumbricals (lateral two), and muscles of the thenar eminence are innervated by the median nerve, except for the FCU and a portion of the FDP, which as previously mentioned are innervated by the ulnar nerve. The median nerve is at risk of trauma if the wrist is hyperextended for prolonged periods of time during physical activity[31] or during periods of repetitive overuse, such as in the development of carpal tunnel syndrome.[3,4,32,33]

The brachial artery crosses anterior to the cubital fossa, passing between the biceps tendon and the median nerve before splitting into the radial and ulnar arteries. Lack of blood flow brought on by trauma increases the risk of compartment syndrome and Volkmann's ischemic contractures,[34] making any compromise to the radial or ulnar artery a medical emergency. In the hand complex, prolonged pressure applied over the hypothenar eminence increases the risk of ulnar artery thrombosis.[20]

LIGAMENTOUS AND SPECIAL TESTS

T he case studies in this chapter may require you to select and use different types of ligamentous and special tests in order to adequately evaluate the injury. The details of how to perform these special tests are beyond the scope of this section; however, Table 6.5 provides a general list of ligamentous tests and special tests that may be required and useful for you to review before beginning the case studies. For a more thorough review of the sensitivity and specificity of each test, please refer to your favorite evaluation text or journal article(s).

TABLE 6.5	Ligamentous and special tests of the wrist and hand complex.
LIGAMENTOUS TESTS	**FUNCTION**
Valgus (UCL) and varus (RCL) stress test of the wrist	Assesses stability of the UCL or RCL ligament of wrist, respectively, with the hand in an anatomical position
Valgus and varus stress test of the IPJ	Assesses stability of the PIPJ and DIPJ collateral ligaments (UCL and RCL) with the hand in an anatomical position
Test for laxity of the collateral ligaments of the thumb	Assesses stability of the UCL and RCL of the thumb at the MCPJ with the hand in an anatomical position
Glide testing (radial, ulnar, superior, and inferior position)	Assesses stability of the collateral or intercarpal ligaments
SPECIAL TESTS	**FUNCTION**
Bunnel-Littler	Distinguishes between tightness of the joint capsule and tightness of the intrinsic finger muscles
Digital Allen	Assesses for partial or complete occlusion of the radial or ulnar artery
Finkelstein's	Assesses for tenosynovitis (de Quervain's Disease)
Flexor tendon avulsion	Assesses integrity of the FDP
Froment's sign	Assesses ulnar nerve pathology, specifically adductor pollicis
Long finger flexor	Assesses integrity of the FDP and FDS
Murphy's sign	Assesses for a dislocated lunate
Phalen's sign	Assesses median nerve pathology and is indicative of carpal tunnel syndrome
Tap or percussion	Assesses for fractures
Tinel's sign	Assesses median nerve pathology and is indicative of carpal tunnel syndrome

REFERENCES

1. Altizer L. Hand and wrist fractures: first part of a 2-part series. *Orthop Nurs.* 2003;22(2):131–138.

2. Altizer L. Boxer's fracture. *Orthop Nurs.* 2006; 25:271–273.

3. Anderson JM. Carpal tunnel syndrome: common, treatable, but not necessarily work-related. *J Controversial Med Claims.* 2007;14(4):1–10.

4. Ashworth NL. Carpal tunnel syndrome. eMedicine [electronic version]. 2006. Available from: http://www.emedicine.com/pmr/TOPIC21.HTM. Accessed January 15, 2008.

5. Boutry N, Lapegue F, Masi L, Claret A, Demondion X, Cotten A. Ultrasonographic evaluation of normal extrinsic and intrinsic carpal ligaments: preliminary experience. *Skeletal Radiol.* 2005; 34(9):513–521.

6. Bowers W. The proximal interphalangeal joint volar plate, II: a clinical study of hyperextension injury. *J Hand Surg [Am].* 1981;6:77–81.

7. Bowers W, Wolf J, Nehil J, Bittinger S. The proximal interphalangeal joint volar plate, I: an anatomical and biochemical study. *J Hand Surg [Am].* 1980;51:79–88.

8. Chan O, Hughes T. Hand. *BMJ* [electronic version]. 2005;330:1073–1075. Available from: http://bmj.com/cgi/content/full/330/7499/1073. Accessed January 17, 2008.

9. Chung KC, Spilson SV. The frequency and epidemiology of hand and forearm fractures in the United States. *J Hand Surg.* 2001;26(5):908–915.

10. Combs JA. It's not "Just A Finger." *J Athl Train.* 2000;35(2):168–178.

11. Freeland AE, Geissler WB, Weiss AP. Operative treatment of common displaced and unstable fractures of the hand. *J Bone Joint Surg.* 2001; 83-A(6):927–945.

12. Hame SL, LaFemina JM, McAllister DR, Schaadt GW, Frederick J, Dorey FJ. Fractures in the collegiate athlete. *Am J Sports Med* [electronic version]. 2004;32:446–451. Available from: http://ajs.sagepub.com/cgi/content/abstract/32/2/446. Accessed May 12, 2007.

13. Hunter D. Diagnosis and management of scaphoid fractures: a literature review. *Emerg Nurse.* 2005;13(7):22–26.

14. Levangie PK, Norkin CC. *Joint Structure and Function: A Comprehensive Analysis.* Philadelphia, PA: F.A. Davis; 2001.

15. Mayfield J. Wrist ligamentous anatomy and pathogenesis of carpal instability. *Orthop Clin North Am.* 1984;15:209–216.

16. McFarland EG, Chronopoulos E, Kim TK. Upper extremity injuries in adolescent athletes. *Athl Ther Today.* 2002;7(6):13–17.

17. Melsom DS, Leslie IJ. Carpal dislocations. *Current Orthop.* 2007;21(4):288–297.

18. Minami A, An KN, Cooney W, Inscheid R, Chao E. Ligament stability of the metacarpophalangeal joint: a biomechanical study. *J Hand Surg [Am].* 1985;10(2):266–260.

19. Moore K, Dalley A. *Clinically Oriented Anatomy* (5th ed.). Baltimore, MD: Lippincott Williams & Wilkins; 2005.

20. Moore R, Levin S. Vascular disorder of the upper extremity. *University of Pennsylvania Orthopaedic Journal.* 1998;11(Spring):52–58. Available from: http://www.uphs.upenn.edu/ortho/oj/1998/oj11sp98p52.html. Accessed January 17, 2008.

21. Morhart M, Tredget EE, Jarman T, Ghahary A. Hand, wrist fractures and dislocations. eMedicine [electronic version]. 2008. Available from: http://www.emedicine.com/plastic/topic318.htm. Accessed December 27, 2009.

22. Otis C. Structure and function of the bones and joints of the wrist and hand. In: *Kinesiology: The Mechanics & Pathomechanics of Human Movement.* Baltimore, MD: Lippincott Williams & Wilkins; 2004:242–277.

23. Prentice WE. *Arnheim's Principles of Athletic Training: A Competency-Based Approach* (13th ed.). Boston, MA: McGraw Hill Publishing; 2009.

24. Rehak DC. Cyclist's hands: overcoming overuse injuries. Hughston Health Alert [electronic version]. 2003;Summer. Available from: http://www.hughston.com/hha/a_15_3_2.htm.

25. Rettig AC. Athletic injuries of the wrist and hand: part I: traumatic injuries of the wrist. *Am J Sports Med.* 2003a;31(6):1038–1048.

26. Rettig AC, Ryan R, Shelbourne DK, McCarroll JR, Johnson F, Ahlfeld SK. Metacarpal fractures in the athlete. *Am J Sports Med.* 1989;17:567–572.

27. Robinson M. Jammed fingers. eMedicine [electronic version]. 2007. Available from: http://emedicine.medscape.com/article/98081-overview. Accessed May 19, 2009.

28. Simpson D, McQueen MM. Acute sporting injuries to the hand and wrist in the general population. *Scott Med J.* 2006;51(2):25–26.

29. Theumann NH, Etechami G, Duvoisin B, et al. Association between extrinsic and intrinsic carpal ligament injuries at MR arthrography and carpal instability at radiography: initial observations. *Radiology.* 2006;238(3):950–957.

30. Theumann NH, Pfirrmann CWA, Antonio GE, et al. Extrinsic carpal ligaments: normal MR arthrographic appearance in cadavers. *Radiology.* 2003;226(1):171–179.

31. Thompson MJ, Rivara FP. Bicycle-related injuries. *Am Fam Physician.* 2001;63(10):2007–2014.

32. Village J, Rempel D, Teschke K. Musculoskeletal disorders of the upper extremity associated with computer work: a systematic review. *Occup Ergon.* 2005;5(4):205–218.

33. von Schroeder HP, Botte MJ. Carpal tunnel syndrome. *Hand Clin.* 1996;12(4):643–655.

34. Wu J, Perron AD, Miller MD, Powell SM, Brady WJ. Orthopedic pitfalls in the ED: pediatric supracondylar humerus fractures. *Am J Emerg Med.* 2002;(6):544–550.

G enki, a certified athletic trainer and strength and conditioning specialist for the United States Track and Field Association (USTFA), has been working at the association's training facilities for the past three weeks. While covering morning clinic hours, a male track-and-field athlete, Ray, reports to the athletic training facility complaining of right wrist pain. The department's secretary instructed Ray to complete some paperwork while she pulled up his medical records from the database.

HISTORY

Genki looks over the paperwork and then begins his evaluation by gathering some general information. Ray states, "The inside of my right wrist began bothering me about ten days ago, and it has progressively gotten worse over the last couple of days." Further questioning by Genki reveals that Ray is a discus thrower who recently modified his throwing technique at his coach's request. Ray demonstrates the new technique, and it appears that he is overemphasizing his wrist snap on release. Ray's record indicates no previous history of wrist, forearm, or elbow trauma, and his pre-participation physical exam was unremarkable.

PHYSICAL EXAMINATION

Ray is alert and in moderate-to-severe discomfort (7/10). A general observation of Ray's right wrist reveals swelling around the carpal rows. A tape measurement between the proximal and distal carpal row demonstrates an extra half-inch on the involved side. Ray is point tender along the palmar and medial joint surfaces (Figure 6.1.1). Active ROM is limited in wrist flexion, extension, and radial deviation secondary to pain and swelling (Table 6.1.1). An isometric break test near the end ranges demonstrates 3+/5 for wrist flexion and ulna deviation. Extension break testing is a 3/5. Stress testing demonstrates increased laxity and pain in the neutral position. Tinel's sign and Phalen's sign are negative, and a wrist glide test is positive. A neurological examination is unremarkable. Genki decides that referral to the association's orthopedic surgeon for further

FIGURE 6.1.1

Palpation of Ray's wrist.

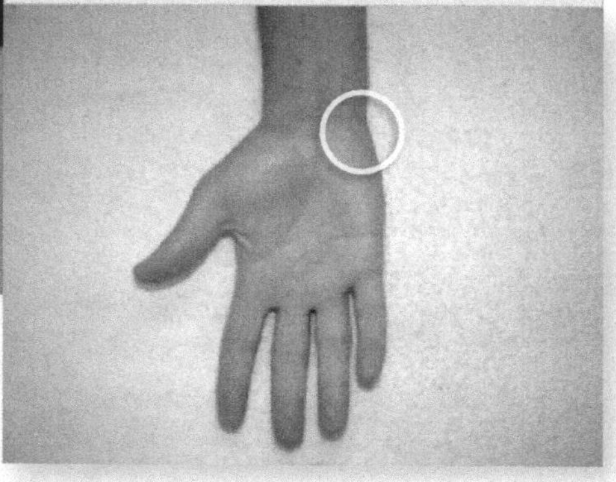

Area of pain is within the circle.

TABLE 6.1.1

Active range of motion in Ray's wrist.

JOINT MOTION	RIGHT	LEFT
Flexion	65°	80°
Extension	55°*	70°
Ulnar Deviation	17°	28°
Radial Deviation	10°*	20°

*Increased pain is noted with this motion.

evaluation and diagnostic testing is warranted. Genki also decides it would be best not to allow Ray to return to throwing the discus. He believes the best initial course of action would be PRICE and a volar splint.

DIAGNOSTIC TESTING

The physician orders standard anteroposterior, lateral, and clenched-fist PA views. They are all unremarkable.

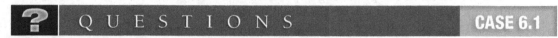

Please answer the following questions based on the above case information.

6.1 / **1.** Based on the information presented in the case, determine (a) the differential diagnoses and (b) the clinical diagnosis.

6.1 / **2.** Ray presented with tenderness along the palmar and medial wrist joint surface as shown in Figure 6.1.1. Identify the structures responsible for providing palmar and medial joint stability.

6.1 / **3.** As part of the physical examination, Genki performed a wrist glide that was positive. Which wrist glide do you think he used and how would you perform it?

6.1 / **4.** Genki decided that referral to the USTFA's orthopedic surgeon was warranted in this case. Do you believe this was an appropriate decision? Why or why not?

6.1 / **5.** Describe how to properly apply a volar splint.

arter, a six-year veteran line worker at Western Technology Industries, was working in the packaging department on Friday afternoon when he injured his right hand. Company policy required him to immediately notify his shift supervisor and then notify the industrial nurse, who ultimately referred him to see Nadal, a certified athletic trainer and occupational therapy assistant working in the Industrial Physical Medicine and Rehabilitation Department. Carter visited Nadal the following Monday. The medical report from the industrial nurse stated, "right, third digit PIP injury." It further read, "evaluate and re-splint as indicated." However, he was unable to get an appointment with Nadal until the Tuesday following the injury.

HISTORY

Nadal begins her evaluation by reviewing the paperwork from the industrial nurse, noting that the injury occurred four days ago. Nothing in the report stands out as unusual given the situation, except that Carter is not wearing a splint today, even though the splint was noted in the medical chart. She then began questioning Carter

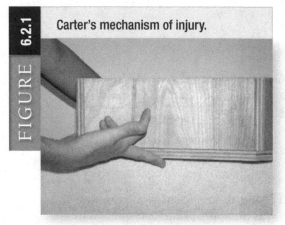

FIGURE 6.2.1

Carter's mechanism of injury.

about the MOI. He reports hyperextending his right middle finger while trying to pack some crates with computer parts. "I was placing some parts into the crates for the afternoon's shipment, and I got distracted. The next thing I realized, I slipped, lost control of some of the equipment, and tried to catch it before it hit the ground. When I did, my finger got caught and pulled backward" (Figure 6.2.1). "It hurt real bad and I grabbed my finger, which helped to decrease the pain." Carter reported experiencing immediate pain and loss of function of the middle finger due to pain.

PHYSICAL EXAMINATION

Carter, a 33-year-old male, is alert and in minor-to-moderate discomfort. Nadal begins by completing an inspection of the attitude and general appearance of Carter's hand and fingers. She notices moderate swelling and ecchymosis at the level of the PIPJ of the third digit. Further observation reveals flexion of the DIPJ and MPJ and hyperextension of the PIPJ of the third digit not consistent with normal hand positioning. Nadal also notes Carter's point tenderness along his involved hand (Figure 6.2.2). Active ROM is painful with extension and flexion, secondary to swelling. Passive ROM causes an increase in pain with extension of the PIPJ. Varus testing is unremarkable. Valgus testing demonstrates 1+ laxity. However, an anterioposterior glide of the proximal middle phalange demonstrates significant (2+) laxity and produces pain, unlike the uninvolved side. Neurological testing is unremarkable. Nadal recognizes the severity of this case and decides it would be best to refer Carter to the company's orthopedic surgeon for further evaluation and diagnostic testing.

ORTHOPEDIC EXAMINATION

Radiographs are unremarkable. The orthopedic surgeon places Carter into another splint and instructs him in the proper use of the splint. She further informs him that if he does not follow her directions, the joint may not heal correctly and that a "more aggressive therapy or treatment may be necessary."

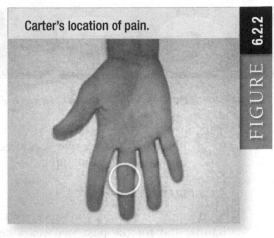

Carter's location of pain.

FIGURE 6.2.2

Pain is located within the circle at the PIPJ.

? QUESTIONS   6.2

Please answer the following questions based on the above case information.

6.2 / 1. Based on the information presented in the case, determine (a) the differential diagnoses and (b) the clinical diagnosis.

6.2 / 2. Given the MOI, why did Nadal find increased laxity when she performed an anterioposterior glide of the proximal interphalangeal joint?

6.2 / 3. Do you believe Nadal adequately evaluated Carter's condition? If not, what would you have done differently as the evaluating clinician?

6.2 / 4. Based on the information presented in the case identify the types of splints the orthopedic surgeon may have recommended for Carter.

6.2 / 5. (a) Do you believe Nadal made the correct decision by referring Carter to the orthopedic surgeon? (b) If this had been an athlete, would you have treated him differently? Why, or why not?

CASE 6.3

by David Draper, Ph.D., LAT, ATC, Brigham Young University, Provo, Utah

This case provides two scenarios that show two completely different mechanisms for the same injury.

SCENARIO ONE

Tom is a 17-year-old wide receiver on a high school football team. He has great hands, and for the past two years he has led the region in reception yardage. At Friday night's game, with no time left on the clock and the team down by 5 points, Tom was thrown a 30-yard pass into the corner of the end zone. At the last second, Tom took his eyes off the ball and glanced down to see if he was still in bounds. As his eyes returned to the ball, it was too late—the ball hit his thumb. Tom couldn't hang on, and the ball fell to the grass. Obviously, Tom was dejected after the game and didn't want to speak to anyone. The assistant coach and anatomy teacher finally caught up with him in the locker room. The coach noticed that Tom was holding his thumb. The coach asked, "May I take a look at that?" Tom responded, "It's just a jammed thumb. I'll ice it, and I'll be ready to practice on Monday. Go look at the guys who have real injuries." Tom thinks it's a minor injury that will keep him out only 72 hours.

SCENARIO TWO

Valerie is in her mid-30s and is a university professor in Colorado. She is in close proximity to several ski resorts, and she decided to take up the sport recreationally. It took only a few seasons for her to become pretty good and quite confident with the sport. One Saturday during one of her runs, she heard someone yell, "Dude, watch out!" A snowboarder crossed directly in front of Valerie. As skilled as she was, Valerie couldn't avoid the huge rut cut out in the snow in front of her. Her ski tips hit the rut and she fell forward into the snow. The only thing that kept her from making a face plant was her outstretched right hand slowing her fall. Valerie got up and gingerly skied down to the bottom of the hill. After a cup of hot chocolate, she decided to try a few more runs. She made it, but her right thumb ached. Before she left the resort, she asked a young man who worked with ski patrol to look at it. He told her, "It's probably just a sprain and will be fine by Monday. Until then, ice it and take some aspirin." She is hoping the sprain will resolve in a few days.

HISTORY

Tom made an attempt to catch a football, but instead of cradling it, the ball hit his thumb. Valerie tried to break her fall with her outstretched hand while skiing. In this case, the ski pole became the force and actually caused the injury. Both Tom and Valerie brush their injuries off as a simple jammed thumb or a mild sprain. In fact, for the next few days, both try to work through the injury. Tom tapes his own thumb and attends practice, but drops a lot of balls. Valerie finds simple tasks at work to be annoying. Hitting the space bar on her computer keyboard is painful, and it appears her thumb is weak. Tuesday night when she tries to use her credit card at the mall, it slips through her thumb and forefinger. Tom and Valerie each call Wildcat Sports Medicine Clinic and are scheduled to be seen by Joel, a certified athletic trainer, the next day.

PHYSICAL EXAMINATION

Joel sees both patients, one after the other, first thing in the morning. Even though the histories are different, the signs and symptoms are quite similar. Both patients present with pain upon palpation and swelling along the ulnar aspect of the meta-carpophalangeal joint (MCPJ). There is also a fair amount of ecchymosis running from the MCPJ into the thenar eminence. Joel asks each patient to perform active ROM of the thumb. All actions are normal except MCPJ flexion, which can go only to 70° instead of the normal 90°. Joel pulls a credit card–sized piece of plastic from his pocket and asks each patient to grip the card between thumb and forefinger. During the respective examinations Joel compares both hands of each patient and notes that, in both cases, the thumb of the injured hand is unable to perform this simple task. Joel writes in his notes, "opposition is weak to absent." Joel then performs a valgus stress test to both hands of each patient. Tom's thumb exhibits pain with increased movement by comparison with the uninvolved thumb. When Joel further examines Valerie's UCL, he finds that it has 30° more laxity than her uninjured thumb.

? | Q U E S T I O N S | **CASE 6.3**

Please answer the following questions based on the above case information.

6.3 / **1.** Based on the information presented in the case, what is the differential diagnosis for both patients?

6.3 / **2.** Based on the information presented in the cases, (a) what is the clinical diagnosis? (b) What is the common term used to describe the clinical diagnosis?

6.3 / **3.** Even though Tom's and Valerie's accidents were very different, (a) why did they both end up with similar injuries? (b) Which of the scenarios shows the more common MOI?

6.3 / **4.** What subjective factors gave Joel the impression that both injuries call for the same clinical diagnosis?

6.3 / **5.** What objective factors gave Joel the impression that both injuries call for the same clinical diagnosis?

6.3 / **6.** If you were in Joel's position, what directions for care would you provide Tom and Valerie at the end of their first visits?

CASE **6.4**

Earlene, a certified athletic trainer, was covering a collegiate water polo strength-training practice when one of the players was injured while weightlifting. Near the end of the practice, Paige, a 21-year-old player, was finishing up performing her cleans when she lost control of the barbell on the catch. She immediately dropped the bar to the ground and began grabbing and pumping her left hand. Eric, the strength and conditioning coach, called Earlene over to evaluate Paige.

HISTORY

Earlene begins her evaluation by trying to determine the MOI by asking Paige, "What happened?" Paige states, "I just finished my clean descent and was about to catch the bar when I started to lose my balance for some reason. As I was moving to my finishing position, I felt a tearing sensation in my wrist. I then dropped the bar to the ground." Further questioning reveals that Paige has moderate pain with wrist flexion and ulnar deviation, along with general volar wrist pain. Paige denies any history of previous wrist injury.

PHYSICAL EXAMINATION

Paige is alert and in moderate discomfort (5/10) without movement of the wrist. Earlene observes the wrist joint and notes no immediate swelling or ecchymosis; however, a notable loss of wrist function is visible. Soft tissue and bony palpation reveal tenderness over the distal end of the medial ulnocarpal joint. Earlene assesses active and passive ROM using a goniometer (Figure 6.4.1). Results of Paige's ROM and resistive muscle testing are found in Table 6.4.1. Ligamentous testing of the wrist is unremarkable. Neurovascular testing is also unremarkable. Earlene discusses the results of her examination with Paige. They agree on the best immediate course of action. Earlene also suggests using a protective wrist strapping procedure when Paige is ready to return to participation.

FIGURE **6.4.1**   Paige's goniometric measurements.

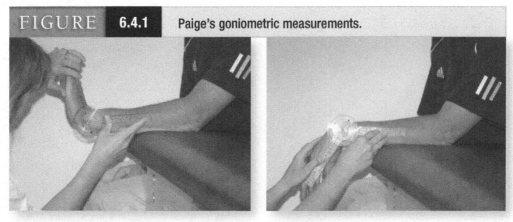

(a) wrist extension

(b) wrist flexion

TABLE	6.4.1	Paige's range of motion results.

| MOTION | MOTION | FINDINGS | |
		RIGHT	LEFT
AROM	Flexion*	80°	50°
	Extension	75°	39°
	Ulnar deviation	42°	20°
	Radial deviation	22°	10°
PROM	Flexion	Minimal-to-no discomfort	
	Extension*	Increased pain at end range motion	
	Ulnar deviation	Minimal-to-no discomfort	
	Radial deviation	Increased pain at end range motion	
RROM	Flexion	3+/5 with pain	
	Extension	4+/5	
	Ulnar deviation	3+/5 with pain	
	Radial deviation	5/5	

*Pain increases to 8/10 with active flexion and passive extension.

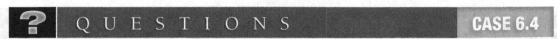

Please answer the following questions based on the above case information.

6.4 / **1.** Based on the information presented in the case, determine the clinical diagnosis.

6.4 / **2.** If Paige also presented with neurological symptoms, what could you conclude about the injury? What type of neurological symptoms may be present?

6.4 / **3.** If you were the evaluating clinician, (a) how would you assess wrist flexion and extension muscle strength? (b) How could you isolate the clinical diagnosis?

6.4 / **4.** Overall, do you believe Earlene adequately evaluated Paige's condition, considering the provided information? If not, what would you have done differently as the evaluating clinician?

6.4 / **5.** As a clinician, discuss how you would explain to a patient or athlete the proper mechanics of performing the weight lifting technique known as a "clean"?

Andy and Randy were best friends and often played racquetball together two or three times a week. Over the course of two years, it was not uncommon for the weekly matches to get a little heated. One particular day, Andy and Randy became very competitive, so much so that when Andy dove for the ball, Randy ended up stepping on Andy's left hand. Andy immediately began to experience pain and tenderness over the end of his middle finger. Not wanting to forfeit the match, Andy taped his fingers together and continued to play for a period of time. After he could no longer play, he decided it would be best to stop. Randy suggested he head over to the physical therapy clinic housed in the athletic club. Amanda, a physical therapist and certified athletic trainer on staff at the Saginaw Tennis Club, often saw club members who injured themselves while playing tennis and racquetball. She asked Andy to fill out some documentation and told him she would be with him in 10 minutes or so.

HISTORY

The physical examination begins with Amanda reviewing the MOI with Andy. Andy states, "I dove for the ball, then Randy stepped on my left hand, crushing the tip of my middle finger." He further states, "I was able to continue playing for about 20 minutes with my finger taped; however, after a while, I think my finger started to swell because it began to throb really bad."

PHYSICAL EXAMINATION

Andy is alert and oriented and is experiencing general discomfort and throbbing throughout his left third phalange DIPJ. A cursory observation of Andy's fingers reveals moderate DIPJ swelling in the third phalange. Further observation of the hand can be seen in Figure 6.5.1. Palpable tenderness is noted along the dorsal and volar aspect of the third phalange DIPJ. Active ROM testing reveals a loss of DIPJ flexion when compared with the other phalanges. Andy experiences increased pain with compression and percussion testing. Neurological testing, including two-point discrimination, is unremarkable.

The results of the physical examination concern Amanda, so she decides it would be best to refer Andy to an orthopedic surgeon for further evaluation. She instructs Andy about how to control the pain and swelling and places him in an Alumafoam splint.

FIGURE 6.5.1

Observation of Andy's hand.

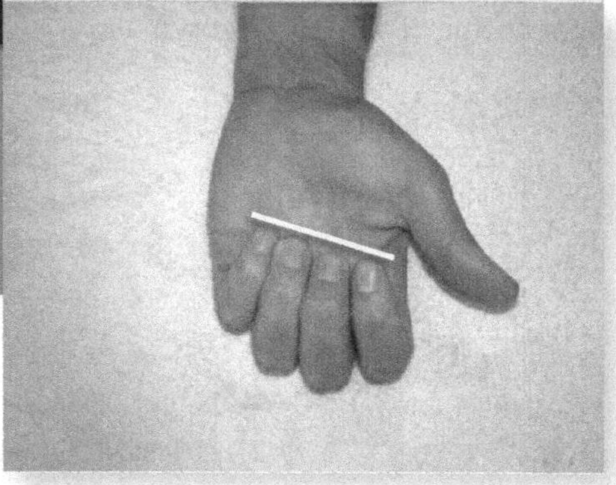

Line indicates angle of fingers while at rest.

Please answer the following questions based on the above case information.

6.5 / **1.** Based on the information presented in the case, determine (a) the differential diagnoses and (b) the clinical diagnosis. What are the distinguishing characteristics of this injury?

6.5 / **2.** Amanda asked a few history questions to guide the physical examination. Based on the information presented in the case, do you believe Amanda took an adequate history? If not, what additional questions would you ask as the evaluating clinician?

6.5 / **3.** Figure 6.5.1 demonstrates Andy's fingers at rest. What is the name of this finger position, and why is it a cause of concern for an athletic trainer observing this position?

6.5 / **4.** Compression and percussion tests are often performed when evaluating the clinical diagnosis, and they were used in this case. Do you believe these are reliable tests? Is there another test that Amanda could have performed?

6.5 / **5.** If you were the evaluating clinician in this case, what if anything would you have done differently or elaborated on?

Bayden, a certified athletic trainer and avid water polo enthusiast, was assigned by his supervisor to cover the National Club Water Polo finals, which were being held at a local university. They were down to the final eight teams and were still running two matches at a time at separate aquatic facilities. Bayden was responsible for covering both pools and was using an undergraduate athletic training intern from the university to help provide coverage. Suddenly Bayden received a call from Alana, the intern. She informed Bayden that she had a player who had just suffered a traumatic injury to his hand. Bayden informed her to keep the player calm and that he would be over in a second.

ON-SCENE ARRIVAL

Arriving on the scene, Bayden is confronted with a perplexing situation. Apparently a bystander from the stands saw the incident occur and came out of the stands to assist in the medical care of this athlete. Alana, not exactly sure what to do, allowed the man, who identified himself as Dr. Smith, to evaluate the player, Paul. After evaluating Paul, Dr. Smith allowed him to return to play. Alana fills Bayden in on what just transpired before he arrived.

HISTORY

Bayden is surprised when Dr. Smith starts relaying Paul's history. He says the player is an 18-year-old freshman on the men's water polo club team. Paul had been attempting to block a pass at short range when the ball struck the tip of his fingers. An injury time-out had been called, and Paul had removed himself from the water and sought medical help. He had reported to Dr. Smith that he felt like his finger was bent backward and to the side and compressed. Dr. Smith remembers Paul saying, "I knew it wasn't right once I got hit."

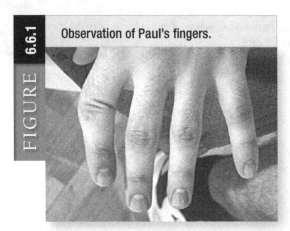

FIGURE 6.6.1

Observation of Paul's fingers.

Source: Millikin University Athletic Training Program.

PHYSICAL EXAMINATION

"Paul was alert and very anxious as he was pacing up and down the pool's deck," Dr. Smith said. "He was in severe discomfort and was holding his left index finger. When I saw the injury (Figure 6.6.1), I immediately knew what was wrong and corrected the problem." Paul's initial pain was relieved, though he was in moderate discomfort. Dr. Smith had taped his fingers together and told him he could get back into the match.

Bayden, clearly upset by the actions of Dr. Smith, confronts him regarding his actions (i.e., assessing, treating, and making RTP decisions) and his medical qualifications. Dr. Smith explains that he is a chiropractor from Utah who came to visit his nephew and watch the water polo match. He continues, "I saw the injury occur and realized that this young lady didn't have a clue how to treat the player. She was going to put ice on the finger. What good is that going to do? He's fine. I told him if his finger still bothers him after the match to put ice on it." Bayden is now extremely upset and calls for the athletic director.

❓ QUESTIONS   CASE 6.6

Please answer the following questions based on the above case information.

6.6 / **1.** Based on the information presented in the case, (a) what is the likely clinical diagnosis? (b) What is the likelihood of perceiving the injury visually as presented in Figure 6.6.1 after the injury has occurred?

6.6 / **2.** (a) Given the MOI, what would you have expected to observe? (b) Is this a common MOI?

6.6 / **3.** If you were the evaluating clinician in this case and you arrived before Dr. Smith, what if anything would you have done differently during the initial evaluation?

6.6 / **4.** Do you believe the actions of Dr. Smith were appropriate? If Paul sustained secondary damage as a result of Dr. Smith's actions, could Dr. Smith be held liable for his actions?

6.6 / **5.** What steps could be taken to minimize the risk of outside interference with an injured athlete occurring at your university or college?

6.6 / **6.** In this case, an on-field event occurred that unfortunately does occasionally occur in the athletic training profession. Putting yourself in the role of Bayden, discuss how you would have wanted the athletic director to assist in handling this situation. In reality, has this or something like this ever occurred to any of your clinical instructors?

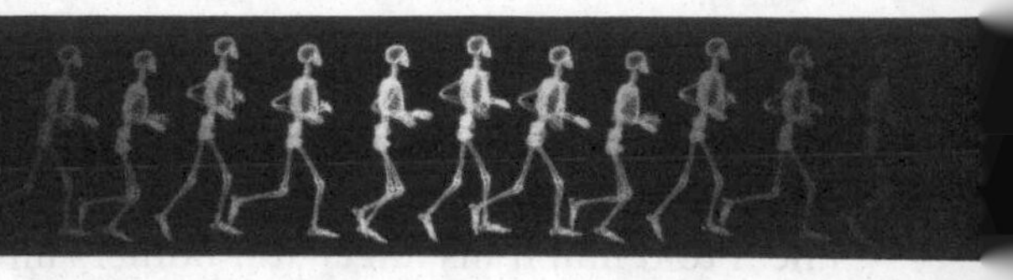

Karen, a certified athletic trainer for the American Professional Motorcross Association (APMA) Pro Racing Circuit, was assigned to cover the APMA Superbike World Classic in Daytona. Karen has been working the APMA Pro Racing Circuit for three years and has really made a name for herself with the medical staff, including the physicians and EMS. During the morning warm-ups, Kal, a rider in his second year on the circuit, was transitioning into curve 2 when he hit an oil spill, lost control of the bike, and fell off the bike backward.

ON-SCENE ARRIVAL

The emergency medical team, including Karen, two EMTs, and an ER physician, are called onto the scene. Upon arrival, the emergency medical team immediately begins to perform a trauma assessment. Kal is alert and oriented and is able to recall the MOI. He states, "I was accelerating into curve 2 when I lost control of the bike and fell off backwards. When I landed, I tried to brace myself." (See Figure 6.7.1.)

FIGURE 6.7.1   Kal's mechanism of injury.

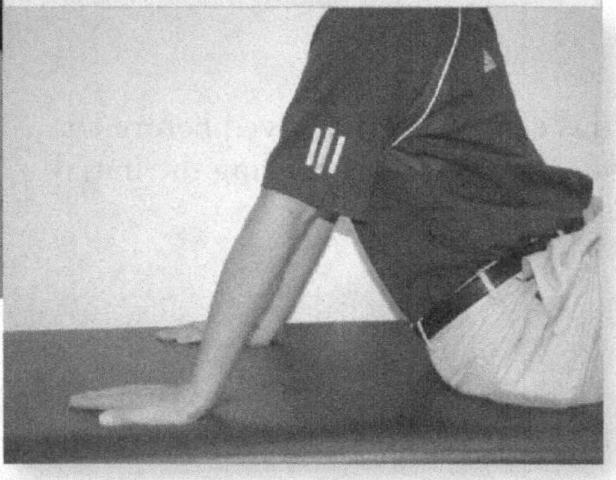

ON-SCENE PHYSICAL EXAMINATION

The trauma assessment reveals a painful, swollen, deformed left wrist, which is immediately splinted. Kal is then packaged and transported back to the track's medical facility for further physical and diagnostic examination.

MEDICAL FACILITY PHYSICAL EXAMINATION

Upon arrival at the facility, Karen and Dr. Todd begin to further examine Kal's left wrist. Kal is alert and in severe discomfort (9/10). A general observation of Kal's wrist reveals swelling and a marked volar deformity along the proximal carpal row. Dr. Todd also notes a positive Murphy's sign. Kal refuses to perform AROM because of pain. A neurological examination by Karen reveals numbness and tingling in the lateral palm and fingers (Figure 6.7.2). Dr. Todd

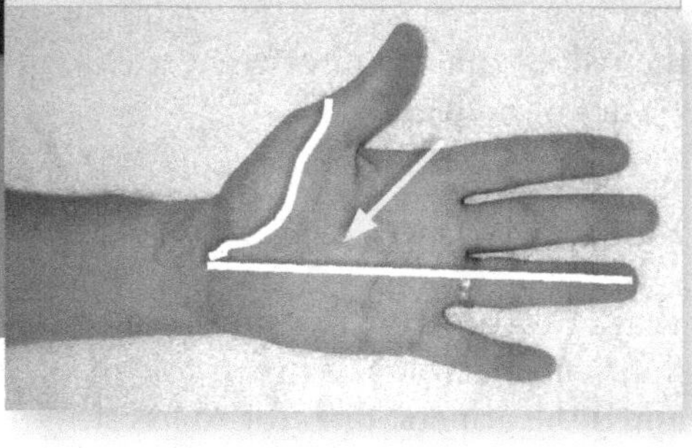

FIGURE 6.7.2   Kal's area of numbness and tingling.

Area of numbness and tingling is the area between the lines.

orders a set of radiographs (posteroanterior, lateral, and 45° angle) to rule
out bony trauma. Results of the radiographs (Figure 6.7.3) reveal a positive
fat carpus sign.

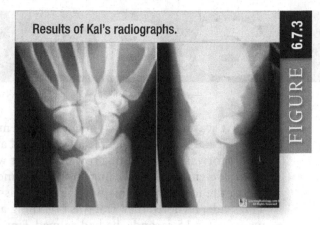

Results of Kal's radiographs.

Source: LearningRadiology.com,
with permission.

FIGURE 6.7.3

? QUESTIONS   CASE 6.7

Please answer the following questions based on the above case information.

6.7 / 1. (a) Based on the information presented in the case, what is the most likely
clinical diagnosis? (b) What is the typical MOI?

6.7 / 2. Do you believe the medical team adequately evaluated the condition? If not,
what would you have done differently as the evaluating clinician?

6.7 / 3. (a) What is a Murphy's sign and a fat carpus sign? (b) How is the Murphy's
sign performed?

6.7 / 4. Karen assessed Kal's neurological status and found numbness and tingling
in the lateral palm and into the second and third fingers. What is/are the
possible cause(s) of this?

6.7 / 5. If you were a collegiate or high school athletic trainer and an athlete presented with wrist pain and swelling over the proximal carpal row, decreased
grip strength, and decreased ROM (i.e., ulnar deviation) with no apparent
history of injury, (a) what clinical diagnosis would you suspect? (b) What
would be the MOI?

I t was a snowy Friday night in November, and Ian was covering his first collegiate ice hockey game as a certified athletic trainer. During the game, Tim, a junior forward, was skating toward the net with the puck when one of the opposing team's defensive players came up from behind and slashed Tim's wrist. Tim instantly fell to the ice grabbing his wrist. Ian was assisted onto the ice, and as he arrived at Tim's side, he noted that Tim was breathing and rolling around on the ice holding his wrist. After 15 seconds, he had calmed Tim down enough to begin to talk with and evaluate him.

HISTORY

Ian begins to question Tim about the injury. Tim states, "The defenseman caught the inside portion of my glove and hit me right across the wrist." (See Figure 6.8.1.) Tim's CCs are pain and tenderness along the lateral distal carpal row and difficulty with the extremes of active extension and radial deviation.

PHYSICAL EXAMINATION

Ian assists Tim to the bench. On the bench, Tim is very alert and in moderate-to-severe discomfort (7/10). A general observation of Tim's wrist reveals immediate swelling around the distal lateral wrist and proximal carpal rows. Active ROM is limited in wrist extension and radial deviation secondary to pain and swelling. Overpressure applied to wrist flexion and radial deviation also produces pain. A quick grip-strength test reveals a moderate (50%) deficiency in the involved hand. Stress testing of the UCL ligament produces pain radially but with no lateral instability. Ian decides it would be best not to allow Tim to return to the game. He believes the best course of action would be RICE and referral to the team's orthopedic surgeon for further evaluation when possible.

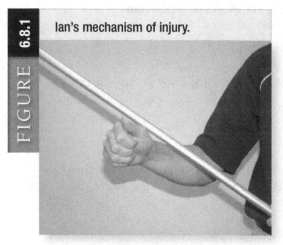

FIGURE 6.8.1

Ian's mechanism of injury.

Please answer the following questions based on the above case information.

6.8 / **1.** Based on the information presented in the case, determine (a) the differential diagnoses and (b) the clinical diagnosis.

6.8 / **2.** If Ian was comparing Tim's wrist bilaterally, the swelling around the radial distal and proximal carpal rows would obscure which anatomical landmark?

6.8 / **3.** The MOI in this case was not typical for the clinical diagnosis. Based on the clinical diagnosis, identify the most common MOI and explain the etiology.

6.8 / **4.** (a) Did Ian make the correct decision in removing Tim from the game? (b) Which, if any other, special test would you have performed?

6.8 / **5.** What type of initial care should Ian provide before Tim sees the orthopedic surgeon?

6.8 / **6.** Based on the case report describe how Ian could have performed a grip strength test while assessing Tim on the sidelines.

6.8 / **7.** What are the special risks of this fracture, and how should this affect any approach to a wrist fracture/sprain?

CASE 6.9

I t was a warm Friday night, and the West Hampton High School varsity foot-ball team was warming up for its rival match against East Hampton High. Inga, West Hampton's athletic trainer, was setting up her treatment area when Cory, a junior wide receiver, tapped her on the shoulder. He was supporting his left arm with the hand held in a slightly flexed and pronated position (Figure 6.9.1) and stated, "I just fell, and now I can't move my wrist." Inga's first thought was, "All Cory ever does is complain about getting injured. I don't have time for this right now."

FIGURE 6.9.1

Cory's position of comfort.

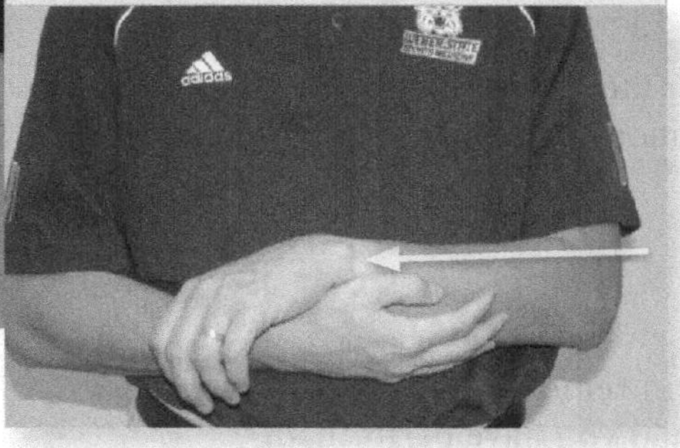

HISTORY

Inga begins her evaluation by trying to deter-mine the exact MOI. She learns that Cory was performing some backpedaling activities when he lost his balance, fell, and landed on an out-stretched hand. She also finds that he is unable to flex and extend his wrist without causing significant pain. Cory states that he has not had a history of left or right wrist trauma.

PHYSICAL EXAMINATION

Inga asks Cory to sit on the plinth she has set up on the field. Cory is alert, in mod-erate-to-severe discomfort (7/10), and is very anxious to get back into warm-ups. Not wanting to take too much time evaluating Cory, Inga quickly performs a general observation of Corey's distal forearm and wrist, which reveals immediate swelling around the distal radius and proximal carpal rows. Cory has palpable tenderness over the distal radius and proximal carpal row. Active ROM is limited in wrist ex-tension and flexion secondary to pain, crepitation, swelling, and a feeling as though there is a restriction. Inga applies overpressure to the wrist extension and flexion, which also produces significant pain. Valgus and varus stress testing of the distal ra-dial and ulnar collateral ligaments produces a significant amount of pain, particularly with valgus stress. Inga decides it would be best not to allow Cory into the game, because of what she feels is a possible wrist sprain. She believes the best course of action would be RICE and referral to the team's orthopedic surgeon the next day for further evaluation.

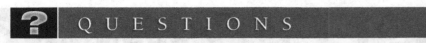

Please answer the following questions based on the above case information.

6.9 / **1.** Based on the information presented in the case, do you agree with Inga's clinical diagnosis? If not, what do you believe is the correct clinical diagnosis in this particular situation?

6.9 / **2.** Because of Inga's indifference to Cory, she missed several key signs. If you were the evaluating athletic trainer, what if any other signs would you have assessed during the general observation component of the physical examination that may have helped you determine the clinical diagnosis?

6.9 / **3.** Based on the clinical diagnosis, which component of the physical examination do you believe Inga forgot to complete, if any? What is the clinical significance of omitting this part of the examination?

6.9 / **4.** Identify the structures comprising the proximal and distal carpal rows. Identify which carpal bones align with each of the five metacarpals.

6.9 / **5.** During the examination, Inga assessed the stability of the radial and ulnar collateral ligaments. If you were the evaluating athletic trainer, would you perform these exams? Why, or why not?

Stephen, a certified athletic trainer for an NCAA Division III men's football team, was at practice Tuesday afternoon helping one of his athletic training students prepare for an oral practical examination. While he and his student were practicing a thumb evaluation, he heard one of the coaches yell his name. He and his athletic training student, Marion, turned and saw the second string quarterback, Art, kneeling holding his thumb. Stephen and Marion both jogged over to Art and knelt down to him. Stephen thought this would be a great learning experience and decided to let Marion begin the exam.

HISTORY

Nervously, Marion begins to question Art about the injury. She learns that Art's throwing hand was struck by the defensive lineman's helmet as he was in the follow-through phase of the throw, causing what would appear to be an adduction force on Art's partially flexed thumb. Further questioning by Marion reveals loss of thumb function in all directions. Art rates his pain as 8/10 and denies any previous history of thumb trauma.

PHYSICAL EXAMINATION

Art is alert, oriented, and starting to become a little agitated. Marion observes what she believes to be a laterally displaced first metacarpal shaft. She also notes the presence of swelling already at the base of the CMCJ. Palpable tenderness and severe pain is noted (Figure 6.10.1). Active ROM is limited and painful, and CMCJ instability is noted. As Marion gently stresses the metacarpal Art reacts loudly to the pain, and his yell causes the football coach to quickly look over. The coach catches what he assumes is an athletic training student hurting one of his players. He responds by screaming at Marion to "get away from him." He proceeds to tell Stephen, "Do your job, I don't want any students touching my players." Taken aback, Stephen steps in and completes the physical examination. Realizing the severity of this injury, Stephen places the thumb in a gutter splint and calls the team's orthopedic surgeon's office to see if he can get an appointment for Art.

After practice, Stephen stops by the coach's office to discuss the events that took place on the field and inform him that Art will be headed for surgery later that night to have his thumb reduced and fixed with percutaneous pins.

FIGURE 6.10.1

Palpation of Art's wrist.

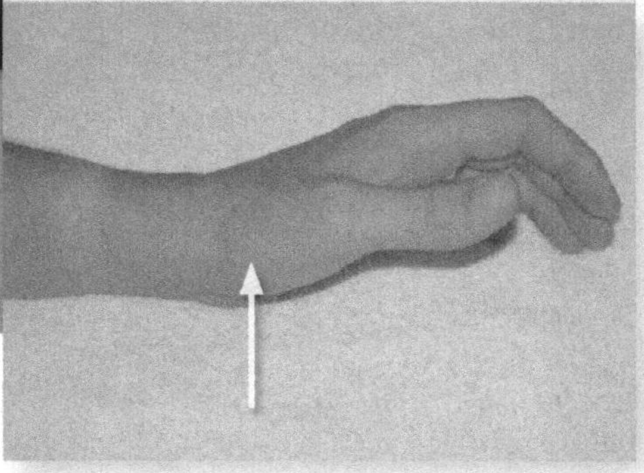

Arrow indicates the location of the pain at the CMCJ.

| ? | Q U E S T I O N S | CASE 6.10 |

Please answer the following questions based on the above case information.

6.10 / **1.** Based on the information presented in the case, determine the clinical diagnosis and describe the injury.

6.10 / **2.** The MOI in this case appeared to be an excessive adduction force applied to Art's partially flexed thumb. What other possible MOI exists for this clinical diagnosis?

6.10 / **3.** In this case, Marion believed she observed a laterally displaced first metacarpal shaft. Based on the clinical diagnosis, what would cause the first metacarpal shaft to be laterally displaced?

6.10 / **4.** Obviously, this case presented with an on-field event that cut short Marion's evaluation of Art's thumb. Identify what, if any, further evaluation would be required in this case.

6.10 / **5.** In this case, an on-field event occurred that unfortunately does occur occasionally in the athletic training profession. Putting yourself in the role of the athletic training student in this case, discuss how you would have responded during and after the coach's outburst. In reality, has this or something like this ever occurred to you? Was the coach right or wrong?

by Brad Franzen, B.S., LAT, ATC, Weber State University, Ogden, Utah

Matt, a factory worker at the local pet food plant, was carrying a box of tools to his station when he accidentally tripped over an exposed metal pipe protruding from the ground. Matt lost his balance and fell forward on the concrete floor while trying to protect the expensive tools (Figure 6.11.1). Matt's fellow co-

FIGURE 6.11.1

Matt's mechanism of injury.

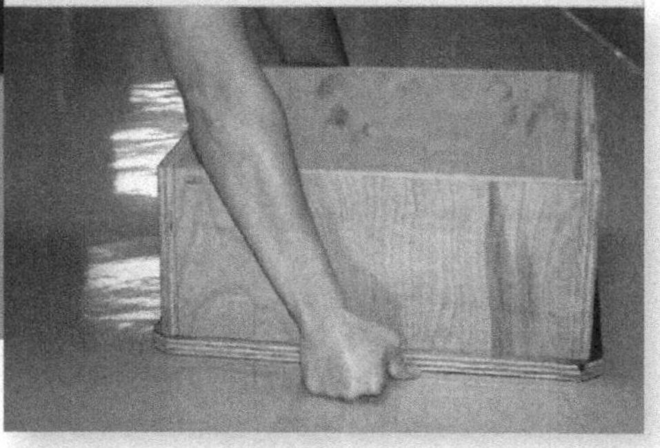

workers witnessed the accident and rushed over to make sure he was alright. When they reached him, he was screaming in pain and protecting his wrist and hand. His co-workers helped Matt over to the office of Kristi, the certified athletic trainer on staff at the plant's physical medicine and rehabilitation facility.

HISTORY

Kristi can see Matt is obviously in a lot of pain and asks him a series of questions to diagnose his injury. Matt states that, "I tripped over a metal pipe sticking out of the floor. I fell forward and landed on the outside of my right hand with a closed fist." He also states that he is getting a "sharp pain" along the border of his little finger. He further reports hearing a "crack" when he landed on the ground. He denies any prior history of wrist or hand injuries and is not currently taking any medications.

PHYSICAL EXAMINATION

An observation of Matt's hand reveals immediate swelling around the knuckle of Matt's fifth phalange. No open wound or deformities are present by comparison with the uninvolved hand. Matt is apprehensive and withdraws his hand when Kristi palpates the shaft of the fifth metacarpal. As a precaution, she also checks his second to fourth metacarpals and notes no tenderness. Active and passive ROM of the fifth MCPJ is limited secondary to pain and Matt's apprehension. Because Matt is experiencing so much pain with all activities, Kristi believes it would be best to refer him to an orthopedic surgeon for an evaluation and diagnostic imaging.

FOLLOW-UP EXAMINATION

After seeing the orthopedic surgeon, Matt returns to the physical medicine and rehabilitation facility, as requested. When Kristi looks at the radiographs (Figure 6.11.2), she immediately knows what she is dealing with. This was confirmed by the physician's note provided by Matt. She proceeds to provide Matt with several exercises to maintain his strength and endurance while the injury heals.

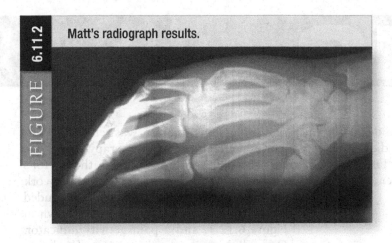

FIGURE 6.11.2

Matt's radiograph results.

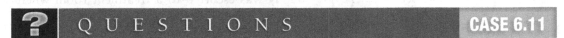

? QUESTIONS   CASE 6.11

Please answer the following questions based on the above case information.

6.11 / **1.** Based on the information presented in the case, determine the clinical diagnosis and identify the layman's term(s) for the diagnosis.

6.11 / **2.** What are the common MOIs associated with this injury?

6.11 / **3.** What special test could have helped Kristi confirm the clinical diagnosis, and how is it performed?

6.11 / **4.** What could Kristi have done to prevent this incident from occurring?

CASE 6.12

S ally, a 49-year-old squash player and professional pianist, was referred to Mt. Blue Sports Medicine, an outpatient athletic and physical therapy clinic, one week after seeing her family doctor for wrist pain. A note faxed from the doctor's office stated "wrist tendinitis, treat accordingly." Sally completed the paperwork provided by the office staff, which included a medical history, the pain profile shown in Figure 6.12.1, and a pain activity indicator. Once all the paper work was completed, Sally was escorted to a treatment room where she was to be evaluated by Ryan, a certified athletic trainer and co-owner of the facility.

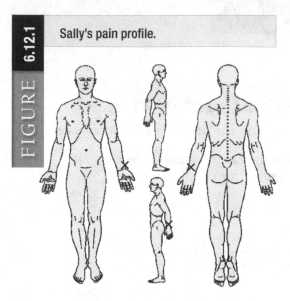

FIGURE 6.12.1 Sally's pain profile.

✗ = denote areas of general pain.

HISTORY

After a few minutes of small talk and introductions Ryan begins his examination by reviewing Sally's past medical history and gathering additional information. He then proceeds by asking, "So tell me what is going on with your wrist?" Sally responds, "I have been preparing for a concert for the last four weeks, playing the piano for up to two or three hours per day. Over the last two weeks I have begun to experience pain in my wrist. The pain tends to be worse when I try to reach for the keys with my thumb. I also play tennis occasionally, and it hurts when I repeatedly snap my wrist at the end of my forehand." She denies any previous history of wrist or thumb pain and is not taking any medication.

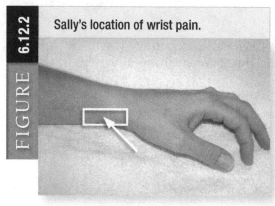

FIGURE 6.12.2 Sally's location of wrist pain.

Area of pain is within the box.

PHYSICAL EXAMINATION

Sally is alert, oriented, and in minimal discomfort with her thumb at rest. Ryan notes swelling and palpable tenderness and pain over the radial side of the wrist (Figure 6.12.2). Sally's wrist and thumb ROMs are presented in Table 6.12.1. Ryan also assesses Sally's thumb strength using a pinch gauge and a multidirectional static dynamometer (flexion, extension, adduction, abduction, and multi-directions). Testing reveals a decrease in pinch grip strength and a decrease in all directions of the static dynamometer, except

TABLE	6.12.1	Sally's range of motion results.

MOTION	JOINT	FINDINGS
AROM	Wrist	Pain primarily with wrist ulnar deviation; some pain with flexion, extension, and radial deviation
	Thumb	Pain primarily with thumb extension and abduction
PROM	Wrist	Limited wrist ulnar deviation secondary to pain
	Thumb CMCJ	Pain primarily with flexion and adduction
	Thumb MCPJ	Pain with proximal MCP flexion
RROM	Wrist	5/5 wrist flexion; 4+/5 ulnar deviation and extension
	Thumb CMCJ	5/5 flexion and adduction; 4/5 extension; 3+/5 abduction
	Thumb MCPJ	5/5 flexion; 4/5 extension

for adduction on the symptomatic side. Ligamentous testing is WNL. A Tinel's sign and Phalen's sign are unremarkable; however, a Finklestein's test is positive.

After completing the physical examination Ryan discusses Sally's options, including referral to another physician for a second opinion if conservative treatment fails. Ryan treats Sally accordingly.

Please answer the following questions based on the above case information.

6.12 / **1.** Based on the information presented in the case, determine (a) the clinical diagnosis and (b) discuss the possible etiology.

6.12 / **2.** In your opinion did Ryan address all the components of a thorough injury assessment? What, if anything, would you have added to the assessment?

6.12 / **3.** Ryan's assessment of Sally's thumb reveals palpable tenderness in tunnel 1. Identify the structures located in tunnel 1. Identify the remaining tunnels and the anatomical structures that lie within them.

6.12 / **4.** If you were the evaluating clinician, how would you have performed the Finklestein test?

6.12 / **5.** Outline a conservative rehabilitation program as if you were the treating clinician.

gt. Rabb, a 35-year-old air force logistic specialist, reported to the Hope Air Force Base Medical Center with a CC of left-wrist and hand pain and numbness. Because all the physicians were in a staff meeting, the triage nurse referred Sgt. Rabb to the physical medicine department for an examination. Sgt. Rabb's vital signs were unremarkable, and she complained of localized discomfort only. Lt. Brown, ATC, EMT, CSCS, was assigned to the case. Before beginning the examination, Lt. Brown asked the secretary to call up Sgt. Rabb's complete electronic medical record from the medical center's database.

HISTORY

Lt. Brown begins her assessment by reviewing Sgt. Rabb's medical history. Before her arrival at the Hope Air Force Base, Sgt. Rabb was treated three years ago for left ulnar neuropathy secondary to a left posterior elbow dislocation during physical training and had a past history of left medial epicondylitis (x 2). The medical records also reveal that Sgt. Rabb was diagnosed with hypothyroidism approximately two years after joining the Air Force. Finally, Lt. Brown reviews Sgt. Rabb's physical training records and notes that at her last PT test her BMI was 27.5, and she had a difficult time passing her last PT test. On this particular day, she is complaining of pain, numbness, and tingling in the area shown in Figure 6.13.1. She reports a decrease in dexterity and also difficulty moving the computer mouse, usually later in the afternoon. She also states, "It has actually gotten worse during the past couple of weeks during PT. I am having a hard time doing gripping activities or flexing my wrist for long periods of time." Further questioning from Lt. Brown reveals complaints of symptoms that are usually worse at night, awakening Sgt. Brown from sleep, necessitating a flick sign. The pain also appears to be radiating up the arm. Sgt. Rabb recalled no acute MOI and is medicating herself with Aleve® (500 mg q.i.d.). She rates her pain as 5/10 at rest, 8/10 while working, and higher during the later evening and early morning.

Sgt. Rabb's location of pain and numbness.

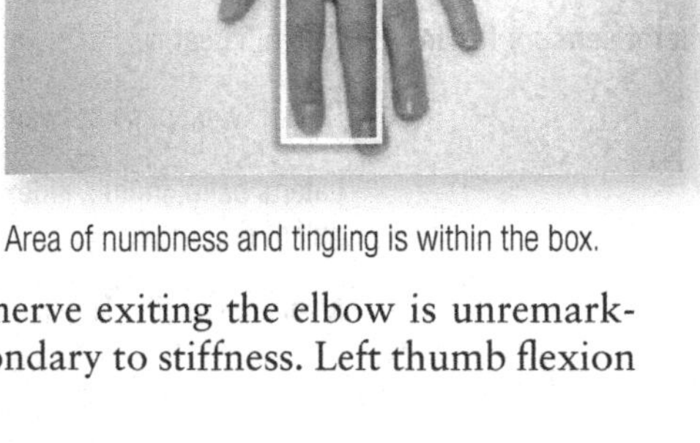

FIGURE 6.13.1

Area of numbness and tingling is within the box.

PHYSICAL EXAMINATION

Sgt. Rabb is alert, oriented, and in minimal discomfort during the physical examination. Lt. Brown notes minor volar carpal swelling and thenar atrophy. She also notes palpable tenderness over the midline of the volar carpal bones; however, direct palpation of the ulnar nerve exiting the elbow is unremarkable. Left wrist AROM is limited in flexion secondary to stiffness. Left thumb flexion and abduction and index and middle finger AROM are also decreased by comparison with the uninvolved hand. Wrist flexion and extension PROM increases Sgt. Rabb's symptoms when moved to the end range. Grip strength measured with a dynamometer at 1, 1.5, 2, 2.5, and 3 inches reveals an overall deficit of 15 percent for the involved hand. Sgt. Rabb's neurological findings are located in Table 6.13.1. Bilateral wrist and elbow ligamentous testing is unremarkable. Radial collateral stress testing at the wrist was negative. Testing for cervical compression, brachial plexus nerve stretch, and TOS is negative. The special test shown in Figure 6.13.2 is negative.

TABLE 6.13.1	Sgt. Rabb's neurological findings.	
TEST	**LOCATION**	**FINDINGS**
DTR	C5	WNL
	C6	WNL
	C7	WNL
Dermatomes	C5	WNL
	C6	WNL
	C7	WNL
	C8	WNL
	T1	WNL
	T2	WNL
Myotomes	C5	WNL
	C6	WNL
	C7	WNL
	C8	WNL
	T1	WNL
Two-point discrimination	Dorsal web space between thumb and index finger	WNL
	Lateral palm, thumb, index, middle finger, and lateral half of ring finger	Positive
	Medial palm, fifth finger, and medial half of ring finger	WNL
Peripheral sensory testing	Lateral forearm	WNL
	Dorsal web space between thumb and index finger	WNL
	Lateral palm, thumb, index, middle finger, and lateral half of ring finger	Hypoesthesia
	Medial palm, fifth finger, and medial half of ring finger	WNL

PHYSICIAN FOLLOW-UP

After completing the physical examination, Lt. Brown documented her findings and sent a copy of the report to Maj. Packer, Chief Orthopedic Surgeon at the base. Dr. Packer called Lt. Brown the next day to discuss her findings. Together they agreed Sgt. Rabb warranted further diagnostic testing and immediate treatment, including the use of pharmacological agents and splinting. She would also be put on profile until further notice.

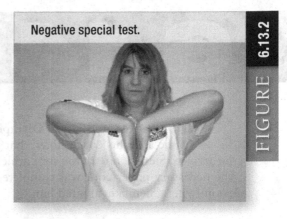

Negative special test.

FIGURE 6.13.2

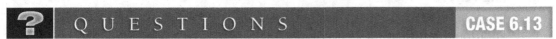

?   Q U E S T I O N S   **CASE 6.13**

Please answer the following questions based on the above case information.

6.13 / **1.** Based on the information presented in the case, determine (a) the differential diagnoses and (b) the clinical diagnosis.

6.13 / **2.** Lt. Brown asked several history questions to guide her physical examination. Based on the information presented in the case, do you believe she took an adequate history? If not, what questions would you have asked as the evaluating clinician?

6.13 / **3.** What is a flick sign, and is it an effective tool for detecting the clinical diagnosis?

6.13 / **4.** Overall, do you believe Lt. Brown adequately evaluated Sgt. Rabb's condition? If not, what would you have done differently as the evaluating clinician and why?

6.13 / **5.** As mentioned in the case, Lt. Brown documented her findings and sent a copy of the report to Dr. Packer's office. Please document your findings as if you were the treating clinician. If the case did not provide information you believe is pertinent to the clinical diagnosis, please add this information to your documentation.

CASE 6.14

Jack, a 20-year-old Junior Olympic cyclist, was referred to the Sports Medicine Clinic after his coach noted that Jack was "not riding to his potential." When he arrived, Sienna, one of the staff athletic trainers, was assigned to his case. Once all the necessary paperwork was completed, Jack was escorted back to an examination room where Sienna evaluated him.

HISTORY

Sienna begins her examination by reviewing Jack's medical history and gathering additional information as necessary. She proceeds by asking, "So what sport and event do you compete in?" Jack, a little irritated that he had to be there, responds, "I am a long-distance cyclist." She follows this up with, "Tell me what is going on." "I have been training for several months, six to eight hours per day for the Olympic Trials and over the last month I have been experiencing numbness and tingling here [Figure 6.14.1]. The pain, numbness, and tingling are worse when I have been on the bike for long periods of time, leaning over my handlebars." Further questioning reveals occasional burning sensation in the same area, as well as a reduction in pain and symptoms during long periods of rest. Jack's current NPS is 5/10. He denies any history of previous trauma.

FIGURE 6.14.1

Jack's location of pain, numbness, and tingling.

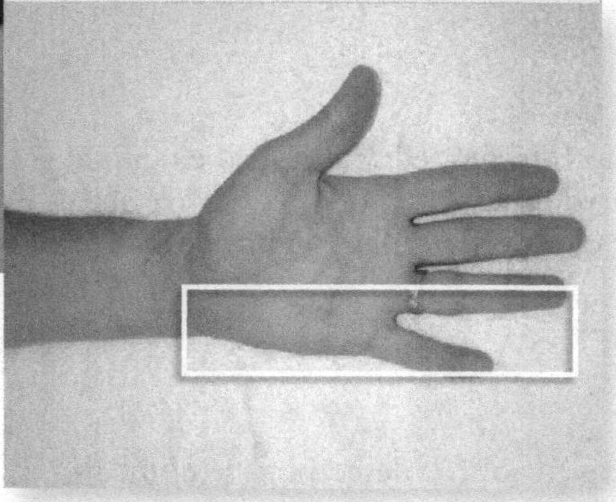

PHYSICAL EXAMINATION

Jack is alert, oriented, and in moderate discomfort at this time. Sienna notes no obvious deformity. Palpable tenderness and pain are noted with forceful compression over the pisiform and hamate. Wrist flexion and extension AROM and PROM are unremarkable. Jack's fifth finger flexion, abduction, and opposition demonstrate a deficit when compared with the uninvolved side. Resisted muscle testing reveals a deficit in fifth MCP flexion (3+/5) and abduction (3+/5). Wrist and hand ligamentous testing is WNL. Neurological testing reveals a positive special test over the area of the pisiform and hamate and a reproduction of sensory deficits (Figure 6.14.2).

FIGURE 6.14.2

Positive special test.

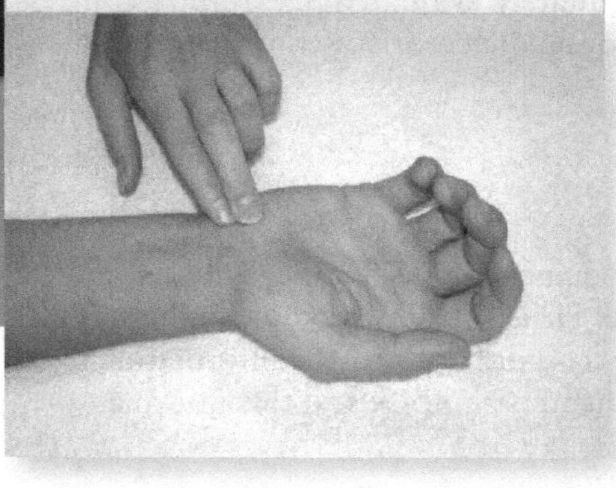

Palpation over the Tunnel of Guyon.

After completing the physical examination, Sienna discusses Jack's clinical diagnosis and his options, including referral to the team's orthopedic surgeon if conservative therapy does not resolve the condition. She also discusses some preventive strategies.

? QUESTIONS   **CASE 6.14**

Please answer the following questions based on the above case information.

6.14 / **1.** Based on the information presented in the case, determine (a) the differential diagnoses and (b) the clinical diagnosis. (c) Identify the common term used to describe the clinical diagnosis.

6.14 / **2.** Sienna assessed AROM and performed muscle testing of the fingers but failed to assess PROM. If you were the evaluating clinician, how would you assess passive flexion and extension ROM and what would you expect to find clinically?

6.14 / **3.** (a) Identify the bony and soft tissue structures Sienna should have palpated as part of her evaluation specific to the wrist and hand. (b) Identify the neurological and vascular structures at greatest risk based on the clinical diagnosis. (c) Identify the anatomical landmarks in Figure 6.14.3.

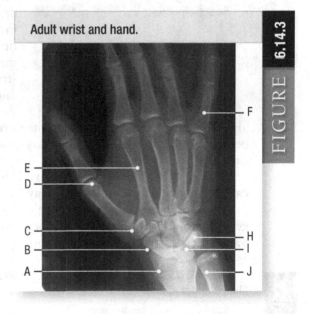

Adult wrist and hand.

FIGURE 6.14.3

6.14 / **4.** Sienna performed the special test shown in Figure 6.14.2. (a) What is the name of this test and what does it assess? (b) Describe how to perform this test.

6.14 / **5.** After completing the physical examination, Sienna discussed Jack's treatment options and prevention strategies. If you were the evaluating athletic trainer, what types of prevention strategies would you recommend?

D avid, an athletic training professor, is sitting at his desk in his office when a middle-aged man knocks on his door. He states that one of David's colleagues referred him to David to see if he could "relocate his finger" that he injured playing basketball.

HISTORY

David begins questioning Mike, a 38-year-old recreational basketball player, about what happened. Mike explains, "We were playing basketball, and I went to catch a pass when the ball hit my finger." He reports experiencing immediate pain and loss of function of the "middle joint" of the index finger.

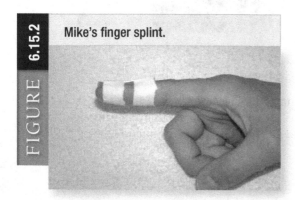

FIGURE 6.15.1

Observation of Mike's finger.

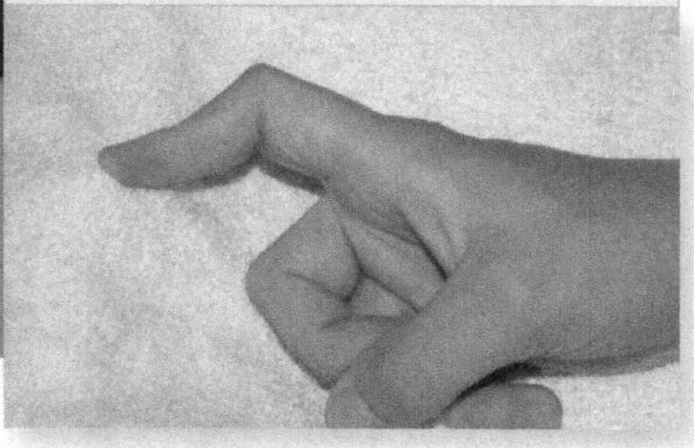

PHYSICAL EXAMINATION

Mike is alert and in moderate discomfort (6/10). He notices that Mike is supporting his right index finger in an attempt to prevent any secondary movement. Figure 6.15.1 demonstrates a general observation of Mike's index finger. No swelling is noted at this time. David identifies point tenderness over the dorsal aspect of the PIPJ. Mike demonstrates limited active extension of his index finger at the PIPJ, with the MCPJ assuming the position of function. However, David is able to passively return the joint to its normal resting position. Resistive ROM is not performed, because of Mike's inability to actively extend the index finger. Neurological testing is unremarkable.

David tells Mike how imperative it is for him to seek out appropriate medical care for his finger, including an X-ray to rule out fracture of the finger. He discusses the need for appropriate splinting in order to limit secondary damage and loss of finger function. David proceeds to place Mike in a splint to stabilize the finger (Figure 6.15.2). He instructs Mike in the correct use of cryotherapy.

FIGURE 6.15.2

Mike's finger splint.

FOLLOW-UP

As David is documenting his evaluation, he realizes he forgot to get a piece of personal information from Mike. He decides to try to find Mike and walks down to the gym where Mike had been playing basketball. When he arrives Mike is taping his fingers together so that he can return to the game. When David asks about what is going on, Mike shrugs and says, "What further damage could I do at this point?"

Please answer the following questions based on the above case information.

6.15 / **1.** Based on the information presented in the case, determine (a) the differential diagnoses and (b) the clinical diagnosis.

6.15 / **2.** What is the common MOI associated with this injury?

6.15 / **3.** David asked only a couple of history questions to guide the physical examination. Based on the information presented in the case, do you believe David took an adequate history? If not, what additional questions would you ask as the evaluating clinician?

6.15 / **4.** Based on the information presented in the case, do you believe David cared for the injury appropriately?

6.15 / **5.** Clearly Mike did not seem concerned about the status of his injury. If a recreational athlete asked you, "What further damage could I do at this point?" how would you respond?

Danni, a high school athletic trainer, was covering a varsity football game. Half-way through the first quarter, an offensive lineman came jogging off the field holding his right hand. When he found Danni, he explained to her, "My finger got stuck in this guy's shirt and when he pulled away it felt like he ripped my finger off. I can't bend the tip of my finger either."

HISTORY

Danni questions Boone, the lineman, about the specific MOI and determines that Boone was blocking the opposing lineman when he got his fingers wrapped in the player's shirt. As the offensive lineman moved away, Boone tried to hold on while his wrapped-up fingers, especially his ring finger, were pulled away. Danni looks down at Boone's finger and is fairly sure of the final clinical diagnosis.

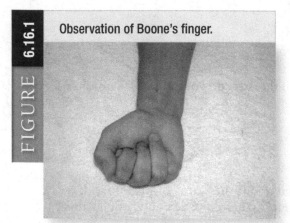

FIGURE 6.16.1

Observation of Boone's finger.

PHYSICAL EXAMINATION

On the bench, Boone is alert and anxious. A general observation of Boone's hand reveals a notable tenderness at the DIPJ of the right hand. Active ROM reveals a reduction in PIPJ motion (Figure 6.16.1) by several degrees bilaterally, with no active flexion of the DIPJ. A neurovascular assessment is unremarkable. Danni applies an ice bag to Boone's finger and decides it is best to consult with the team physician. Before she allows him to return to play she applies a splint to the finger.

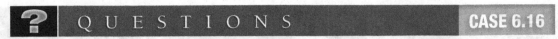

Please answer the following questions based on the above case information.

6.16 / **1.** Based on the information presented in the case, determine the clinical diagnosis.

6.16 / **2.** What test(s) could a clinician add to Danni's evaluation to assist in determining the clinical diagnosis? How would you perform the test(s)?

6.16 / **3.** (a) How would performing a PROM test assist in determining the clinical diagnosis? (b) If you were the evaluating clinician how would you perform PROM testing on the DIPJ and PIPJ?

6.16 / **4.** Which finger is the most susceptible to this injury?

6.16 / **5.** Why is it necessary for a clinician to recognize this injury and refer the athlete as early as possible?

Madison, a 12-year-old female basketball player, was at the local athletic club playing in a youth league basketball tournament. As she moved down the court, a teammate passed her the ball while she was not paying attention. Realizing the pass was for her, Madison attempted to catch the ball; however, it hit the tip of her fingers instead. She immediately grabbed her finger and began crying. The referee called a time-out, and her coach went to see what was wrong. Her coach saw that her finger was deformed and immediately placed ice on the finger. The coach called the front desk and requested further medical care. Tyler, a certified strength and conditioning coach and certified athletic trainer who worked for the athletic club, was asked to evaluate Madison's finger.

HISTORY

As Tyler begins his history, he notes that Madison is supporting her left index finger. Madison explains to Tyler that the basketball ball "jammed" her index finger. Further questioning by Tyler reveals that when the ball struck the index finger of the involved hand, the finger was straight. Madison denies hearing any popping or unusual sounds; however, she rates her pain as 7/10.

PHYSICAL EXAMINATION

Upon physical examination, Madison presents with moderate-to-severe discomfort. Madison's second DIPJ appears to be in a flexed position. No swelling or ecchymosis is present at this time. Tyler determines that Madison is point tender on the dorsum of the DIPJ. Passive ROM is WNL, and MMT reveals 0/5 during DIPJ extension. Tyler's assessment of the ligamentous stability is unremarkable. Neurologically, Madison is intact.

Tyler calls Madison's parents. While waiting for her parents, Tyler splints Madison's finger. When Madison's dad arrives, Tyler explains what has occurred and the required immediate and follow-up care. Madison's dad completes some necessary paperwork and takes Madison home.

Please answer the following questions based on the above case information.

6.17 / 1. Based on the information presented in the case, determine (a) the differential diagnoses and (b) the clinical diagnosis. (c) What is the colloquial term for this injury?

6.17 / 2. Tyler asked several history questions to guide the physical examination. Based on the information presented in the case, what one question do you believe he should have asked to guide the physical examination?

6.17 / 3. According to the case report, no special tests were performed—only PROM and muscle testing. Describe how Tyler might have assessed Madison's inability to extend her finger.

6.17 / 4. A component of Tyler's care was to splint Madison's finger. Based on the information provided in the case, describe the splinting procedure proper to this clinical diagnosis.

6.17 / 5. Would radiographic studies be useful in this case? Why, or why not?

CONCLUSION

G ross traumatic injuries to the wrist and hand complex can be very easy to detect and will normally correlate well with a clinician's physical examination findings. On the other hand, when an athlete or patient presents with spontaneous onset of wrist pain with no apparent MOI, or distant history of trauma, or the patient's activities consist of repetitive loading, the injury evaluation becomes complicated. Further complicating the injury evaluation and management process are the clinicians who take a nonchalant approach to the management of wrist and hand injuries and perpetuate the concept that wrist and hand injuries "are no big deal." As you have learned in your injury evaluation courses and through some of the cases presented here, the wrist and hand complex is an extremely intricate and complicated area. Proper recognition and management requires taking a thorough history, particularly the MOI and pattern of pain, and having a strong foundation in wrist and hand anatomy and function.

The injuries presented in this chapter for the most part were detected early and treated appropriately. Early identification is essential because early detection and appropriate management normally lead to full recovery and full function of the wrist or hand upon resolution of the injury. Delayed care or a missed diagnosis (because it was "just" a jammed finger) can lead to a severe disability. Case in point, one of the authors learned from his undergraduate students about the case of a collegiate athlete who thought he had jammed his finger. Unfortunately, he had actually suffered a Jersey finger and ignored the signs and symptoms for two weeks before he sought care from the athletic trainer. Intraoperatively, the FDP was found scarred down to the FDS, requiring a palmaris longus graft to repair the damage. Postoperatively, the athlete lost his ability to flex not only his DIPJ but also his PIPJ and his MCPJ of the finger. The moral of the story is that, as athletic trainers, we need to be competent at evaluating a wide array of musculoskeletal injuries and at educating athletes and patients about the rewards and consequences of correctly and incorrectly managing these injuries.

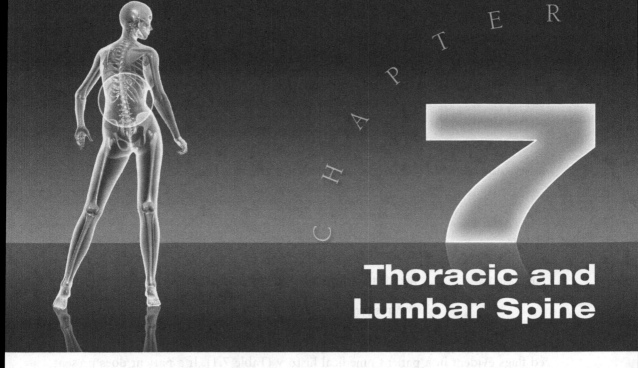

INTRODUCTION

I n this chapter we will examine the clinical evaluation and management of
eight different thoracic and lumbar spine pathologies. They will be presented
in a variety of settings, using both on-field and off-field scenarios and a diverse patient population. The pathologies presented in this chapter include both
acute and chronic conditions and are a good representation of injuries encountered
by a certified athletic trainer or commonly reported in the literature. In fact, one of
the authors has encountered all eight of these injuries during his career as a certified athletic trainer. Remember that some of the cases presented in this chapter may
have been intentionally written with inappropriate actions, procedures, treatments,
and general mismanagement of the case by the clinician in order to allow you to
critically analyze the cases, identify the inappropriate decision(s), and state what
you believe is the current gold-standard treatment. Additional information such as
special tests will be discussed to help you remember previous course materials or
clinical experiences. If at any time you feel that a more in-depth review is needed,
please refer to your favorite anatomical, assessment, and/or stress/special-tests reference guides or articles.

You may have learned in previous classes that the goal of the physical examination is to establish the clinical diagnosis in order to make the appropriate referral
and initiate a course of treatment. When dealing with the lumbar spine, however, it is
always necessary to identify patients who may also require immediate surgical evaluation and those whose symptoms suggest a more serious underlying pathology.[14] This
is because certain medical conditions, such as malignancies and spinal infections,
may present as low back pain (LBP).[13] Therefore, it will be necessary to also inquire
and determine whether or not a patient is at increased risk by identifying lumbar pain

TABLE 7.1	Acute low-back pain red flags.
RED FLAGS	**QUESTIONING**
Cancer	Ask about the patient's age (>50 or <20 years), history of cancer or strong suspicion of cancer, unexplained weight loss, progressive motor or sensory deficits, unrelenting night pain, or failure to improve after six weeks of conservative therapy.
Cauda equina syndrome	Ask about any progressive motor or sensory deficits, saddle anesthesia, bilateral weakness, new difficulty urinating, or new fecal incontinence. Of all the red flags, this syndrome is considered a surgical emergency and requires referral to the emergency room.[11]
Fracture	Ask about the patient's age, significant trauma, history of osteoporosis, chronic oral steroid use, and substance abuse.
Spinal infection	Ask about a history of fever, chills, unrelenting night pain, recent urinary tract or skin infection, penetrating wound near spine, IV drug use or drug abuse, or immunosuppression.

red flags evident in a patient's medical history (Table 7.1). If a patient does present with one or more of the red flags appearing in Table 7.1, he or she must be immediately referred to a physician for further diagnostic evaluation.

Acute thoracic or lumbar trauma is normally the result of some type of direct compression force applied to the back (e.g., falling from a height, being struck with a blunt object),[16] elongation of static and dynamic stabilizers of the spine,[10,24,26] cyclic loading or prolonged and sustained loading of the spine in an abnormal position (e.g., disc herniation),[3,18] or repeated motion with and without compression and/or shear forces.[19] Chronic injuries to the thoracic and lumbar spine include spondylopathies, facet syndrome, spinal stenosis, degenerative joint disease, nerve root impingement, centrally herniated discs, degenerative spondylolisthesis, trauma/fractures, epidural abscess, sacroiliac dysfunction, piriformis syndrome, and facet syndrome.[1,9,25] Repetitive joint loading, muscle imbalance, poor flexibility, decreased muscle endurance of the abdominal and back muscles, and poor training techniques and mechanics are only some of the 100 risk factors associated with chronic back pain.[2,3,6,18–20]

Injuries to the thoracic and, especially, the lumbar spine can be prevented by following three simple rules[7]: (1) Keep your head level to maintain your spine's three curves (cervical, thoracic, and lumbar) when lifting or sitting. (2) Keep your load close to the body while lifting or carrying anything. (3) Do not twist your spine when lifting or when in a seated position; turn the body as a unit.

ANATOMICAL REVIEW

The spinal or vertebral column consists of 33 vertebrae and is divided into 5 regions: 7 cervical, 12 thoracic, 5 lumbar, 5 fused bones of the sacrum, and 4 fused bones of the coccyx (Figure 7.1). Our focus in this chapter is the thoracic and lumbar vertebrae, which work together to provide a base of support for the attachment of ligaments, bones (ribs), and muscles of the thorax (ribcage) and pelvis. The vertebral or spinal column is responsible for four major functions: (1) to provide a base of support of the body in an upright posture; (2) to allow for locomotion and movement; (3) to protect the spinal cord as it resides in the spinal canal; and (4) to provide shock absorption during sitting, standing, and moving via the intervertebral discs.[8,13,15,19,22]

Thoracic Vertebrae

The thoracic spine is considered to be the least mobile area of the spine (compared with the cervical and lumbar spine). In an anatomical position, the thoracic spine's curvature is concave anteriorly and convex posteriorly, extending from the T2 to T12 (Figure 7.2).[22] It consists of 12 thoracic vertebrae, labeled as T1 through T12, with T1 being located below C7 around the base of the neck and T12 located before L1 at rib 12. Each vertebra is separated by an intervertebral disc. Both the thoracic vertebrae and the lumbar vertebrae consist of a vertebral body (located anteriorly), a pedicle, and a lamina that form the vertebral arch, the transverse and spinous processes, and the inferior and superior facets, which increase in size from T4 to T12 (Table 7.2). The vertebral arch forms the circular vertebral foramen, which houses and protects the spinal cord. The vertebral foramen is narrowest at T6.

Costospinal joints

The thoracic vertebrae are unique among the vertebrae in that they have two special joints, the costovertebral joint and costotransverse joint. Together these two joints are often referred to as costospinal joints.

The costovertebral joint, a synovial plane joint, is the articulation between the ribs, the costal facet or two lateral hemifacets on the vertebral bodies, and the disc that lies between each vertebral segment (Figure 7.3). The joint is supported by a fibrous joint capsule and the radiate ligament. Ribs 1, 11, and 12 articulate fully with the costal facets on the body of T1, T11, and T12, respectively. Ribs 2 through 10 attach to the hemifacets of the vertebral body that are above and below the associated rib. For example, rib 3 is attached to the T2 inferior hemifacet and the T3 superior hemifacet.

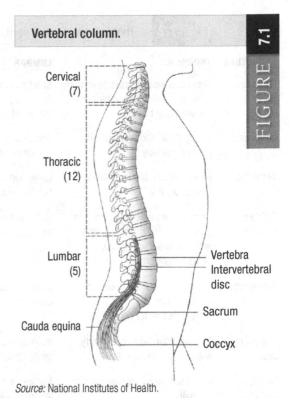

Vertebral column.

FIGURE 7.1

Cervical (7)

Thoracic (12)

Lumbar (5)

Cauda equina

Vertebra
Intervertebral disc

Sacrum

Coccyx

Source: National Institutes of Health.

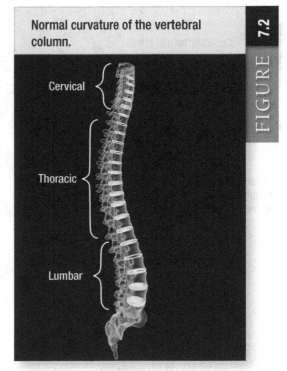

Normal curvature of the vertebral column.

FIGURE 7.2

Cervical

Thoracic

Lumbar

The lumbar and cervical spine create a lordotic position; the thoracic spine creates a kyphotic position.

TABLE 7.2	Thoracic and lumbar vertebral structural characteristics and function.[8,15,22]		
STRUCTURE	**THORACIC**	**LUMBAR**	**FUNCTION**
Pedicles	Short and stout, passes posteriorly from the posterolateral aspect of the vertebral body	Short and stout, passes posteriorly from the posterolateral aspect of the vertebral body	Together the pedicles and laminae form the posterior arch that encloses the vertebral foramen
Laminae	Short, thick, and broad, faces posteromedially	Short and broad, faces posteromedially	The pair of lamina meet at midline to form the spinous process
Vertebral body	Heart shaped, medium sized, facets for ribs	Large, kidney shaped, no costal facets on body	Resists compressive forces
Spinous process	Long and narrow, protrudes in a posteroinferior direction, aligns with the lower vertebral body, limits extension	Short and large, aligns with corresponding vertebral body	Resists compressive forces and transmits to laminae; serves as attachment site for muscles and ligaments
Transverse process	Long, progressively becomes smaller from T1 to T12, most contain facets for rib articulation	Long and slender, L3 is usually the broadest of the lumbar vertebrae	Serves as attachment site for muscles and ligaments
Superior facet	Thin and flat, faces posteriorly, superiorly, and laterally	Vertical and concave, faces posteriomedially	Work together as a facet joint to resist shear, compressive, tensile, and rotational forces; transmits forces to the laminae
Inferior facet	Faces anteriorly, inferiorly, and medially	Vertical and convex, faces anterolaterally	

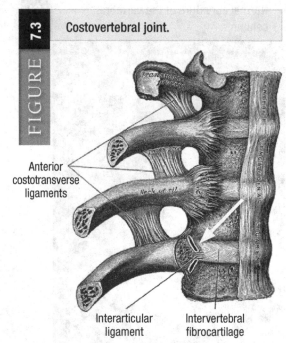

FIGURE 7.3   Costovertebral joint.

Anterior costotransverse ligaments

Interarticular ligament

Intervertebral fibrocartilage

Arrow indicates the area of the hemifacets.

Source: Gray's Anatomy.

At the costotransverse joint (another synovial joint) is the articulation between the tubercle of the ribs and the thoracic transverse spinous process. Each thoracic transverse process contains a costal facet for the tubercle of the rib and is supported by a fibrous capsule, a costotransverse, superior costotransverse, and lateral costotransverse ligament. Costal facets of T1 through T6 are found anteriorly on the transverse process, while the facets of T7 through T12 are located more superiorly on the transverse process. However, ribs 11 and 12 do not articulate with the thoracic transverse processes.

Lumbar Vertebrae

The lumbar spine consists of five lumbar vertebrae, labeled as L1 to L5, each separated by an intervertebral disc. Structurally, each lumbar vertebral body gradually increases in size from L1 through L5 in order to assume a greater weight-bearing role, and the lumbar spine is functionally more mobile than the thoracic spine.[8,15,21,22] The most mobile vertebra is L5, which has a distinctive, stout transverse process and blunt spinous process.[21,22] In an anatomical position, the lumbar spine's curvature is convex anteriorly and concave posteriorly, extending from T12 to the lumbosacral junction.[22] This posteriorly concave curve is often referred to as a lordotic curve or lumbar lordosis and is most noticeable when observing a patient laterally.[15,22] Adaptive muscle shortening or lengthening will cause a decrease or increase in this curve, possibly predisposing a patient to LBP.

Similar to the thoracic vertebrae, the lumbar vertebrae consist of a vertebral body, a pedicle and lamina, transverse and spinous processes, and inferior and superior facets (Figure 7.4). The vertebral foramen is triangular in the lumbar spine,[8] and it is larger than the thoracic spine but smaller than the cervical spine.[22] This section still houses the spinal cord and also supports the cauda equina. The cauda equina is a bundle of spinal nerve roots arising from the lumbosacral region and is comprised of the roots of all the spinal nerves below the first lumbar. It is most distinguishable at the L5 level. Narrowing of the foramen (stenosis), a result of either degeneration, space occupying lesion, or congenial abnormality, can result in neurological signs and symptoms of compression of the lumbar nerve roots or cauda equina.

Facet Joints

The formal term for these joints is apophyseal or zygapophyseal joint. They occur at the articulation between the inferior articular process of the superior vertebra and the superior articular facet of the inferior vertebra both on the right and left side of the spine (Figure 7.5). The orientation of the joints varies between the thoracic and lumbar spine (Table 7.3), but all influence

FIGURE 7.4

Structures of the vertebra.

Ligamentum flavum
Spine
Vertebral foramen or spinal canal
Vertebral arch
Spinal cord
Lamina
Facet joint
Pedicle
Nerve root
Posterior longitudinal ligament
Anterior longitudinal ligament
Intervertebral disc

Source: National Institutes of Health.

FIGURE 7.5

Lateral view of the vertebral column and facet joints.

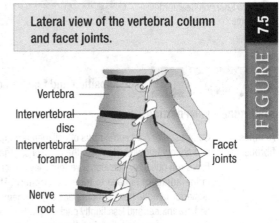

Vertebra
Intervertebral disc
Intervertebral foramen
Facet joints
Nerve root

Source: National Institutes of Health.

TABLE 7.3	Orientation of the thoracic and lumbar facet joints.[8,15,22]	
FACET	**THORACIC**	**LUMBAR**
Superior facet	Thin and flat, faces posteriorly, superiorly, and laterally	Vertical and concave, faces posteromedially
Inferior facet	Faces anteriorly, inferiorly, and medially	Vertical and convex, faces anterolaterally

ROM and function. Facet joints are synovial, plane joints surrounded by a fibrous capsule that allows gliding motions between joints. Richly innervated with free endings, each facet joint is supplied by two nerves and thus is a common source of back pain.[4,5,17] In the lumbar spine, the facet joints are responsible for assisting in the transmission of weight-bearing forces, for stabilizing the spine, and for preventing injury by limiting motion in all planes of movement.[5] In an upright posture, the thoracic vertebral bodies and discs are responsible for load bearing forces; however, when the thoracic spine is placed in flexion, rotation of the spine will increase the compressive forces on the facet joints.[22]

Location of the vertebral body and vertebral disc within the body.

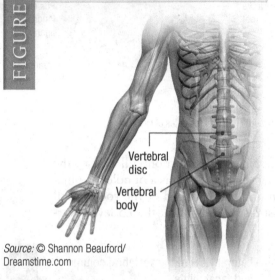

Vertebral disc

Vertebral body

Source: © Shannon Beauford/ Dreamstime.com

Intervertebral Discs

Located between the vertebral bodies in both the thoracic and lumbar spine are the intervertebral discs. Accounting for 25 percent of the spinal column height, each intervertebral disc acts primarily to bear the weight of the body, absorb compressive forces applied to the spine, and provide strength to the spinal column during movement (Figure 7.6).[15,21,22] The discs also act to maintain the opening between the intervertebral foramina, allowing for passage of the spinal nerve roots from the spinal cord. Composed primarily of water, each disc has an inner gelatinous portion called the nucleus pulposus, an outer fibrocartilage portion called the annulus fibrous, and two vertebral end-plates (Table 7.4). The disc

TABLE 7.4	Composition and function of intervertebral discs.[8,15,21,22]	
STRUCTURE	**COMPOSITION**	**FUNCTION**
Annulus fibrous	Composed of concentric rings of collagen arranged into sheets known as lamella, the parallel collagen fibers run obliquely between 2 vertebra, laying across in the adjacent lamella to form an X pattern. The posterior lamella have a more parallel arrangement and are thinner and less tightly packed, predisposing them to trauma and degeneration.	This encapsulates the nucleus pulposus, permitting angular movement while providing stability against shear and torsion forces.
Nucleus pulposus	Core of the intervertebral disc is composed of semifluid gel of water, proteoglycans, and collagen. The proteoglycans are responsible for attracting and retaining water. The percentage of the water in the nucleus pulposus gradually decreases with age.	Acts as shock absorber for axial forces and semifluid ball bearing during flexion, extension, rotation, and lateral flexion of the spinal column. Disc herniations are commonly seen in the lumbar spine at the levels of L4 to 5 and L5 to S1.
End-Plate	Composed of thin layers of cartilage covering the superior and inferior surface of the vertebral body, the end-plate is sometimes considered part of the disc.	This acts as a growth plate, transfers nutrients from the vertebral body to the disc, and prevents the nucleus pulposus from bulging into the vertebral body.

becomes thicker from the thoracic to the lumbar region and is thickest in the anterior section of the disc in the lumbar region. Ruptures of the lumbar intervertebral disc in the general adult population are very common. A herniated nucleus pulposus in children and adolescents appears to account for less than 2 to 6 percent of all reported cases of lumbar disc herniations,[12,23] though the true incidence rate is not known.[23]

Ligaments

Several ligaments play an important role in stabilizing the spine by limiting excessive spinal motion (Figure 7.7).[8,21] These include the anterior and posterior longitudinal ligaments, the ligamentum flava, and the supraspinous and interspinous ligaments (Table 7.5).

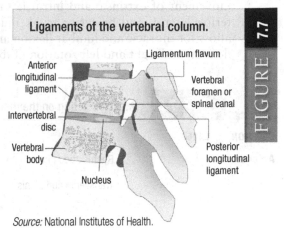

Ligaments of the vertebral column.

FIGURE 7.7

Ligamentum flavum

Anterior longitudinal ligament

Vertebral foramen or spinal canal

Intervertebral disc

Vertebral body

Posterior longitudinal ligament

Nucleus

Source: National Institutes of Health.

TABLE 7.5	Ligaments of the thoracic and lumbar spine.[8,15,21,22]	
LIGAMENT	**LOCATION**	**FUNCTION**
Anterior longitudinal ligament (ALL)	Broad fibrous band, extends from C1 and occiput to sacrum; firmly fixed to the anterior aspect of all the vertebrae bodies and discs	Maintains stability of vertebral joints and limits hyperextension
Posterior longitudinal ligament (PLL)	Narrow and weaker than ALL, extends from C2 to sacrum; fixed to intervertebral discs and posterior edge of the vertebral bodies in the spinal canal	Prevents hyperflexion of spinal column and any posterior protrusion of discs with noted lack of support in the lumbar area
Ligamentum flava	Located between anterior margins of superior and inferior vertebral lamina from C2 to sacrum, are strongest in lower thoracic region	Straightens spinal column after it has been flexed; maintains normal curvature of spinal column; limits spinal flexion, rotation, and lateral flexion
Interspinous	Short ligament connecting the adjacent spinous processes; more pronounced in lumbar region	Limits spinal flexion, rotation, and lateral flexion, stretches in the flexed position and is slacked in extension
Supraspinous	Extends along posterior margin of spinous processes of C7 through L3/L4.	Limits spinal flexion
Intertransverse	Paired intertransverse ligaments connect transverse processes above and below; more pronounced in the lumbar region	Compresses/stretches in response to lateral bending with ligaments on left side stretched during lateral bending to the right while right ligaments are slack, and vice versa when bending in the opposite direction

Muscles

Motion of the thoracic and lumbar spine is accomplished through the coordinated movement of extrinsic and intrinsic muscles acting on the spine. Together the anterior, lateral, and posterior trunk musculature maintain lumbar stabilization and allow for thoracic and lumbar flexion and extension of the spine, right and left lateral flexion, and right and left rotation (Table 7.6).

TABLE 7.6		Muscles acting on the thoracic and lumbar spine.[15,21,26]	
POSITION	**LAYER**	**MUSCLE**	**ACTION**
Anterior		Rectus abdominis	Flexion of the lumbar spine against gravity
		Transverse abdominis	Rotation and lateral flexion of the trunk (opposite side)
			Compression of the abdominal content and lumbar spine stabilization
		Psoas major	Superior portion, flexes the vertebral column laterally
			Inferior portion with the iliacus muscle flexes the trunk
		External abdominal oblique	Acting together, lumbar flexion
			Unilaterally, contralateral rotation of the trunk and ipsilateral lateral flexion of the trunk
		Internal abdominal oblique	Acting together, lumbar flexion
			Unilaterally, ipsilateral rotation and flexion of the trunk
Lateral		Quadratus lumborum	Acting together, depression of thoracic rib cage
			Unilaterally, extension and lateral flexion of the vertebral column
Posterior	Extrinsic	Latissimus dorsi	Trunk extension, stabilization of spine through the thoracolumbar fascia
		Trapezius (middle and lower one third)	Fixation of thoracic spine
		Rhomboids major	Fixation of thoracic spine
		Rhomboids minor	Fixation of the thoracic spine
	Intrinsic, superficial	Splenius cervicis	Acting together, extension of head and neck
			Unilaterally, lateral flexion and rotation to the same side
	Intrinsic, intermediate	[a]Iliocostalis (lumborum, thoracis)	Acting together, extension of vertebral column
			Unilaterally, lateral flexion of vertebral column
		[a]Longissimus (thoracis)	Acting together, extension of vertebral column
			Unilaterally, lateral flexion of vertebral column
		[a]Spinalis (thoracis)	Acting together, extension of vertebral column
			Unilaterally, lateral flexion of vertebral column

POSITION	LAYER	MUSCLE	ACTION
	Intrinsic, deep	[b]Multifidus	Acting together, extension of the trunk and stabilization of the vertebral column
			Unilaterally, flexes the trunk laterally and rotates to the opposite side
		[b]Rotatores	Acting together, extension of the trunk and stabilization of the vertebral column
			Unilaterally, rotation of the vertebral column to the opposite side
		[b]Semispinalis (thoracis)	Acting together, extension of vertebral column (cervical and thoracic)
			Unilaterally, rotation toward the opposite side

[a]Commonly referred to as the erector spinae, each muscle is divided into three sections that act on different sections of the spine and cranium.

[b]Commonly referred to as the transversospinal muscle, because these short muscles course in an oblique direction between the spinous processes and the transverse processes of the spine.

Nerves

The spinal cord has 31 pairs of nerves: 8 cervical, 12 thoracic, 5 lumbar, 5 sacral, and 1 coccygeal nerve. These nerves combine to form a network of intersecting nerves called a nerve plexus (e.g., brachial plexus, lumbar plexus, sacral plexus). Only the lumbar plexus will be discussed in this section; the brachial plexus is discussed in Chapter 4, and the sacral plexus is discussed in Chapter 9. At the inferior end of the spinal cord, roughly around L2, the spinal nerves exit through the vertebral canal to form the cauda equine (horse's tail). The 12 thoracic spinal nerves divide into ventral and dorsal rami, with the ventral rami of T1 through T11 forming the intercostal nerves and the ventral ramus of T12 forming the subcostal nerve. The dorsal rami nerves innervate the muscles, bones, joints, and skin of the back. Each of the 12 thoracic spinal nerves supplies a cutaneous branch to the skin. These are called dermatomes and are arranged segmentally from T1 to T12.

The lumbar plexus is formed from the T12 through L4 or L5 nerve roots and is found behind the psoas major and in front of the transverse processes of the lumbar vertebrae (Figure 7.8). The first lumbar nerve divides

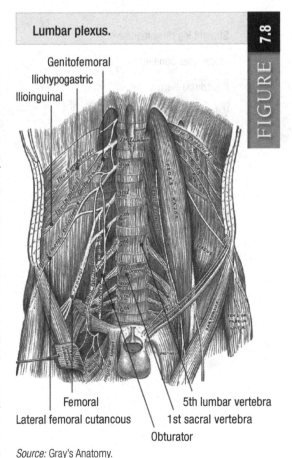

Lumbar plexus.

FIGURE 7.8

Genitofemoral
Iliohypogastric
Ilioinguinal

Femoral
Lateral femoral cutaneous
Obturator
5th lumbar vertebra
1st sacral vertebra

Source: Gray's Anatomy.

into an upper branch, which forms the iliohypogastric and ilioinguinal nerves, and a lower branch, which connects with the L2 branch to form the genitofemoral nerve. The remaining portion of the L2, L3, and L4 nerves divides into ventral and dorsal divisions. The ventral division forms the obturator nerve, and the dorsal division of L2 and L3 splits into other branches; a smaller branch to form the lateral femoral cutaneous nerve and a larger branch that connects with L4 to form the femoral nerve.

SPECIAL TESTS

The case studies in this chapter may require you to select and utilize special tests in order to adequately evaluate the injury. The details about how to perform each special test are beyond the scope of this section; however, Table 7.7 provides a general list of special tests that may be required and would be useful for you to review before beginning the case studies. For a more thorough review, please refer to your favorite evaluation text or journal article(s).

TABLE **7.7** Special tests of the lumbar spine.

SPECIAL TEST	FUNCTION
Slump	Dural lining, spinal cord, and spinal nerve root impingement
Straight leg raise maneuver	Disc herniation/nerve pathology of leg
Prone knee bending	L2 and L3 nerve roots
Brudzinski-Kernig	Meningeal irritation, nerve root(s)
Valsalva	Intrathecal pressure
Femoral nerve traction	Irritation of nerve roots of L2–L4
One-leg standing with lumbar extension	Par interarticularis (spondylolisthesis)
Milgram's	Nerve root compression
Hoover	Malingering test
FABER (flexion, abduction, external rotation)	Lumbar spine/SI pathology
Bowstring	Irritation of sciatic nerve

REFERENCES

1. Alverez JA, Hardy RH. Lumbar spinal stenosis: a common cause of back and leg pain. *Am Fam Physician* [electronic version]. 1998;59:1825–1834, 1839–1840. Available from: http://www.aafp.org/afp/980415ap/alvarez.html.

2. Arne B, Brandseth K, Fretheim S, Tvilde K, Ekeland A. Back injuries and pain in adolescents attending a ski high school. *Knee Surg Sports Traumatol Arthrosc.* 2004;12(1):80–85.

3. Bono C. Low back pain in athletes. *J Bone Joint Surg Am.* 2004;86-A(2):382–396.

4. Cavanaugh J, Lu Y, Chen C, Kallakuri S. Pain generation in lumbar and cervical facet joints. *J Bone Joint Surg Am.* 2006;88-A(Suppl 2):63–67.

5. Cohen SP, Raja SN. Pathogenesis, diagnosis, and treatment of lumbar zygapophysial (facet) joint pain. *Anesthesiology.* 2007;106:591–614.

6. Cole M, Grimshaw P. Low back pain and lifting: a review of epidemiology and aetiology. *Work.* 2003;21:173–184.

7. Downing D. Three simple rules for back safety. 2009. Available from: http://www.backsafe.com/newsroom/threerules.html. Accessed September 12, 2009.

8. Ebraheim NA, Hassan A, Lee M, Xu R. Functional anatomy of the lumbar spine. *Semin Pain Med.* 2004;2(3):131–137.

9. Furman MB, Puttiliz KM, Pannullo R, Simon J. Spinal stenosis and neurogenic claudication. *eMedicine* [electronic version]. 2009. Available from: http://emedicine.medscape.com/article/310528-overview. Accessed June 9, 2009.

10. Gallaspy JB, May JD. *Signs and Symptoms of Athletic Injuries.* St. Louis, MO. Mosby; 1996.

11. Heck JF, Sparano JM. A classification system for the assessment of lumbar pain in athletes. *J Athl Train.* 2000;35(2):204–211.

12. Hoffman H. Childhood and adolescent lumbar pain: differential diagnosis and management. *Clin Neurosurg.* 1980;27:553–576.

13. Humphreys SC, Eck JC. Clinical evaluation and treatment options for herniated lumbar disc. *Am Fam Physician.* 1999;59(3):575–582.

14. Kinkade S. Evaluation and treatment of acute low back pain. *Am Fam Physician.* 2007;75:1181–1188, 1190–1182.

15. Levangie PK, Norkin CC. *Joint Structure and Function: A Comprehensive Analysis.* Philadelphia, PA: F.A. Davis; 2001.

16. Lischyna N, Karim R. Thoracic spine compression fractures following a snowboarding accident: a case study. *J Can Chiropractic Assoc.* 2003;47(2):110–115.

17. Manchikanti L, Boswell M, Singh V, Pampati V, Damron K, Beyer C. Prevalence of facet joint pain in chronic spinal pain of cervical, thoracic, and lumbar regions. *BMC Musculoskeletal Disorders* [electronic version]. 2004. Available from: http://www.biomedcentral.com/1471-2474/5/15. Accessed September 28, 2009.

18. McGill S. The biomechanics of low back injury: implications on current practice in industry and the clinic. *J Biomechan.* 1997;30(5):465–475.

19. McGill S. Functional anatomy of the lumbar spine. In: *Low Back Disorders: Evidence-Based Prevention and Rehabilitation.* Champaign, IL: Human Kinetics; 2002:45–86.

20. McGill S. Linking latest knowledge of injury mechanisms and spine function to the prevention of low back disorders. *J Electromyogr Kinesiol.* 2004;14:43–47.

21. Moore K, Dalley, A. *Clinically Oriented Anatomy* (5th ed.). Baltimore, MD: Lippincott Williams & Wilkins; 2005.

22. Oliver J, Middleditch A. *Functional Anatomy of the Spine.* Oxford: Butterworth-Heinemann Ltd; 1991.

23. Ozgen S, Konya D, Toktas OZ, Dagcinar A, Ozek MM. Lumbar disc herniation in adolescence. *Pediatr Neurosurg.* 2007;43(2):77–81.

24. Schultz SJ, Houglum PA, Perrin DH. *Examination of Musculoskeletal Injuries* (2nd ed.). Champaign, IL: Human Kinetics; 2005.

25. Schwellnus MP. A clinical diagnostic approach to chronic low back pain in athletes. *Int SportMed J.* 2000;1(4):1.

26. Starkey C, Ryan J. *Evaluation of Orthopedic and Athletic Injuries* (2nd ed.). Philadelphia, PA: F.A. Davis; 2002.

CASE **7.1**

aroline, a licensed, certified athletic trainer and massage therapist, was in her office early on a spring morning when the head football coach at the large state university walked into her office. He was hunched over, with his right hand on his low back. Sixty-nine-year-old Coach Post was a legend at the university and was known for his hard work ethic and commitment to the student-athlete. Caroline immediately went over and helped Coach Post find a comfortable position on the treatment table. Coach Post was clearly in discomfort, and Caroline knew she was going to need to evaluate some sort of spine injury.

HISTORY

Caroline begins by asking Coach Post, "What happened? Don't you get enough exercise on the field?" Coach Post says, "I do, I actually hurt myself in the garden yesterday. I went to pick up a 50-pound bag of fertilizer, and as I lifted the bag, my lower back went into spasm. I dropped the bag to the ground and have been in pain ever since. Sitting, standing, and driving here this morning were all painful and uncomfortable." After some further questioning, Caroline determines that Coach Post's symptoms are (1) diffuse pain to the right lateral side of the low back musculature, with some pain radiation into the buttock but not to the lower extremity (bilaterally) and (2) an increase in pain with extension and right lateral flexion. Coach Post denies any history of lumbar disc pathology, but he does report a history of facet syndrome. His pain is rated as a 6/10 at rest and 8/10 with active movements.

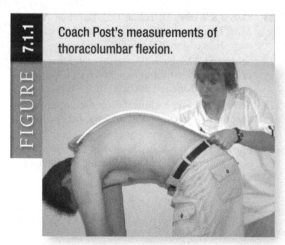

FIGURE 7.1.1
Coach Post's measurements of thoracolumbar flexion.

Tape measure applied from S2–C7.

PHYSICAL EXAMINATION

Coach Post is alert and in moderate discomfort with and without movement of the lumbar spine. Caroline's observation of the lumbar spine reveals right paraspinal spasms (L2–L5) and palpable tenderness. There is no point tenderness over the spinous processes of the lumbar vertebrae. Caroline notes some warmth and swelling over the involved area when compared with the uninvolved side. Caroline assesses thoracolumbar mobility using a tape measure (Figures 7.1.1 and 7.1.2). Results reveal a deficit in forward flexion, which is painful, and right lateral flexion, which is also painful. Active thoracolumbar extension is also limited and reproduces Coach Post's pain. Caroline grades trunk extension manual muscle testing as 3/5. A spring test to the individual segments of the lumbar spine is unremarkable. Neurological testing, including assessment of the lower extremity dermatomes, myotomes, peripheral nerves, and deep tendon reflexes, is unremarkable.

Caroline and Coach Post discuss the results of the physical examination. They agree the best immediate course of action would be referral to the coach's family physician without delay. Caroline also suggests the use of cryotherapy while at home.

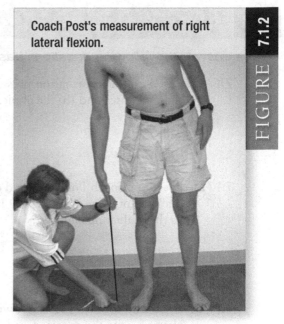

Coach Post's measurement of right lateral flexion.

FIGURE 7.1.2

Tape measure applied from fingertips to floor.

Please answer the following questions based on the above case information.

7.1 / 1. Based on the information presented in the case, determine (a) the differential diagnoses and (b) the clinical diagnosis.

7.1 / 2. Based on Coach Post's age and clinical presentation, do you believe Caroline's history was appropriate? If not, what would you have done differently as the evaluating clinician?

7.1 / 3. If Coach Post also presented with neurological symptoms such as sensory changes over the anterior middle-thigh, over the patella, and the medial lower-leg to the great-toe, along with weakness in ankle dorsiflexion, (a) what could you conclude about the injury? (b) What deep-tendon reflex should be assessed with this clinical presentation?

7.1 / 4. Based on the clinical presentation, Caroline rated Coach Post's thoracolumbar extension strength as 3/5. Describe the test position required to make this determination.

7.1 / 5. If you were the treating clinician, besides providing basic conservative therapy (i.e., cryotherapy, OTC anti-inflammatory medicine, muscle strengthening), what information should be included as part of Coach Post's rehabilitation plan?

CASE 7.2

A 38-year-old construction worker was referred from his orthopedic surgeon to Vanderkay Physical Therapy and Fitness for evaluation and treatment. When Eric arrived at the outpatient physical therapy center, the staff found that his prescription simply stated "treat for LBP 3 x 3." He explains to the administrative staff that the physician really wanted him to be seen today if possible. Kenrick, the ATC, PT assigned to the case, attempts to contact the physician for a clarification of the diagnosis, but the answering service informs him the office is closed for the day. Kenrick decides to evaluate Eric and call the physician first thing in the morning for further clarification.

HISTORY

Eric begins by stating that he has had LBP for several days now and that this is not his first time experiencing this pain. Kenrick asks about the MOI; however, Eric does not remember any specific event or activity that caused his current problem. When asked about his past medical history, he states, "About a year ago I was lifting an 85-pound bag of concrete, and as I picked it up, I rotated to the right and felt a sharp pain in my low back. I immediately dropped the bag. I went to therapy for a while, but it really did not help much. The pain eventually went away, but now it's returned." Further questioning reveals that when Eric moves the wrong way, his back does flare up for a couple of weeks, causing a decrease in strength along with numbness and tingling from the center of his low back down to his right leg. He further states, "The last time I was at therapy, they gave me some exercises that seemed to help, but this is the worst the pain has ever been." Kenrick asks Eric to fill out a McGill Pain Questionnaire. The present pain intensity is 4. No red flags are noted.

PHYSICAL EXAMINATION

Eric is alert and in moderate-to-severe discomfort, and this is noticeable as Eric continues to shift in his chair while talking with Kenrick. An observation of Eric's posture demonstrates an increased lumbar lordosis and left lateral shift. Palpation reveals tenderness around the L4–L5 and L5–S1 joint spaces. Muscle guarding is also noted over the right erector spinae muscle group. Active ROM produces minimal discomfort with all lumbar and thoracolumbar movements. However, repeated movements, particularly into flexion and right-side glide (left-side lateral flexion) begin to significantly increase pain, and this reproduces the neurological symptoms reported in the history. Interestingly, repeated extension actually reduces Eric's symptoms. Muscle testing identifies abdominal weakness, particularly in the transversus abdominis. There was also weakness in the tibialis anterior and extensor hallucis longus on the right side. A straight leg raise test is painful at 30°, and

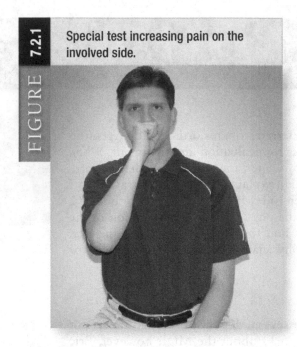

FIGURE 7.2.1

Special test increasing pain on the involved side.

the test in Figure 7.2.1 increases pain on the involved side. Eric's L4 DTR is 1+ on the involved side.

Before Eric leaves the clinic, Kenrick prescribes several exercises for Eric to complete at home and asks him to keep track of his pain location and intensity upon getting up in the morning, before and after exercise, and before going to bed. Some of the exercises Kenrick prescribes include repeated extension in standing and repeated extension in lying (prone position). Figure 7.2.2 shows Eric's VAS pain pattern in the morning, pre-exercise, post-exercise, and in the evening.

FIGURE   7.2.2   Eric's VAS pain pattern.

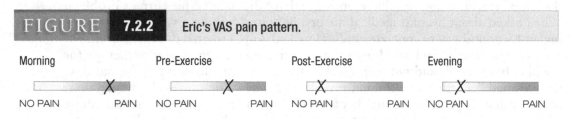

QUESTIONS   CASE 7.2

Please answer the following questions based on the above case information.

7.2 / **1.** Based on the information presented in the case, determine (a) the differential diagnoses and (b) the clinical diagnosis.

7.2 / **2.** The injury in this case is typically seen in the adult population, often as a result of twisting of the trunk while carrying or lifting weight. For adolescent athletes, (a) what is the likelihood of this injury? (b) What would be the MOI?

7.2 / **3.** During the physical examination, Kenrick notes that Eric is constantly shifting in his chair. As the evaluating clinician, what conclusion can you draw regarding this behavior?

7.2 / **4.** (a) What is the difference between lumbar and thoracolumbar motion? (b) How would you as the evaluating clinician assess lumbar motion? (c) Thoracolumbar motion?

7.2 / **5.** As part of the physical examination, Kenrick performed a neurological examination. Complete Table 7.2.1, which shows the sensory and motor deficits associated with nerve root involvement at each of the lumbar and sacral levels identified in the chart.

TABLE	7.2.1	Sensory and motor deficits in association with nerve root involvement at individual lumbar and sacral levels.

DISC LEVEL	LOCATION OF DERMATOME SYMPTOMS	MOTOR DEFICITS
L1	Back, over greater trochanter and groin	
L2		Hip flexion and adductors, diminished patellar tendon reflex
L3		Knee extension, diminished patellar tendon reflex
L4	Anterior medial lower leg	
L5		Great toe extension
S1	Lateral side and plantar surface of the foot	
S2		Knee flexion and great toe flexion

7.2 / **6.** (a) Why is Eric's pain worse in the morning and improved after exercise? (b) If you were treating Eric, what activities would you have him perform during his exercise phase to reduce his discomfort?

CASE 7.3

J ustin, a 38-year-old project manager for a large construction company, started noticing left-side lumbar pain. However, he figured it was just old age and he ignored the pain. As his pain level kept worsening, he decided he would ask the athletic trainer who worked at his son's high school to take a look at his back. After he dropped his son at school for his basketball practice, Justin walked into the athletic training room to find Steve, the high school's certified athletic trainer. Steve said he would be glad to evaluate Justin's back.

HISTORY

Steve begins by asking several general questions about the injury, including onset of the symptoms, pain characteristics, and general medical history. Justin states that about 14 days ago he was playing ball with his friends (he called them "the over 30 club") when he got knocked into the wall. He struck an object protruding from the wall on his left posterior flank. When he awoke the next morning he reported

FIGURE 7.3.1

Justin's location of pain.

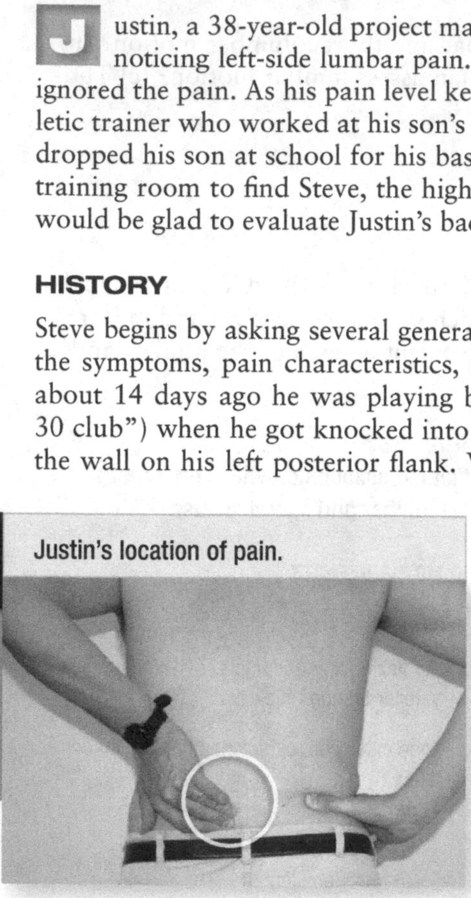

Area of pain is within the circle and by the left fingers.

increased pain on his left side (Figure 7.3.1). He initially thought he just hit the wall hard and his age was starting to catch up with him, but the pain remained localized, progressively worsening. He describes the pain as a dull aching pain (5/10). He states that side-bending or rotation (to the involved side) causes a significant increase in his LBP and limits his movement. Further questioning reveals no history of previous cervical, thoracic, or lumbar spine trauma and no history of osteoporosis, chronic oral steroid use, urinary incontinence, or substance abuse. Justin also reports the use of a heating pad for the last couple of days, with no great relief in pain.

PHYSICAL EXAMINATION

Justin is alert, but apprehensive and deliberate in his movements. Steve's general observation of Justin reveals carrying a posture to lessen his pain (slightly flexed and rotated to the right). He also notes palpable tenderness, pain, and spasm over the left paravertebral muscle. Range of motion is limited (Table 7.3.1). Steve elicits pain with PROM of the trunk to the involved side. A provocative test is positive for pain and hypomobility at the L4 and L5. Steve performs an SLR and a slump test, which yield negative results. During his neurological evaluation, Steve notes that lower quadrant sensory and motor testing demonstrate results WNL, as does the neurological testing performed in Figure 7.3.2.

| TABLE | 7.3.1 | Justin's ROM results. |

AROM*	LEFT	RIGHT	PROM	LEFT	RIGHT
Extension		15°	Extension		N/A
Flexion		75°	Flexion		80°
Rotation	30°	45°	Rotation	35°	50°
Lateral flexion	13°	36°	Lateral flexion	16°	40°

*Combined extension, left rotation, and left lateral flexion are decreased and cause increased pain.

Based on the results of the physical exam, Steve suggests to Justin that he seek further medical assistance from an orthopedic physician. He explains that a definitive diagnosis of this condition is normally made through diagnostic testing or injecting the area with an anesthetic and noting the changes in the symptoms. Justin asks Steve if he could send a note to the doctor after an appointment has been made. Steve also recommends that Justin use an ice pack rather than an electric heating pad on his back, along with some sort of anti-inflammatory drugs to assist in pain control.

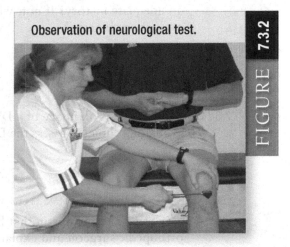

Observation of neurological test.

FIGURE 7.3.2

? QUESTIONS   CASE 7.3

Please answer the following questions based on the above case information.

7.3 / **1.** Based on the information presented in the case, determine (a) the differential diagnoses and (b) the clinical diagnosis.

7.3 / **2.** Steve asked several history questions to guide his physical examination. Based on the information presented in the case, do you believe he acquired an adequate history? If not, what questions would you have asked as the evaluating clinician?

7.3 / **3.** Figure 7.3.2 is an image of a DTR. What is a DTR? How would you as the evaluating clinician assess the DTR in Figure 7.3.2?

7.3 / **4.** Steve suggested to Justin that he seek further medical assistance from an orthopedic surgeon and explained how the clinical diagnosis may be confirmed. How does injecting the area with an anesthetic and noting the changes in the symptoms assist in making the clinical diagnosis?

7.3 / **5.** After completing the physical examination, Steve documented his findings electronically and sent a copy of the report to Justin's orthopedic surgeon. Using your athletic training room's computer tracking software, document your findings electronically as if you were the treating clinician. If the case did not provide information you believe is pertinent to the clinical diagnosis, please add this information to your documentation. If you do not have access to injury-tracking software, consider downloading a trial version from CSMI Solutions (Sportsware) by going to www.csmisolutions.com/cmt/publish/service_software_dl.shtml and following the on-screen directions.

A 17-year-old female collegiate gymnast reported to the athletic training room on an early fall morning before practice. Rochelle's CCs were low back cramps (LBC) and stiffness, with increased pain after practice the previous day. Tim, the athletic trainer covering women's gymnastics, has never dealt with her before. Before evaluating Rochelle, Tim opens up her electronic medical record. A review of the record indicates a long history of medical and orthopedic problems dating back to junior high, including multiple bilateral sprained ankles, several cases of recurrent knee pain, stress fractures (right foot, left tibia), and LBP, with the most recent episode one year ago. As Tim scans the pre-participation physical exam, he identifies a previous diagnosis of spondylolysis at L5. After a big sigh, Tim begins his examination of Rochelle.

HISTORY

Tim says, "Tell me what seems to be the problem this time?" Rochelle stated, "Over the last couple of weeks, I began noting an increase in low back pain that gets worse after activity. Practice typically lasts 2.5 to 3 hours, and during the last half of practice the pain typically increases. By the time practice is over it is really bad, and in the morning I am really stiff." Tim questions Rochelle about her past medical history, and she informs Tim that during her senior year in high school she developed a stress fracture in her back that caused her to miss about six weeks of practice. Rochelle states, "When I had this problem before, I went to therapy, and basically all they did was heat, massage, and something that made my skin feel like I had ants crawling across it." Tim determines that Rochelle's specialty is tumbling and balance beam, both of which Rochelle says place a lot of stress on her back, especially when she extends. During the history, Tim notices that Rochelle continually shifts in her chair while talking with him.

PHYSICAL EXAMINATION

Tim begins the evaluation by asking Rochelle to stand up. A postural assessment identifies genu recurvatum and an anteriorly titled pelvis. There is localized tenderness and pain, with increased tenderness in response to deep palpation above the landmark in Figure 7.4.1. Active ROM during trunk flexion is limited but pain free, with some hesitation, when moving into flexion. As Rochelle moves back to an upright position (extension) she reports an increase in

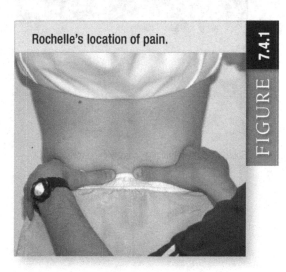

Rochelle's location of pain.

FIGURE 7.4.1

Tim's hands are located on Rochelle's iliac crests.

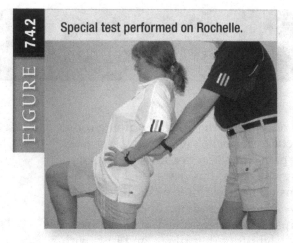

FIGURE 7.4.2

Special test performed on Rochelle.

pain. Tim also notes pain during lumbar rotation. Muscle testing identifies abdominal weakness and muscular imbalance between the abdominal muscles and hamstrings. In fact, hamstring muscle length reveals 65° of ROM to the right hip and 68° to the left hip with the knee in an extended position. The special test performed in Figure 7.4.2 is positive bilaterally. A lower quarter screen was unremarkable. Tim applies an ice bag and high TENS and decides it is best to consult with the team physician, believing that Rochelle probably needs radiographs and a possible MRI.

DIAGNOSTIC IMAGING

After seeing Rochelle, the team physician at the sports medicine clinic agrees with Tim and recommends a series of radiographs. Rochelle is sent to the student health clinic. Figure 7.4.3 shows a copy of the radiographs taken at the health center.

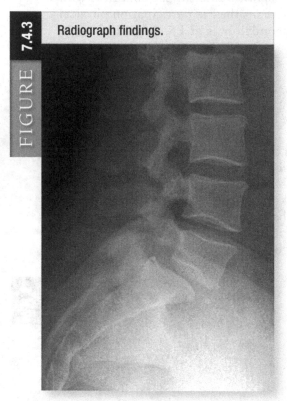

FIGURE 7.4.3

Radiograph findings.

Source: LearningRadiology.com, with permission.

? Q U E S T I O N S   **CASE 7.4**

Please answer the following questions based on the above case information.

7.4 / 1. Based on the information presented in the case, determine (a) the differential diagnoses and (b) the clinical diagnosis.

7.4 / 2. Overall, do you believe Tim took an adequate history? What if anything would you as the evaluating clinician have done differently?

7.4 / 3. (a) Based on the clinical diagnosis, what else may have Tim noted during his palpation of Rochelle, particularly if the injury had a significant progression? (b) Is this a reliable clinical indicator of the clinical diagnosis?

7.4 / 4. (a) What is the name of the special test performed in Figure 7.4.2? (b) What is considered a positive finding?

7.4 / 5. Based on Figure 7.4.3 how would the clinical diagnosis be graded?

D utch, a certified athletic trainer and physical therapist, is a long-time employee and part owner of the MedCare Rehabilitation and Fitness Center. Dutch has been employed in this capacity for 25 years and is well respected by the area physicians for his reputation for providing quality clinical care. Dr. McMurray is no exception and often refers many of his spine patients to MedCare. On this particular day, 67-year-old Doris is referred to Dutch from Dr. McMurray. After completion of the standard paperwork, Doris is escorted to an exam room.

HISTORY

As he does with all new patients, Dutch begins with a review of Doris's chief complaints, medical history, living environment, social, work, and functional status. He determines that Doris is an elderly individual, who is fairly active, participating in community exercise groups, walking clubs, and aqua classes. She volunteers at the information booth at the local hospital two days a week and lives with her husband of 40 years. Doris and her husband watch their four grandchildren three days a week for 4 hours in the afternoon. She states that she saw Dr. McMurray because of occasional numbness and weakness in her lower legs and mild pain when performing her normal exercises, especially walking and chasing the grandchildren. She states, "My legs are always fatigued. My pain started some time ago but was bearable; however, the pain is becoming worse and the numbness and weakness are also getting worse." When Dutch asks about an MOI, Doris cannot remember anything in particular. Her medical history reveals a history of slightly elevated blood pressure, which Doris has been controlling through diet and exercise. She also has a history of osteoarthritis in her knees and lumbar spine. Her pain is rated at 7/10 while exercising and 3/10 under normal conditions. Her pain patterns can be found in Figure 7.5.1.

PHYSICAL EXAMINATION

Upon inspection, Dutch observes no obvious deformities of the extremities, back, or thorax and normal spinal curvatures. Doris is sinewy and well toned. An observation of Doris's skin reveals no presence of any cutaneous signs of occult spinal dysraphisms. Dutch does note some apparent discomfort in Doris's facial expression during ambulation, but the pain appears to be relieved when she ambulates with a slight stoop and when lying down. Palpation of the low

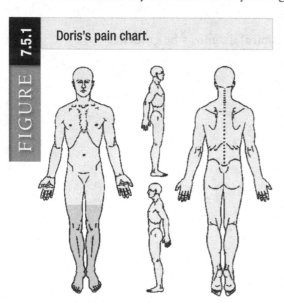

FIGURE 7.5.1

Doris's pain chart.

The area of compromise is shaded.

back, spine, pelvis, and thigh regions do not elicit any pain. Reflexes are normal. Range of motion is limited and painful with active lumbar extension but relieved with flexion. When assessing PROM, lumbar extension again is limited and painful, reproducing her neurological symptoms. Doris does have some sensory disturbances of her thigh and lower legs. Muscle grading of her involved extremities revealed a 4/5 for knee flexion, knee extension, hip flexion, and hip extension when compared with the left side. A Hoover test, Milgram's test, and Kernig test are negative. The test shown in Figure 7.5.2, however, produces some discomfort and neurological symptoms. A neurological exam reveals no significant sensorimotor deficits at rest or in a neutral position; however, Dutch notes bilateral sensory deficit and motor weakness after a period of ambulation.

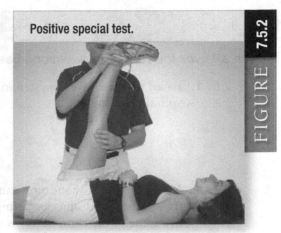

Positive special test.

FIGURE 7.5.2

Following the physical examination, Doris and Dutch sit down to discuss Doris's treatment options based on her physical examination, diagnostic report, and medical records from Dr. McMurray's office.

? QUESTIONS   CASE 7.5

Please answer the following questions based on the above case information.

7.5 / **1.** Based on the above case scenario, what do you suspect is wrong with Doris's spinal column?

7.5 / **2.** Many times, this condition can be found in other regions of the spine and may cause other signs and symptoms. If other problems were to occur, what are some of the complications that you as the evaluating clinician may need to observe or determine as part of the history?

7.5 / **3.** Based on the clinical diagnosis, what are some of the most common diagnostic tests used when diagnosing this condition?

7.5 / **4.** If you were the treating clinician, what types of conservative therapy would you consider for this clinical diagnosis to help alleviate pain and discomfort?

7.5 / **5.** As the evaluating clinician, if Doris asked about her options and wanted you to elaborate on the three most common surgical techniques, how would you respond?

CASE 7.6

Gene, a certified athletic trainer, and his athletic training student Maria were covering an NCAA Division I collegiate tennis match when one of the players, Sig, began demonstrating signs of a possible shoulder injury during his match. Sig, the number two player on the team, served two more times before requesting a medical time-out.

MEDICAL TIME-OUT HISTORY

Being aware of the medical time-out rule, Gene immediately attends to Sig, who states that while he was serving, he felt a "strong twinge" in the middle of his back. He says that the next two serves increased his pain during the middle of wind-up and the middle-to-late follow-through phase. He demonstrates right-sided point tenderness. Gene massages and stretches the area for the remainder of the time-out and instructs Sig about what he can do to alleviate the pain. Sig completes the remainder of his set, but unfortunately he is unable to complete the match, because he is not allowed to receive any more assistance from Gene and the pain keeps getting worse.

POST-MATCH HISTORY

After coming off the court in observable discomfort, Gene asks Maria to complete an injury assessment. Maria begins her evaluation by trying to determine the MOI by asking Sig, "What happened?" Sig stated, "During the follow-through of one of my serves, I realized I was in the wrong position and tried to correct for my poor foot position by slightly rotating and flexing my torso further than normal. All of sudden, I felt a pulling sensation in the middle of my back. I tried playing through the pain, but every time I extend and flex my back, I get these spasms. In fact, breathing is getting harder." Further questioning reveals that Sig has moderate-to-severe, stabbing thoracic pains (8/10). Sig denies any history of previous back or shoulder injury and is not taking any medication.

PHYSICAL EXAMINATION

Sig is alert and appears to be guarding the right posterior thoracic wall. Further observation of the posterior thoracic spine reveals no immediate swelling; however, an increase in muscle tone is evident to the right of the thoracic spine (Figure 7.6.1). Bony palpation reveals no tenderness over the spinous process; however, soft tissue palpation reveals pain and increased muscle tone between the ribs and around the transverse process of

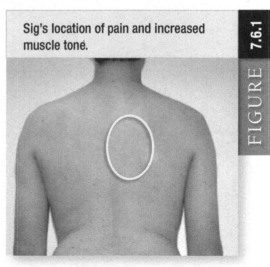

Sig's location of pain and increased muscle tone.

FIGURE 7.6.1

Area of pain is located within the circle.

T6 through T9. Sig's AROM testing reveals a deficit in trunk extension and right trunk side flexion; shoulder extension and flexion are limited secondary to thoracic pain and spasm. Active trunk flexion on the involved side with the arm hanging to the side also increases thoracic pain.

Maria discusses the results of her examination with Gene, and they both agree on the sideline clinical diagnosis. They also both agree on the best immediate course of action and discuss this with Sig. Gene instructs Maria to apply cryotherapy to Sig's injury, and he heads over to discuss the findings of the exam with the coach. While Maria fills an ice bag, a spectator strikes up a conversation with her. After a few minutes of small talk, the spectator inquires into the status of Sig. Maria proceeds to recap the findings of the physical examination and informs the spectator that Sig will most likely miss the conference finals.

The next morning, Gene is called into the athletic director's office and is confronted by a very unhappy tennis coach who throws the local newspaper onto the table. The sports section headline reads, "Northsouth University Tennis Team Loses Key Player for Conference Finals."

Please answer the following questions based on the above case information.

7.6 / **1.** Based on the information presented in the case, (a) what is the likely clinical diagnosis? (b) What is the normal MOI?

7.6 / **2.** In this case, Sig was initially evaluated and treated by Gene during a medical time-out. However, Sig was forced to retire from the match because he could not receive any additional care. Why?

7.6 / **3.** (a) Identify the posterior extrinsic muscles acting on the spinal column that Maria should have palpated as part of her evaluation. (b) Identify the different layers of the intrinsic muscles acting on the posterior spine. (c) Identify the muscles that make up the erector spinae muscle group, and describe the technique used to identify this muscle group.

7.6 / **4.** The tennis coach in this case was obviously unhappy when he confronted Gene in the athletic director's office the morning after the game. What was he upset about? How could this situation be prevented?

CASE 7.7

S amantha, an athletic training student, was working with her clinical supervisor, Lauren, at an invitational high school track meet. Both were busy this particular day, treating muscle strains and blisters and performing various evaluations for injuries, covering many of the participating teams that did not have an athletic trainer on staff at their respective schools. Just as there seemed to be a break, Lauren and Samantha were summoned over to the pole vault pit where a male pole vaulter was injured.

HISTORY

As Lauren and Samantha approach the scene, bystanders describe the incident. Seventeen-year-old Paul, a student at the high school where Lauren works, successfully cleared 12 feet but, in the process, landed slightly off the mat on the left side (Figure

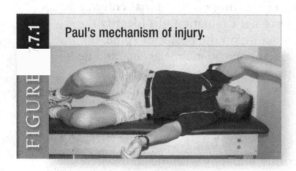

FIGURE 7.7.1

Paul's mechanism of injury.

7.7.1). The pole was not broken. Samantha and Lauren notice that Paul is sitting upright, but his head is bent over. Luckily he does not appear to be seriously injured. Paul denies losing consciousness and reports no sensory or motor deficits of the upper or lower extremity. He does report feeling a weird sensation of intense pain and cracking in the middle of his back when he contacted the ground after missing the mat.

PHYSICAL EXAMINATION

Paul is alert but apprehensive and deliberate in his movements. Lauren observes Paul's carrying posture, which appears designed to lessen his pain. Palpation of the posterior ribs, scapula, and cervical and thoracic spine does not indicate abnormal pathologies. He is able to walk and move all extremities equally, and he states that he is feeling better. Based on no abnormal signs and symptoms and confident that there is not a cervical spine issue, Lauren decides to ice the upper back and prohibit further pole vaulting that day, with follow-up instructions to see her the next day in the athletic training room.

FOLLOW-UP EXAMINATION

About 18 hours after the initial injury, Paul reports to the athletic training room, experiencing increased stiffness and pain in his upper back and slight discomfort when trying to take a breath. Lauren notices spasm of the paraspinal muscles in the thoracic region, slight tenderness of the ribs near the thoracic spinal column, and difficulty breathing (increased pain with inhalation). Neurologically, Paul appears to be intact.

Lauren decides that because of pain and spasms associated with the thoracic area and difficulty breathing, the athlete needs to be referred for diagnostic evaluations with the local orthopedic group in town.

Please answer the following questions based on the above case information.

7.7 / **1.** Based on the information presented in the case, determine (a) the differential diagnoses and (b) the clinical diagnosis.

7.7 / **2.** Why do you think that the condition did not manifest itself acutely after the incident?

7.7 / **3.** The literature lists catastrophic injuries to pole vaulters as rare. Please describe the common MOIs that athletic trainers must nevertheless be aware of, and closely prepared for, when supervising pole vaulters.

7.7 / **4.** Based on the case, if the pole vaulter was suspected of having a catastrophic injury, what management steps should Lauren and Samantha follow in order to spineboard the athlete?

by Joel Beam, Ed.D., LAT, ATC, University of North Florida, Jacksonville

J im, a 20-year-old cross-country athlete, has been experiencing posterior hip and buttock pain and numbness for three weeks and decided to go to the athletic training room for help.

HISTORY

Hannah, the head athletic trainer, observes Jim as he enters, and after he sits down, she begins to ask him questions regarding the pain. Jim states that the pain gradually began three weeks ago during the conclusion of the competitive season, and he does not remember any specific MOI. Jim tells Hannah he is training for a triathlon and has recently increased the mileage of both running and cycling. Jim states, "The pain and numbness start in my right hip and continue down into the back of my upper leg, and I sometimes get a burning sensation." He adds, "It gets worse after I finish a hard run or bike-training session or if I sit down for a long time. I just began a summer job that requires me to sit at a desk 5 to 6 hours each day." Hannah and Jim discuss Jim's past medical history, which is unremarkable except for a right third metatarsal stress fracture last year during the season.

FIGURE 7.8.1

Freiberg sign.

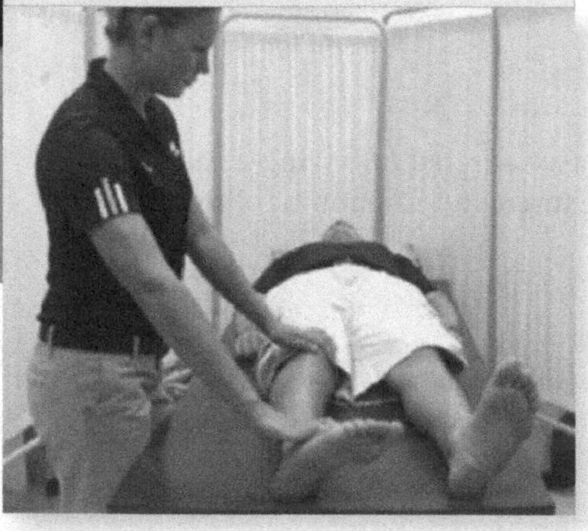

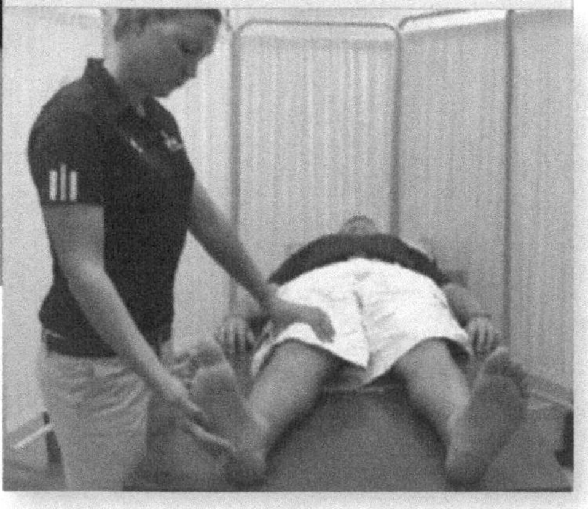

PHYSICAL EXAMINATION

Jim is alert and in mild discomfort (1/10–3/10 on a numerical pain scale). Hannah begins the physical examination by observing the soft tissue and bony structures of the thoracic and lumbar spine, pelvis, thigh, and lower extremities. A 7 mm right leg length discrepancy is noted. Upon palpation, moderate pain (6/10–7/10) is produced over the right gluteus maximus and piriformis. Focal palpation over the piriformis near the sciatic notch elicits mild numbness into the right posterior thigh. Active and passive ROM and special tests for the thoracic and lumbar spine and pelvis are WNL. Hannah places Jim in a supine position on a table and is able to recreate the posterior hip and buttock pain with passive internal rotation of the right hip (Freiberg sign), resisted external rotation of the right leg, and the straight leg test (Lasegue's test) (Figures 7.8.1, 7.8.2, and 7.8.3,

FIGURE 7.8.2

Resisted external rotation.

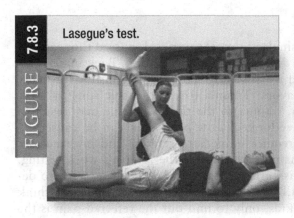

Lasegue's test.

FIGURE 7.8.3

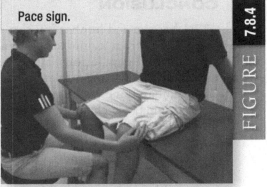

Pace sign.

FIGURE 7.8.4

respectively). Resisted hip abduction (Pace sign) in a seated position produces the posterior pain in the right hip and buttocks (Figure 7.8.4) and also reveals muscular weakness (3/5). All neurological tests are WNL. Based on the findings, Hannah refers Jim to the team's orthopedist for further evaluation and diagnostic testing. The orthopedist finds that plain radiographs of the lumbar spine, pelvis, and hip are normal.

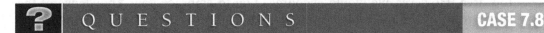

? **Q U E S T I O N S**   **CASE 7.8**

Please answer the following questions based on the above case information.

7.8 / **1.** Based on the information presented in the case, determine (a) the differential diagnoses and (b) the clinical diagnosis.

7.8 / **2.** Hannah assessed several body areas during the physical examination. Based on the information presented in the case, do you believe it was necessary for her to perform all of these tests?

7.8 / **3.** Which findings in the history and physical examination possibly led Hannah and the team orthopedist to the clinical diagnosis above?

7.8 / **4.** Describe the etiological anatomical factors in the development of the clinical diagnosis.

7.8 / **5.** If you were Hannah, and Jim asked, "What is the plan for treatment and rehabilitation of my condition," what would be your response?

CONCLUSION

Thoracic and lumbar injuries, similar to most injuries discussed thus far, can range from a mild strain to a debilitating disc herniation. Back injuries affect all populations, ages, and work settings and are responsible for many missed workdays and athletic endeavors. Trauma to the thoracic spine is rarer than lumbar spine trauma; however, trauma to the thoracic spine may result in chest trauma, which must not be overlooked. Low back pain can be caused by numerous medical conditions that require immediate referral and intervention, and the prevalence of the conditions may depend on the athlete's work setting. Therefore, an understanding of at-risk athletes/patients is crucial in order to deliver proper care. Imagine suffering LBP when you are 55 years old that you think is caused by playing with the grandkids, only to find out the referred pain is the result of a malignancy.

The cases in this chapter demonstrate the complexities of completing a thorough physical examination of the thoracic and/or lumbar spine. In the authors' experiences, the spine, particularly the lumbar spine, is probably one of the most complicated areas of the body to evaluate. The difficulty of grasping the complex interaction between each spinal level and how spinal mechanics affect joint mobility and stability scares many clinicians from learning about and treating this area. However, we would encourage you to embrace your knowledge of the spine: read, study, and remain up to date on current spine research, including the mechanics of and treatment of various pathological conditions. One semester of injury evaluation is not going to make you an expert—you must get out there and practice, practice, practice. Find mentors who feel competent evaluating the spine, and learn from them.

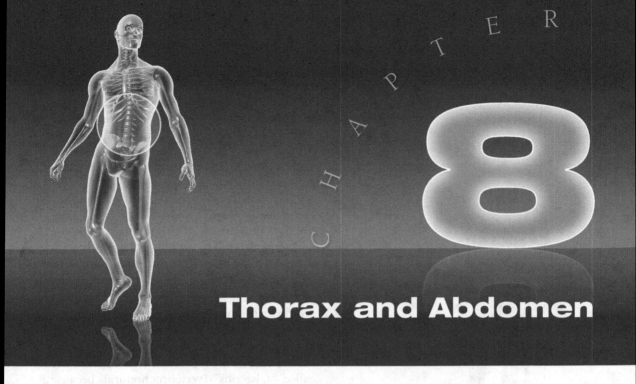

Thorax and Abdomen

INTRODUCTION

T his chapter will provide ten different scenarios that will cover injuries to the thorax and abdominal regions. Particular emphasis will be placed on the major thoracic and abdominal organs of these regions, but other conditions and injuries will also be presented. As with all scenarios in this text, they are presented in a manner to provide enough crucial information to answer the questions. However, some information will be intentionally omitted, and presented sometimes in the wrong order, to promote critical thinking skills. Although a multitude of pathologies could be presented, most of these cases focus on common conditions found in the literature. We did select some that are rare, but life threatening.

In order to decipher and solve the case scenarios effectively, a brief overview of the anatomy, including the bones, muscles, abdominal organs, and nerves, will be presented. Additional information, such as special tests, will also be briefly discussed to help you remember previous course materials or clinical experiences.

ANATOMICAL REVIEW

A n outer skeletal framework (ribs and sternum) and strong abdominal muscles function together for protection of the internal organs and other anatomical structures (Figure 8.1). One of the main bones of the thorax region is the sternum. The sternum is a flat bone that forms the anterior section of the thoracic cage and consists of three distinct parts: manubrium, body, and xiphoid (Figure 8.2). The manubrium is typically found at the level of T3 (T stands for thoracic) and T4 vertebral level and has a triangular shape, with a jugular notch on the superior portion and

FIGURE 8.1

Musculoskeletal framework of support for the internal organs of the thorax and abdomen.

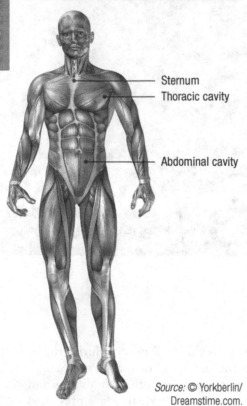

Sternum
Thoracic cavity

Abdominal cavity

Source: © Yorkberlin/
Dreamstime.com.

clavicular notches on both sides just below the jugular notch. The sternal angle (also known as the angle of Louis) is found roughly at the T4 and T5 vertebral region and separates the manubrium from the body of the sternum.[7] The body of the sternum is found in the T5 to T9 vertebral region. At the base of the sternal body is the xiphoid process, which is cartilaginous until roughly the age of 40.

The ribs make up the thoracic cavity. They are generally curved, narrow, flat bones (Figure 8.3) that attach to the thoracic vertebrae and wrap around to articulate anteriorly with the costal cartilage of the sternum, with the last two ribs "floating," meaning they are not attached to the sternum. Typically, the 12 ribs are divided into sections (Figure 8.4). Ribs 1 through 7 are called "true ribs" (vertebrosternal) because they attach directly to the sternum via the costal cartilage. Ribs 8 through 10 are called "false ribs" (vertebrochondral) because they attach to the cartilage of the rib superior to them. Ribs 11 and 12 are considered "floating ribs" because they do not attach to the cartilage and float in the posterior/lateral abdominal cavity.[1,3,4] A typical rib consists of articular facets on the head that attach to the vertebrae, a neck, a tubercle that articulates with the transverse process, and a body (shaft)

FIGURE 8.2   Anterior view of the sternum.

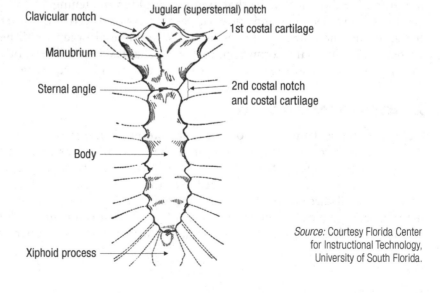

Clavicular notch

Jugular (supersternal) notch

1st costal cartilage

Manubrium

Sternal angle

2nd costal notch
and costal cartilage

Body

Xiphoid process

Source: Courtesy Florida Center
for Instructional Technology,
University of South Florida.

that has an angle curving around in an anterior direction (Figure 8.3). The tenth through the twelfth ribs have one facet, and the eleventh and twelfth ribs have no necks or tubercles.

Thoracic and Abdominal Muscles

The muscles of the thorax and abdomen aid in respiration, protect internal organs, or are used for movement (Table 8.1; see also Table 7.6, Chapter 7, for additional abdominal muscle action).[5]

Muscles of the thorax

Starting superficially, the thorax has similarly functioning muscles covering the chest region, the pectoralis ("pect" for short) major and minor. Below these muscles, located between the ribs, are the intercostal muscles (external and internal). The external intercostal muscles are found on the inferior border of the ribs and attach to the superior border of the rib below; the internal intercostal muscles are found on the inner surface and costal cartilages of the ribs and insert to the superior border of the rib below. The external intercostal muscles help elevate the ribs, and the internal intercostal muscles help depress the rib cage during

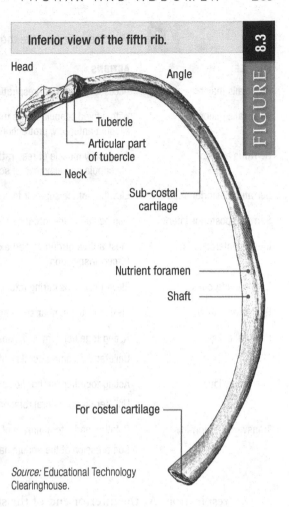

FIGURE 8.3

Inferior view of the fifth rib.

Head
Angle
Tubercle
Articular part of tubercle
Neck
Sub-costal cartilage
Nutrient foramen
Shaft
For costal cartilage

Source: Educational Technology Clearinghouse.

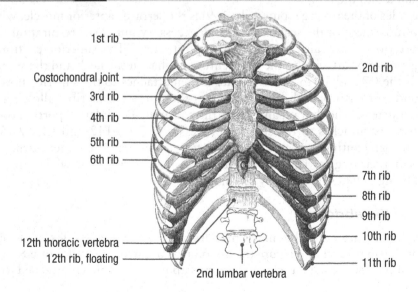

FIGURE   8.4   Thoracic cavity.

1st rib
2nd rib
Costochondral joint
3rd rib
4th rib
5th rib
6th rib
7th rib
8th rib
9th rib
10th rib
12th thoracic vertebra
12th rib, floating
11th rib
2nd lumbar vertebra

Source: Gray's Anatomy

TABLE 8.1	Muscles acting on the thoracic and abdominal regions.[1,5]
MUSCLE	**ACTIONS**
Pectoralis major	Accessory muscle of respiration, horizontal shoulder adduction, medial rotation of arm
Pectoralis minor	With a fixed scapula raises the third to fifth rib during forced inspiration, tilting of scapula anteriorly, protraction and medial rotation of scapula
Serratus anterior	Accessory muscle of respiration, abduction and lateral rotation of scapula, depression of scapula and elevation of scapula
Serratus posterior superior	Elevation of the superior four ribs
Serratus posterior inferior	Depression of the inferior four ribs
Internal intercostals	Most active during forced expiration, portion acts with external intercostals during forced inspiration
External intercostals	Elevation of ribs during forced inspiration
Rectus abdominis	Flexion of the lumbar spine against gravity and compression of abdominal content
External oblique	Acting together, lumbar flexion Unilaterally, contralateral rotation of the trunk and ipsilateral lateral flexion of the trunk
Internal oblique	Acting together, lumbar flexion Unilaterally, ipsilateral rotation and flexion of the trunk
Transverse abdominis	Rotation and lateral flexion of the trunk (opposite side) Compression of the abdominal content and lumbar spine stabilization

respiration. At the inferior end of the sternum/xiphoid process region and extending throughout the inferior region of the rib complex is the diaphragm. The diaphragm assists with respiration by increasing the size or cavity of the thorax region, allowing air to be pulled into the lungs.

On the sides of the rib cage (outer ribs 1–9) is the serratus anterior muscle, which assists with movement of the scapula and is an accessory muscle of respiration. The serratus posterior muscle also assists with inspiration.[2,3,7] The superior portion of the serratus posterior attaches to the ligamentum nuchae in the neck and the spinous processes of the C7 and T1 to T3 vertebrae. It then attaches to the superior borders of the second to fourth or fifth ribs. It elevates the inferior four ribs, allowing for increased diameter of the thorax, and raises the sternum. The inferior portion of the serratus posterior attaches to the spinous processes of T11–T12 and L1–L2 (8th–12th ribs). It then continues to attach to the inferior borders of the inferior three or four ribs near their angles. This muscle depresses the inferior ribs, which prevents them from being pulled superiorly by the diaphragm.

Muscles of the abdomen

In the abdominal region, the abdominal muscles act to flex, laterally flex, and rotate the trunk and help protect and secure the abdominal organs in place (Figure 8.5).[1,2,5] The largest of the abdominal muscles is the rectus abdominis, which is attached to the

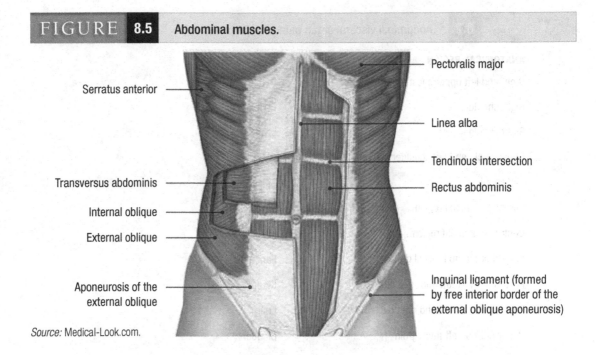

FIGURE 8.5 Abdominal muscles.

Pectoralis major

Serratus anterior

Linea alba

Tendinous intersection

Transversus abdominis

Rectus abdominis

Internal oblique

External oblique

Aponeurosis of the external oblique

Inguinal ligament (formed by free interior border of the external oblique aponeurosis)

Source: Medical-Look.com.

rib cage superiorly and the pubic region inferiorly. A line (called the "linea alba") runs down the middle of the rectus abdominis. The linea alba divides the muscle into left and right portions, and three transverse lines divide the muscle into separate sections running superiorly to inferiorly. The internal and external oblique muscles assist with lateral flexion and rotation. The external oblique attaches to the lower ribs and runs inferiorly and obliquely to the ilium, pubic crest, and fascia of the rectus abdominis. The internal oblique arises from the iliac crest, inguinal ligament, and lumbar fascia and runs superiorly and obliquely to ribs 10 through 12 on each side. The transverse abdominis primarily holds abdominal contents in place. It attaches to the outer inguinal ligament and iliac crest and other structures and inserts onto the linea alba, xiphiod process, and pubis.

Thoracic and Visceral Organs

The thorax and abdominal cavity houses numerous organs, all of which are needed to sustain life (Figure 8.6). Each organ has special features and functions, but only a general overview of the organ's main function, its location in the body, and any pain-referral pattern will be presented. A brief synopsis of organ pain-referral patterns in this area of the body is provided in Table 8.2 and Figure 8.7.

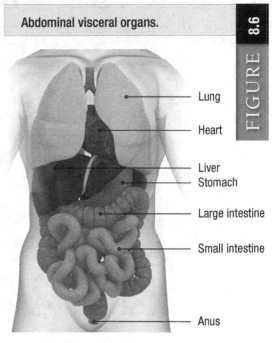

Abdominal visceral organs.

FIGURE 8.6

Lung

Heart

Liver
Stomach

Large intestine

Small intestine

Anus

Source: Eraxion/Dreamstime.com.

TABLE 8.2 Abdominal visceral organ pain referral patterns.[1-3]

ANATOMICAL REGION	ORGAN REFERRAL
Right and left upper chest and shoulders	Diaphragm
Right shoulder	Gallbladder
Right shoulder	Liver
Chest, neck, and left shoulder and arm	Heart
Left shoulder	Spleen
Throat/abdominal region	Stomach
Central abdominal region	Intestine
Central or left abdominal region	Pancreas
Posterior lower left and right back	Kidney
Posterior upper left and right back	Lung
Upper right or left thigh/groin	Bladder

Reported pain referral patterns may vary slightly among sources.

FIGURE 8.7 Anterior thorax and abdominal pain referral patterns.

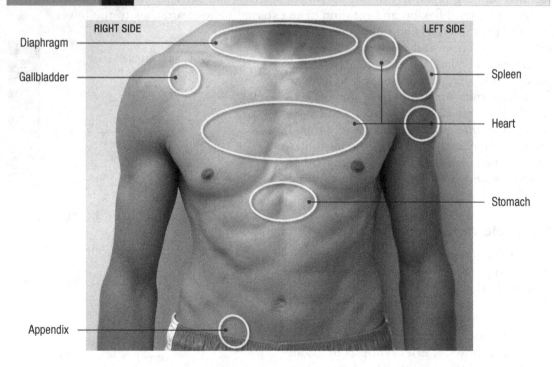

Circles indicate generalized locations of selected pain referral patterns.

Lungs

Within the thoracic cavity are the lungs: a right lung with three lobes, and a left lung with two lobes. Each lung is surrounded by a pleural sac, with the parietal pleura surrounding the chest cavity and the visceral pleura surrounding the lungs. The lungs have an apex, three surfaces (costal, mediastinal, and diaphragmatic), and three borders (anterior, inferior, and posterior). Running from the trachea to the lungs are the right and left bronchi, and these divide into smaller passageways. Within each lung are alveoli (air sacs), the smallest divisions in the lung. They branch off the bronchi and expand and contract with each ventilation.

Heart

The heart is positioned just to the left of and underneath the sternum, and it is surrounded by a sac called the pericardium. The heart is composed of four chambers, multiple valves, arteries, and veins and is about the size of a clinched fist. The walls of each chamber have three distinct layers: endocardium (internal), myocardium (middle), and epicardium (external). The right atrium collects the venous blood that flows through the tricuspid valve between the right atrium and right ventricle. The deoxygenated blood is pumped out of the right ventricle to the lungs via the pulmonary artery. After the blood receives oxygen in the lungs, it flows back to the left atrium via the pulmonary vein. The blood exits the left atrium through the mitral valve to the left ventricle. Blood is pumped from the left ventricle to the aorta, where it branches off to deliver oxygenated blood throughout the body. Damage to the heart has pain-referral patterns to the left shoulder and neck, upper arm and forearm, and sternum.

Liver

On the right side of the body, just below the right lung, is the liver. The liver is found in the upper right quadrant of the abdomen area and is the largest internal organ. The liver is divided into two separate lobes and serves to assist in digestion, glucose regulation, and filtration of chemicals within the body. Injury or damage to the liver will refer pain to the right shoulder.

Gallbladder

Located inferiorly to the liver is the pear-shaped gallbladder. The gallbladder stores the bile that is secreted from the liver and releases it into the small intestine for digestion. The pain-referral pattern for this organ is to the top right shoulder.

Stomach and intestines

The stomach is located to the middle and left of the esophagus and small intestine. It mixes and stores food and secretes gastric acids needed for digestion. Only small amounts of absorption occur in the stomach, though caffeine and alcohol are readily absorbed. Pain can be referred via the throat and abdominal region.

Food leaving the stomach passes into the small intestine, which is a hollow organ. It has three distinct sections: duodenum, jejunum, and ileum. Despite its name, the small intestine can be as long as 20 feet. Nutrients from food are absorbed primarily in the small intestine. The pain-referral pattern is usually located to the central abdomen.

Extending from the small intestine is the large intestine. The large intestine is approximately seven feet in length and divided into three distinct sections; cecum, colon, and rectum. Pain referral is usually to the lower abdomen area.

Spleen

The spleen, the largest lymphatic organ, lies inferior to the diaphragm on the left side, at approximately the ninth through eleventh ribs. The spleen stores red blood cells, helps regulate the release of blood cells into the body, and produces antibodies. Injury to the spleen will refer pain to the left shoulder, referred to as the Kehr's sign.

Pancreas

Between the small intestine and the spleen is the pancreas. The main function of the pancreas is the production of secretions to aid in the digestion of foodstuff and the production of insulin and glucagon to control the amount of glucose or amino acids in the bloodstream. Pancreatic pain can be referred to the anterior abdomen, at the center or left side.

Kidneys

The kidneys are located approximately in the center of the back, one on either side of the spine. They function as filters of the bloodstream and expel waste products via the urine. Pain can be referred to the posterior lower back.

Appendix

The appendix is located in the lower right quadrant of the abdomen at the anatomical landmark called "McBurney's point" (Figure 8.8). The size of the appendix is approximately 10 cm long on average. The appendix is generally thought to have no major function within the human body, but an infection to the appendix (appendicitis) may cause severe pain and even death, necessitating its removal. Pain from the appendix is usually referred to the umbilicus and lower right abdomen.

FIGURE 8.8

McBurney's point.

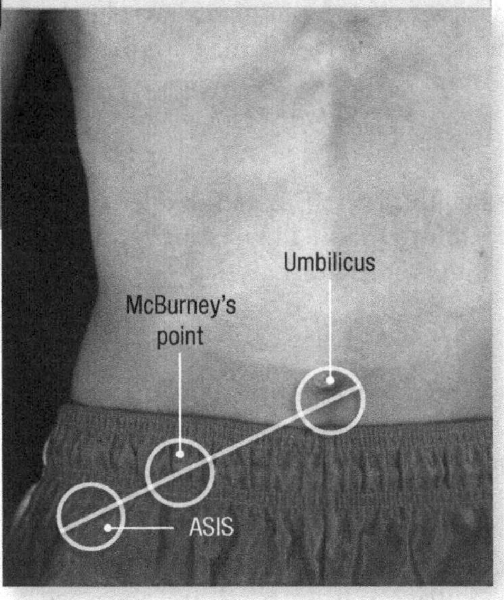

Umbilicus

McBurney's point

ASIS

McBurney's point is one third of the way between the right ASIS and the umbilicus.

Bladder

The bladder is located behind the pubic symphysis bone. It stores urine from the kidneys to be eliminated from the body. Most often, the pain-referral pattern is found in the inner thigh and groin area.

Reproductive organs

The male and female reproductive organs are found both inside and outside (male) the abdominal cavity. The specific functions and anatomical markings can be found in other reference materials.

Abdominal and Thorax Quadrants

The abdominal organs can be classified into regions or quadrants for ease of identification. Usually the abdominal and thorax region is divided into the four quadrants (Figure 8.9) used in this text, but it may also be divided into nine sections (Figure 8.10). To divide the abdomen into four quadrants, a vertical line is drawn through the umbilicus region to divide the abdominal/thoracic region into right and left halves. Another line is then drawn transversely through the umbilicus to divide the abdominal region into an upper or lower half. The right upper quadrant (RUQ) houses organs such as the liver, gallbladder, head of the pancreas, kidney, and right lung. The left upper quadrant (LUQ) houses organs such as the spleen, stomach, body and tail of the pancreas, kidney, left lung, and heart. The right lower quadrant (RLQ) houses organs such as the appendix, cecum, ascending colon, right ovary or right spermatic cord, right ureter, and part of the bladder. The left lower quadrant (LLQ) houses organs such as the descending colon, sigmoid colon, rectum, left ovary or left spermatic cord, left ureter, and part of the bladder.

Abdominal Organ Assessment

Assessing the abdominal organs is difficult because the athletic trainer cannot visually inspect the organs. Instead, the athletic trainer must rely on palpation, referred pain patterns, and auscultation to help evaluate potential injuries.[1]

Palpation

Palpating the abdominal or thoracic region should be conducted in a systematic fashion, beginning at the superior thoracic region and working inferiorly. The patient should be placed in a supine position, with the arms to the side and the knees and hips slightly flexed to alleviate stresses on the thorax and

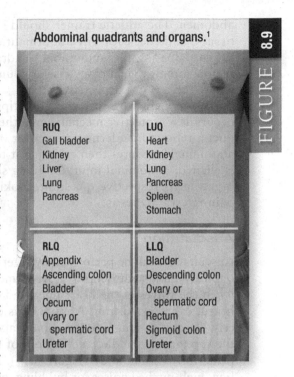

Abdominal quadrants and organs.[1]

FIGURE 8.9

RUQ	LUQ
Gall bladder	Heart
Kidney	Kidney
Liver	Lung
Lung	Pancreas
Pancreas	Spleen
	Stomach

RLQ	LLQ
Appendix	Bladder
Ascending colon	Descending colon
Bladder	Ovary or
Cecum	spermatic cord
Ovary or	Rectum
spermatic cord	Sigmoid colon
Ureter	Ureter

Together the abdominal cavity (houses the visceral organs) and the pelvic cavity (houses the reproductive organs, bladder, and rectum) comprise the abdominopelvic cavity.

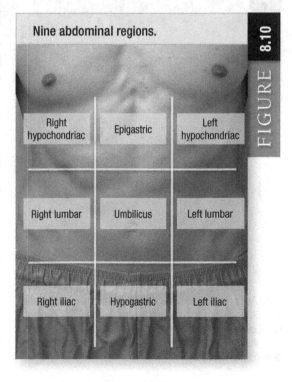

Nine abdominal regions.

FIGURE 8.10

Right hypochondriac	Epigastric	Left hypochondriac
Right lumbar	Umbilicus	Left lumbar
Right iliac	Hypogastric	Left iliac

abdomen. The athletic trainer should palpate all bony tissue first, followed by soft tissues, and check for any abnormalities (e.g., abdominal rigidity and distention). When palpating the abdominal quadrants, the athletic trainer should begin at a region and move in a clockwise or counter-clockwise fashion, starting from an area where there is no suspected injury.

When palpating, use the fingertips and feel for abdominal rigidity. Rigidity occurs as a protective mechanism of the body to splint the area that is injured. Conduct a rebound tenderness maneuver by pressing the tissue firmly down (to create abdominal pressure) then releasing it to relieve the pressure. Upon release, if pain is elicited, abdominal injury/bleeding should be suspected. Be sure to palpate each organ in its respective quadrant, looking and feeling for rigidity, tenderness, and pain-referral patterns.

Auscultation

Auscultation can be performed by listening to the sounds of thoracic and abdominal organs with a stethoscope. Heart sounds are distinctive, having a "lub-dub" sound when the valves of the heart open and close. Sometimes a soft or blowing sound is heard, called a murmur. A murmur is caused by a valve that does not work properly. Breath or lung sounds should also be examined. Place the stethoscope over the top (apex), middle, and bottom of the lungs on both sides, both anteriorly and posteriorly on the body (Figure 8.11). Abnormal sounds, such as wheezing, crackling, high-pitched noises, or bubbling, may indicate injury or illness, and proper care and medical referral may be required. Bowel sounds are more difficult to decipher. Bowels normally have gurgling or peristaltic sounds, and in many cases, there may be no sounds at all. A stethoscope can be placed anywhere within the bowel region to assess bowel sounds. Percussion of the organs, which identifies the sound of the organ, should be conducted on each internal organ when appropriate. A solid organ has a dull, thumping sound; a hollow organ may have a resonant or tympanic sound.

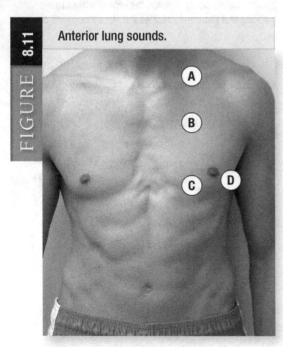

FIGURE 8.11

Anterior lung sounds.

Note: Auscultation should be performed comparing right to left at each position before moving lower. A = Apex, B = Middle, C = Lower, D = Midaxillary position. Consult a text on lung auscultation procedures for more locations and an explanation of abnormal sounds.

SPECIAL TESTS

There are relatively few special tests used for assessing injuries of the thoracic and abdominal regions. When injuries do occur in these regions, pain and pain-referral patterns should be used as a guide for care and to determine medical referral. Rib tests include compression in both an anterior and posterior direction and from the lateral sides.[6] For abdominal organs, percussion and auscultation examinations are required.[6] In addition, examination of urine color for blood and abdominal walls for discoloration, and assessment of breathing for abnormalities are all important, because these are indicators for serious internal trauma. For a more thorough review, please refer to your favorite evaluation text or journal article(s).

REFERENCES

1. Anderson MK, Hall SJ, Martin M. *Foundation of Athletic Training: Prevention, Assessment, and Management.* Philadelphia, PA: Lippincott Williams & Wilkins; 2005.

2. Behnke RS. *Kinetic Anatomy.* Champaign, IL: Human Kinetics; 2001.

3. Clemente CD. *Anatomy: A Regional Atlas of the Human Body.* (4th ed.). Baltimore, MD: Lippincott Williams & Wilkins; 1997.

4. Evans RC. *Illustrated Essentials in Orthopedic Physical Assessment.* St. Louis, MO: Mosby; 1994.

5. Kendall FP, McCreary EK. *Muscles Testing and Function.* (3rd ed.). Baltimore, MD: Lippincott Williams & Wilkins; 1983.

6. Magee DJ. *Orthopedic Physical Assessment.* (4th ed.). Philadelphia, PA: Saunders; 2002.

7. Moore KL, Agur AMR. *Essential Clinical Anatomy.* Baltimore, MD: Lippincott Williams & Wilkins; 1995.

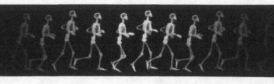

Billy, a 21-year-old lacrosse player at a midwestern Division II University, collided with a teammate during practice. He was hit in the chest region by his teammate's shoulder. Billy did not seek immediate medical attention, because the discomfort was minimal. He waited until the day after this event to seek treatment from Monica, the certified athletic trainer for the team.

HISTORY

Monica asks Billy to explain the event leading up to his CC. Billy relates the history of the event, explaining the contact with his teammate's shoulder, and proceeds to describe chest discomfort, mild pain, and dyspnea. Although his symptoms are not severe, Billy is worried because they are not getting better. He rated his pain as 5/10. Billy denies any prior health or medical conditions related to this incident and any other medical conditions.

PHYSICAL EXAMINATION

Billy is alert and in minor-to-moderate discomfort. Monica observes no obvious evidence of significant trauma other than some ecchymosis on his chest wall. Palpation of the ribs on the side of the injury reveals no point tenderness, only slight discomfort. Monica assesses Billy's respiration at 21 per minute, and he has heart rate and blood pressure values within normal limits. Range of motion of the upper extremity of the affected side is unremarkable, and all dermatomes, myotomes, and peripheral nerves are within normal limits.

Later that same day, Billy's condition is no better, and even worsening. Breathing is becoming more shallow and labored. Monica refers Billy to the team physician. He auscultates the lungs and determines an abnormal result. Percussion testing to the affected side also reveals an abnormal finding, a hyperresonance sound. The physician determines Billy needs to be sent to the hospital immediately for further evaluation and examination for a suspected injury. Radiographs are negative for fracture of the ribs, scapula, or sternum; however, an abnormal shadow is noticed on the radiographs.

Please answer the following questions based on the above case information.

8.1 / **1.** Based on the information presented in the case, determine (a) the differential diagnoses and (b) the clinical diagnosis.

8.1 / **2.** What is the immediate management for this condition?

8.1 / **3.** (a) What other signs and symptoms may be presented with this injury?
(b) What precautions should an athletic trainer take?

8.1 / **4.** After Billy is diagnosed and treated appropriately, (a) when should he be allowed to return to play? (b) Should any other restrictions be put in place?

8.1 / **5.** This condition often is classified by two separate causes: one is spontaneous; the other traumatic. Please describe both.

Andrew and Tara, certified athletic trainers, were contracted to cover an amateur track and field event sponsored by a local sports medicine clinic. It was a beautiful day, with temperatures hovering around the middle 80s and a full sun. The medical tent where Andrew and Tara were stationed was at the corner of the track, about 100 meters from the start/finish line. The athletic trainers informed all coaches of the exact location of the medical tent and told the coaches to refer all athletes to them at the tent if necessary. The day was passing uneventfully, with most athletes presenting with blisters or slight dehydration problems.

HISTORY

At the end of the 1,500 meter run, one of the athletes, a 19-year-old male, collapsed about 5 meters past the finish line. The athlete's coach was at the finish line and approached the athlete only to find him unresponsive. The coach immediately contacted Andrew and Tara, who were on the scene in approximately 30 seconds.

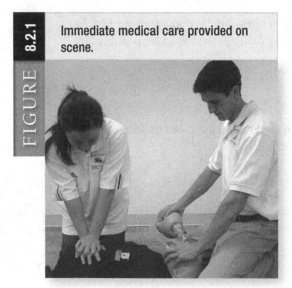

FIGURE 8.2.1

Immediate medical care provided on scene.

ON-SCENE ARRIVAL

On initial assessment, Andrew found the athlete to be unresponsive. Immediate medical care was initiated (Figure 8.2.1), along with activating EMS. When paramedics arrived about 3 minutes later, Andrew and Tara were still providing care. EMS immediately connected the athlete to an AED, and three shocks were administered without resolution. The athlete was packaged and transported to the local medical facility, following local EMS protocol.

FOLLOW-UP

After the scene cleared, Andrew and Tara began completing their paperwork. An interview with the coach revealed that the athlete had no previous injury or medical history of significance that he was aware of, and he never had an incident involving a heat-related emergency before. Medical personnel at the facility informed Andrew and Tara that the athlete died at the hospital.

Please answer the following questions based on the above case information.

8.2 / **1.** Based on the information presented in the case, identify the clinical diagnosis.

8.2 / **2.** Andrew and Tara initiated immediate medical care, as identified in Figure 8.2.1, after the primary assessment. Looking at the figure, (a) what is the name of this procedure? (b) Do they appear to be performing the procedure correctly?

8.2 / **3.** (a) Did Andrew and Tara handle the situation appropriately? (b) Outline the management steps you would employ in this same situation.

8.2 / **4.** What are some associated medical conditions that may be involved in the outcome of the above scenario?

8.2 / **5.** It has been postulated that pre-participation examinations (PPE) should screen for heart-related irregularities. What are some screening questions and tests that should be used to help detect abnormalities? When should an athlete be restricted from athletic participation?

CASE 8.3

Antwan's location of pain.

Antwan's location of palpable tenderness.

The palpable tenderness falls along the line and under the fingers.

Suko, an athletic training student at a National Association of Intercollegiate Athletics (NAIA) Division II college, was working with her certified athletic trainer, Will, to cover fall football practice. Heavy rain had made for a miserable practice, and players were slipping in the mud. While Will was taping an athlete's sprained ankle on the sideline, Suko was watching the wide receivers' drills. Antwan, one of the wide receivers, dove for a ball with his left arm over his head and landed on his left side. She noted that he was slow to get up, but he eventually went back in line for his next rotation. During his next rotation, Antwan did not perform to his usual physical abilities. Afterward, he approached Suko to inform her that his left side hurt.

HISTORY

Suko starts by saying, "I saw you land pretty hard on that left side, how do your ribs feel?" Antwan replied, "My ribs feel ok, a little sore, but you know most of my pain is up in here (Figure 8.3.1) but I guess that's just from falling on the shoulder." He denies any previous history of rib or chest trauma. He reports no changes to his neurological status.

PHYSICAL EXAMINATION

Antwan is alert, is in minor-to-moderate discomfort, and has some difficulty removing his shoulder pads. Suko's observation of Antwan is unremarkable, and she does not notice any discoloration or distention at the site of injury. She begins palpating the thorax (anterior and posterior) and notices some palpable tenderness (Figure 8.3.2) on the left flank. He also has some slight rebound tenderness in the upper left quadrant. She records his pulse at 92 and strong, his respiration at 20 and normal, and his blood pressure at 114/70. Suko also examines his left shoulder for pathology and does not find any abnormal indications or shoulder pathology when compared with his right shoulder. Suko escorts Antwan over to see Will on the other side of the field.

FOLLOW-UP EXAMINATION

A re-evaluation 10 minutes later by Will finds similar signs and symptoms; however, Antwan's vital signs are changing (Table 8.3.1a and b). Will suspects something is going on, and Antwan is immediately transferred to the local medical facility, arriving 45 minutes after the initial injury.

TABLE	8.3.1	Antwan's vital signs.

(a) Side-Line baseline.

VITAL SIGNS	FINDINGS
Pulse	92, regular, and strong
Respiration	20 and normal
Blood pressure	114/70
Mental status	Alert and oriented

(b) Side-Line follow-up.

VITAL SIGNS	FINDINGS
Pulse	110 and thready
Respiration	25, shallow and labored
Blood pressure	102/60
Mental status	Alert and disoriented

Please answer the following questions based on the above case information.

8.3 / **1.** Based on the information presented in the case, determine (a) the differential diagnoses and (b) the probable clinical diagnosis.

8.3 / **2.** The literature suggests that this injury is made worse if a specific illness is present before sustaining a traumatic event. What is the illness?

8.3 / **3.** Management of injuries to the abdominal region is based on signs, symptoms, severity, location, and what other factor(s)?

8.3 / **4.** What are the special tests or signs used to assess this injury?

8.3 / **5.** After completing the physical examination, Will helped Suko to document her findings electronically and sent a copy of the report to Antwan's physician. Using your athletic training room's computer tracking software, document your findings electronically as if you were the treating clinician. If the report does not provide information you believe is pertinent to the clinical diagnosis, please add this information to your documentation. If you do not have access to injury tracking software, consider downloading a trial version from CSMI Solutions (Sportsware) at

www.csmisolutions.com/cmt/publish/service_software_dl.shtml

and following the on-screen directions.

CASE

8.4

imothy, a 23-year-old volleyball player for a collegiate team in the southwest, was having a great game as a blocker. He has led the conference in the number of blocks per game, thanks in part to his 6'5" height and his 180 pound weight, with a 42-inch vertical jump. He is physically fit and spends a great deal of time working on conditioning and balance exercises.

HISTORY

During the game, Timothy jumps in the air to block a shot. Since he is out of position, his jump comes too far back from the net, exposing a four-foot gap between him and the net. An opposing player, seeing this opportunity, drills a spike directly at Timothy, smashing him in the upper right thorax. Timothy immediately grabbed the area and winces in pain. The coach calls a time-out, and Timothy goes to the bench to see Rochelle, the certified athletic trainer.

PHYSICAL EXAMINATION

Timothy is leaning slightly forward, using his hands to cover his right thorax on the lateral side where the ribs angle around the body (Figure 8.4.1). He reports his pain as 8/10. His respirations are noticeably shallow and rapid. He feels very uncomfortable moving his hand over his head or making excessive body movements. Rochelle palpates this site of injury and notices point tenderness over the area. There is no immediate discoloration or swelling and no obvious deformity. Timothy does not have any referred pain pattern to his right shoulder or flank or groin areas, and he is not coughing or spitting blood. Rochelle decides to apply pressure to the area (rib compression test), and Timothy winces in pain.

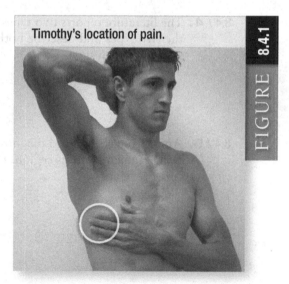

Timothy's location of pain.

FIGURE 8.4.1

Pain and tenderness is located within the circle.

? | Q U E S T I O N S   CASE 8.4

Please answer the following questions based on the above case information.

8.4 / **1.** Based on the information presented in the case, determine (a) the differential diagnoses and (b) the clinical diagnosis.

8.4 / **2.** What is the immediate management for this type of condition?

8.4 / **3.** Injuries to this area often are associated with other potentially damaging injuries. Please list some possible associated or secondary injuries.

8.4 / **4.** The literature reports two types of classifications for the injury. Please name the two types and describe both the MOIs and sports that may be associated with each type.

8.4 / **5.** Apart from the clinical diagnosis, stress fractures can also occur within the bony segments of this region. Please describe the etiology of how these fractures develop.

Fernandez, a certified athletic trainer, works at a local sports medicine clinic in the morning and at an industrial factory providing outreach in the afternoon. He was approached during the early evening by an employee, Tina. Tina, a 42-year-old female, had been working at the plant for 10 years. Her position in the assembly line entails long periods of standing and being under extreme pressure to assemble parts at a rapid pace. She is paid by the amount of parts fabricated correctly. Tina's current assignment is making parts for doors used in automobiles. Her chief complaint when she found Fernandez is of chest pain. Fernandez immediately has her begin completing the required OSHA and employer injury documentation, including a pain chart (Figure 8.5.1).

HISTORY

Fernandez pulls Tina's medical file and reviews her medical background while she is completing the documentation. Tina has no prior significant medical history conditions, except for a fractured ulna when she was 12. She reports no known medical diseases but has a family history of heart disease and high blood pressure. Tina's CCs are chest tightness and some pain in her left shoulder. She had been experiencing this pain for about a month, with the pain more pronounced during her working shifts than in her non-employed time, though the pain never seems to go away completely. She explains that when she takes a deep breath or coughs, her chest feels uncomfortable. Tina rates her pain as about 7/10.

| FIGURE | 8.5.1 | Tina's pain profile. |

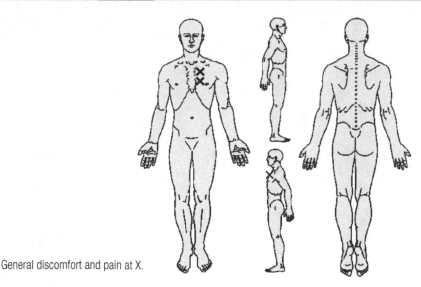

General discomfort and pain at X.

FIGURE   8.5.2

Special test eliciting pain near the sternum.

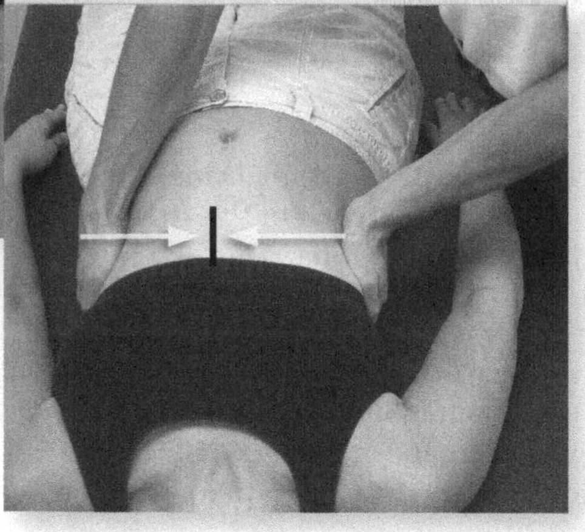

Arrows indicate the direction of force applied to the lateral rib cage. Thick single line indicates location of pain elicited by the test.

PHYSICAL EXAMINATION

Tina is alert and oriented. Her blood pressure is 120/80, pulse rate is 80, and respiration is 14 per minute. Tina cannot recall any particular incident of chest trauma or blow to the chest. Upon palpation, Fernandez is able to elicit pain at the rib/sternal junctions of the upper ribs, predominately around ribs two through five. Compression on the sternum also elicits pain. The test shown in Figure 8.5.2 elicits pain near the sternum. All shoulder and upper extremity ROM is within normal limits, but elevated movements cause slight discomfort in her chest.

Because many of her signs and symptoms suggests a heart-related pathology, Fernandez immediately refers Tina to the hospital for further analysis. Two days later, Tina visits with Fernandez. All heart-related conditions were ruled out. Instead, the diagnostic X-rays reveal another chest pathology that commonly mimics chest pain.

Please answer the following questions based on the above case information.

8.5 / **1.** Based on the information presented in the case, determine (a) the differential diagnoses and (b) the clinical diagnosis.

8.5 / **2.** This condition is sometimes confused with a similar disorder that affects the same region. (a) Please identify and describe this similar disorder. (b) How can a clinician differentiate between the two disorders?

8.5 / **3.** Aspegren, Hyde, and Miller have found that several treatment methods have been effective for managing this disorder. Please (a) describe the methods, and (b) discuss which methods may be most appropriate in managing this condition.

8.5 / **4.** Palpation is an important part of the assessment of this condition. A good understanding of the anatomy is important for successful palpation. Describe the anatomy of the structures involved in this condition and the bony structures you would have palpated.

8.5 / **5.** Overall, do you believe Fernandez performed an adequate evaluation? What, if anything, would you as the evaluating clinician have done differently?

CASE

8.6

P lacido is a male athletic trainer working part-time for the Bullets, a semi-professional men's ice hockey team. Placido has been the club's athletic trainer for four
years. His full-time position is Director of Rehabilitation for a sports medicine clinic.

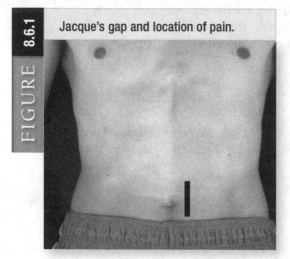

FIGURE 8.6.1

Jacque's gap and location of pain.

Thick line indicates location of the gap and pain.

FIGURE 8.6.2

Positive functional test.

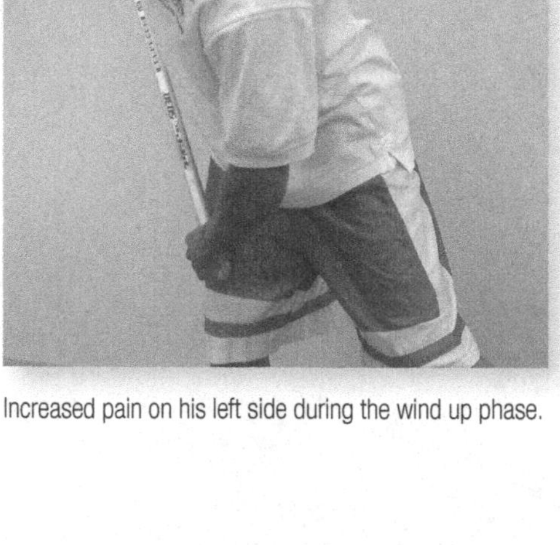

Increased pain on his left side during the wind up phase.

HISTORY

At practice, one of the offensive players,
24-year-old Jacque, approaches Placido during a break. Jacque states that his abdominal
region is painful and sore. His discomfort has
increased over the past three days, but he decided to seek medical attention only today
because his pain is limiting his shot. Jacque
does not recall any direct contact to the abdominal area in the last several days, but he
has been practicing his slap shot more frequently over the past week, often shooting 50
to 100 times a night after practice to improve
his shooting.

PHYSICAL EXAMINATION

Placido meets with Jacque after practice
for a thorough examination. Jacque is alert
and in moderate discomfort. He has already
showered and is wearing shorts and a shirt.
Placido immediately notes that Jacque is in
obvious discomfort when he is asked to remove his shirt. He is slow at removing the
shirt, with an increase in pain as he raises
his arms overhead. Initial inspection reveals
no gross abnormalities. There are no signs
of swelling or discoloration. Palpation of
the area is normal except for a slight gap in
Jacque's left lower abdominal musculature,
about two inches to the left of his umbilicus
(Figure 8.6.1). Jacque also reports tenderness
with pressure at the site. Placido has Jacque
lie supine and asks him to pick each leg up
independently, which he does, but with slight
difficulty keeping his abdomen tight in these
motions. In addition, when Placido asks him
to mimic a slap shot motion (Figure 8.6.2),
Jacque winces while in the windup phase.

Jacque's upper extremity strength is normal, but he has slight discomfort with all muscle grading and when the abdominals are used in accessory motions. He says there is no obvious blood in his urine and no referred pain to his shoulders or flank.

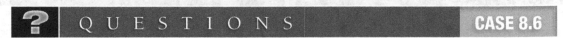

? QUESTIONS   **CASE 8.6**

Please answer the following questions based on the above case information.

8.6 / **1.** Based on the information presented in the case, determine (a) the differential diagnoses and (b) the clinical diagnosis.

8.6 / **2.** What is the major function of the muscle(s) in this region?

8.6 / **3.** What is the major MOI for this injury and the associated signs and symptoms?

8.6 / **4.** Based on the information presented in the case, (a) why didn't Placido perform any special tests? (b) What, if anything, would you have done differently as the evaluating clinician? (c) How would you manage this condition?

8.6 / **5.** What are some common sports in which this injury occurs?

CASE 8.7

T wenty-one-year-old Jennifer is a female college gymnastic athlete who has been involved in the sport since she was five. Jennifer was practicing on the uneven bars when she missed a dismount and landed flat on her stomach. Her head did not touch the ground. She got off the mat and walked over to the side of the gymnasium, obviously in some discomfort. Brad, the senior athletic training student, was sent over by the supervising athletic trainer, Leona, who was busy taping other athletes in the gymnastics room and could not examine Jennifer's injury.

HISTORY

Brad approaches Jennifer and asks about the injury. Jennifer explains that she fell off the beam, landing on her stomach and chest. She explains, "My chest, particularly my left side, is throbbing." Brad questions Jennifer about head or neck pain, which she denies. She reports no pain or discomfort to her extremities. Her only symptom is left breast pain.

PHYSICAL EXAMINATION

Brad begins his assessment by palpating the whole spine. He notes no abnormality, pain, or other neurological signs and symptoms (myotome, dermatome, and peripheral nerves appear intact throughout the upper and lower extremity). He notes that Jennifer is not gasping for breath but that inspirations appear slightly painful. Brad then proceeds to palpate Jennifer's left breast area looking for tenderness or deformity of the underlying ribs. Jennifer only reports tenderness to the breast itself.

Meanwhile, Leona, the supervising athletic trainer, comes over to Brad while he is assessing Jennifer's injury. Leona immediately intervenes and tells Brad to go wait in her office. Leona reviews the MOI and signs and symptoms with Jennifer. She also notes that shoulder ROM (active, passive, and resistive) and vital signs appear WNL. Leona decides to allow Jennifer to return to activity based on comfort and instructs her to report to the athletic training room after practice in order to ice the area to help reduce swelling and bruising.

QUESTIONS

Please answer the following questions based on the above case information.

8.7 / **1.** Based on the information presented in the case, determine (a) the differential diagnoses and (b) the clinical diagnosis.

8.7 / **2.** Please describe the anatomy of the structure involved in the clinical diagnosis.

8.7 / **3.** Based on the clinical diagnosis, what are the most common athletic injuries to the involved anatomical structure, and how should they be treated?

8.7 / **4.** A contusion to the affected tissue can lead to a rare benign disease. Please describe this disease.

8.7 / **5.** Clearly, Brad engaged in an act that caught Leona off guard. Based on the information presented in the case, (a) what if anything did Brad do that was inappropriate or unethical? (b) How would you have handled the situation if you were the evaluating athletic trainer?

Amanda, a certified athletic trainer, has been working for the X Games, covering many of the winter sporting events. She has been covering the events for the last three years and has really enjoyed her position. This year, Amanda was covering the games in Aspen, Colorado, and because of the extreme nature of the sports, had been extremely busy, often managing traumatic injuries such as fractures and dislocations. During a snowboarding competition, Punch, one of the female snowboarders, fell on her back after a difficult jump. She was slow to get up but finished her routine without another incident. Amanda was not present at the time of the incident, but Punch sought her out for treatment the next day because she needed to compete again and her back was aching.

HISTORY

When Punch finds Amanda, she retells what happened during the jump. Punch also states that in addition to the pain caused by yesterday's fall, her back has been hurting for about one month but was not painful enough to seek treatment. Punch attributes that pain to the consistent blows to her body when falling and thinks this soreness is common for her type of activity. Usually her pain at rest is graded as 3/10. However, during some upper body motions while snowboarding, her pain increases to 7 or 8 or higher if she falls on her back. She describes the pain in her left shoulder as intermittent. Her pain is classified as a dull ache. Although Punch has good ROM of the shoulder, all motions cause pain and discomfort.

FIGURE 8.8.1

Punch's location of palpable tenderness.

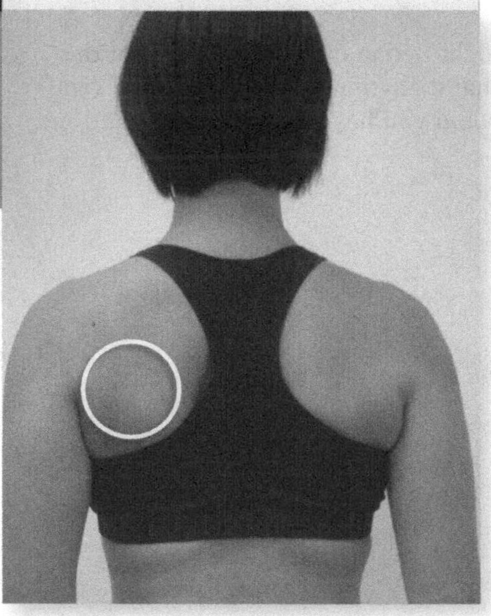

Area of pain is within the circle.

PHYSICAL EXAMINATION

Upon examination, Punch is alert and in good spirits. Palpation of the back reveals some point tenderness around the inferior border/fossa region of the scapula but no associated pain around the fourth to tenth ribs on that side (Figure 8.8.1). Shoulder AROM is slightly restricted in abduction; adduction is weak, and there is slight evidence of scapular winging by comparison with the right shoulder area. Sensory evaluation is unremarkable. Ligamentous testing is unremarkable, and an impingement test was also negative. Amanda decides it is best to refer Punch for diagnostic imaging at the local hospital after consultation between Amanda and a medical director for the games.

DIAGNOSTIC IMAGING

Plain radiographs are negative. Since Punch is still complaining of pain, the medical director and Amanda discuss other options. Punch is placed in a sling, restricted from activities for several days, and prescribed NSAIDs to relieve pain. Punch is upset about not being able to compete, but she complies.

FOLLOW-UP EXAMINATION

Two weeks later, Punch meets with Amanda because she still has a dull ache and feels pain during her overhead activities in the same area (Figure 8.8.1). The medical director is informed of the prognosis, and Punch is sent for further diagnostic tests. Results from these tests reveal a not-so-common pathology of the posterior thoracic region.

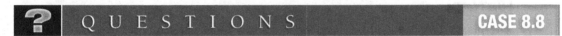

❓ QUESTIONS   CASE 8.8

Please answer the following questions based on the above case information.

8.8 / **1.** Based on the information presented in the case, determine (a) the differential diagnoses and (b) the clinical diagnosis.

8.8 / **2.** What are the recommended diagnostic tests to confirm the condition?

8.8 / **3.** What is the average healing time for this injury, and why?

8.8 / **4.** If the injury in this case is non-displaced, it can be treated non-operatively. Outline the treatment/management you would provide to Punch as the treating clinician.

S am, a female athletic training student, was working with her certified athletic trainer, Joey, during a fall practice for women's field hockey. During practice, one of the players was hit in the abdomen with an opponent's stick. The player immediately fell to the ground in obvious discomfort. Both Joey and Sam approached the scene immediately.

HISTORY

The player is 16-year-old Tisha. She is a sophomore starter and has never been injured before. From what Sam and Joey gather, an opposing player swung for the ball and missed. The follow through of the field hockey stick hit Tisha on the right side of her abdomen (Figure 8.9.1). Tisha is in pain but does not report any other lower- or upper-extremity pain or discomfort. Tisha is not coughing up blood and feels no nausea or dizziness.

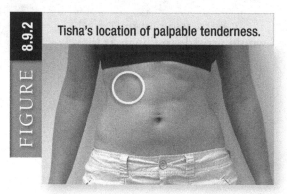

FIGURE 8.9.1

Tisha's mechanism of injury.

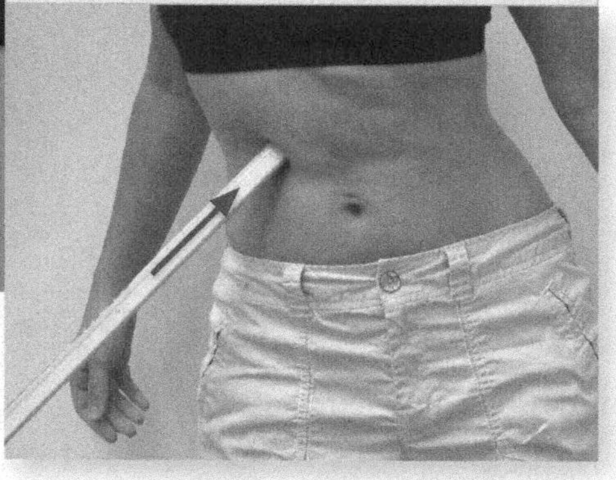

Arrow indicates direction of force applied to the body.

FIGURE 8.9.2

Tisha's location of palpable tenderness.

Circle indicates location of pain and tenderness.

PHYSICAL EXAMINATION

When she reaches the side of the field, Tisha complains of pain on her right side and slight discomfort in her right shoulder. She rates her pain about 6/10. During palpation of the affected side, Tisha reports discomfort at about ribs eight through twelve, mostly in the intercostal spaces. Pain is increased with palpation just below the diaphragm (Figure 8.9.2). There are no visible signs of bleeding at the site and no apparent rib deformity. Pulse is 88 and regular, respiration is 18 and normal, and blood pressure is WNL. Tisha is also examined around her right shoulder for pathology, which reveals nothing remarkable.

The coach questions Joey about Tisha's status and Joey responds, "She should be fine." Practice is almost over, so Joey decides to let Tisha rest on the sidelines because he believes Tisha just had the wind knocked out of her. About 30 minutes later, Tisha begins to vomit and loses consciousness.

Please answer the following questions based on the above case information.

8.9 / **1.** Based on the information presented in the case, determine (a) the differential diagnoses and (b) the clinical diagnosis.

8.9 / **2.** What are the most common MOIs for this injury?

8.9 / **3.** Any injury to the abdominal region requires the athletic trainer to examine all internal organs for injury. List the organs of the abdominal region by quadrant, and indicate the referred-pain sites for the major organs.

8.9 / **4.** When an athlete is complaining of abdominal trauma, palpation of the area is recommended while the athlete assumes the hook-lying position in order to relax the abdominal muscles. In addition, palpation is conducted specifically to assess for what three items?

8.9 / **5.** Clearly, Joey handled the situation inappropriately. If you were the evaluating clinician, what would you have done differently, and why?

Jeremy is the starting running back for a collegiate Division I football team in the Pacific Northwest. He has been a starter and team captain for two years, and this is his last season playing football at the collegiate level. During the second quarter of a tense game, Jeremy took a handoff for 6 yards and was tackled near the sidelines. He got up slowly, obviously in slight discomfort and pain, and came off the field. Jeremy was approached by Amanda, who has been the head athletic trainer for football the last eight years.

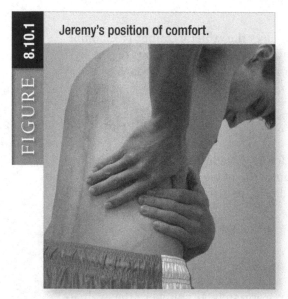

FIGURE 8.10.1

Jeremy's position of comfort.

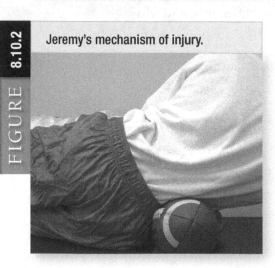

FIGURE 8.10.2

Jeremy's mechanism of injury.

HISTORY

Jeremy is bent forward slightly, grasping his right side with his left hand (Figure 8.10.1). Amanda proceeds to ask Jeremy what happened during the tackle that may have caused his distress. Jeremy states that when he was tackled, he landed on the ball on his right side, just below the chest area (Figure 8.10.2). Amanda assists Jeremy in removing his jersey and shoulder pads for better inspection of the area. Amanda does notice that Jeremy moves his right arm overhead with caution because of pain and discomfort.

PHYSICAL EXAMINATION

Upon inspection, Amanda does not see any discoloration or obvious deformity to the chest or abdomen region. Suspecting a rib or internal organ injury, Amanda palpates the lower ribs for crepitus or abnormalities, with unremarkable findings. Pressure to the right flank elicits pain in that area but no referred pain to the right shoulder. Sensation to the abdomen and chest is equal bilaterally. Overhead motions of the right shoulder elicit discomfort in the right flank area. Sensation and reflex testing of Jeremy's right shoulder is normal. Right shoulder ROM, strength in abduction, and forward flexion are diminished as compared with the left, because of flank pain. Heart rate and BP are within normal limits. Jeremy's breathing is a little rapid and shallow, but Amanda attributes this to his recent activity.

FOLLOW-UP EXAMINATION

Amanda takes away Jeremy's helmet, and he is kept out of the game for the remainder of the quarter, with a re-assessment during halftime. The re-evaluation approximately 20 minutes later reveals the same findings. Jeremy is asked to void and the color of his urine is checked, with no obvious hematuria. Amanda consults with the team physician, and they decide that Jeremy should not play for the rest of the game.

After the game, Jeremy is re-assessed by Amanda and the team physician. To rule out rib fractures, Jeremy is sent for diagnostic imaging along with a CT scan of the internal organs of that area. Urinary analysis at the hospital now demonstrates a slight trace of blood; however, imaging studies show no lacerations or major bleeding of the right-side organs.

? QUESTIONS   CASE 8.10

Please answer the following questions based on the above case information.

8.10 / **1.** Based on the information presented in the case, determine (a) the differential diagnoses and (b) the clinical diagnosis.

8.10 / **2.** What is the recommended treatment for the injury, and what are some signs and symptoms to observe over time?

8.10 / **3.** According to the American Association for the Surgery of Trauma Grading System (AASTGS), what are the five injury classifications for this injury?

8.10 / **4.** If this player's organ had to be removed, can he still play professional football or other contact sports after successful surgery and healing of the area?

8.10 / **5.** Neither the physician nor Amanda conducted a complete abdominal organ evaluation. If either had, what should they have done?

CONCLUSION

I n this chapter, the scenarios presented are more traumatic in nature because the injuries that occur have greater likelihood of damaging vital internal organs. As an athletic trainer, it is important to understand that careful follow-up and re-assessment is vital in ensuring positive outcomes, because the signs and symptoms of an internal injury may not be immediately apparent. When an injury occurs to the thorax or abdominal region, thorough knowledge of the MOI and pain-referral patterns is often the key to determining the proper clinical diagnosis. For example, an athlete reporting to you about pain in the right shoulder may quickly be assessed as having a contusion or slight muscle strain if no apparent signs are visible, but this may in fact be an injury to the liver. In addition, cartilage or bony injuries to the thorax region can lead to life-threatening conditions if displacement occurs. As with all evaluations, scrutiny and attention to detail in assessing thoracic and abdominal injuries are paramount.

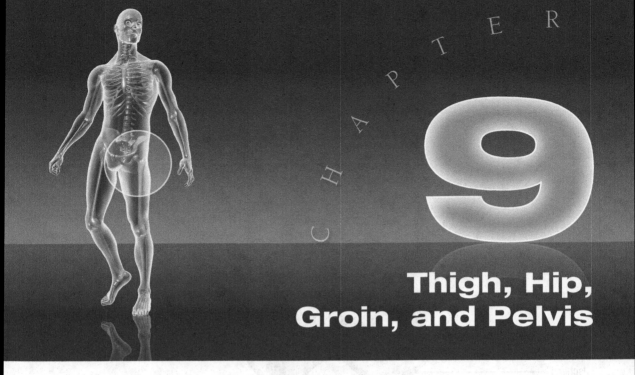

Thigh, Hip, Groin, and Pelvis

INTRODUCTION

In this chapter, we will examine the clinical management of 13 different thigh, hip, groin, and pelvis pathologies in a variety of settings with a diverse patient population. In many instances, the scenarios are actual pathologies or modifications of injuries presented in the literature. The scenarios are written to provide information needed for you to determine the pathology presented. However, some information may be missing, and some information is included that may or may not help you decipher the injury.

The purpose of providing these scenarios is to heighten your awareness of different types of conditions associated with this area of the body and to exercise your clinical skills and other techniques learned by answering the questions provided. As a reminder, some of the cases presented in this and other chapters have intentionally been written with inappropriate actions/procedures/treatments and general mismanagement of the case by the clinician in order to allow you to critically analyze the cases, identify the inappropriate decision(s), and then provide the appropriate gold-standard treatment.

ANATOMICAL REVIEW

The pelvis is comprised of three distinct bones fused together: the ilium, ischium, and pubis[8] (Figure 9.1). Together they form an irregular shape, with the ilium at the top, the ischium in the posterior, and the pubis in the anterior portion of the pelvis. The ilium has two bony prominences: one located anteriorly called the anterior superior iliac spine (ASIS) and one located posteriorly called the posterior

FIGURE 9.1   Anterior view of the male pelvis.

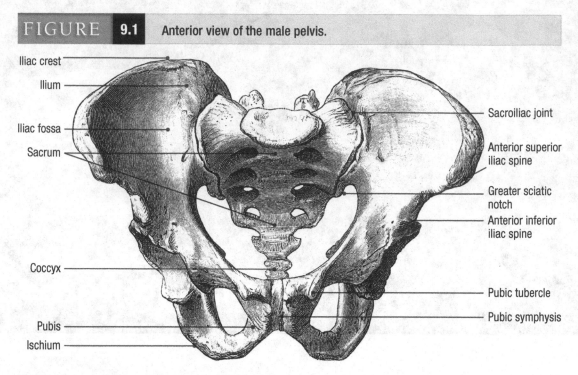

Iliac crest

Ilium

Iliac fossa

Sacrum

Coccyx

Pubis

Ischium

Sacroiliac joint

Anterior superior iliac spine

Greater sciatic notch

Anterior inferior iliac spine

Pubic tubercle

Pubic symphysis

The pelvis is constructed of two ischial, two pubic, and two ilial bones bordered posteriorly by the sacrum.

Source: Courtesy FCIT, http://etc.usf.edu

superior iliac spine (PSIS). The iliac crest runs between these two prominences. Just below the ASIS and PSIS are the anterior inferior iliac spine (AIIS) and the posterior inferior iliac spine (PIIS), respectively (Figure 9.2). The greater sciatic notch is located inferior to the PIIS. The ischium is the most inferior of the pelvic bones and has a large prominence called the ischial tuberosity, which provides a major muscle attachment for the hamstrings and is the bone on which we commonly sit. Finally, the pubic bone, located anteriorly in the pelvis, articulates with the ischium via the inferior pubic ramus and the ilium via the superior pubic ramus. The pubic symphysis connects the left and right pubic bones in the center. The acetabulum is formed at the interaction of all three bones and faces inferolaterally and anteriorly, housing the head of the femur. The right and left sides of the pelvis are connected posteriorly via the sacrum and anteriorly at the pubic symphysis. The shape and function of the pelvis depends on the patient's gender (Table 9.1).

Articulating with the acetabulum is the head of the femur, creating a ball and socket joint with 3° of freedom[6] (Figure 9.3 and Table 9.2). The head of the femur is separated from the shaft of the femur by the anatomical neck. At the base of the femur's neck are two bony projections called the greater trochanter and the lesser trochanter.[8] These two bony prominences act as landmarks for muscle and ligamentous attachments. The lesser trochanter is found distally and medially to the greater trochanter. An intertrochantric ridge runs between the greater and lesser trochanters. Running longitudinally down the femur shaft on the posterior aspect is the linea aspera, which is also used as a muscular attachment site.

FIGURE **9.2** **Lateral view of the pelvis.**

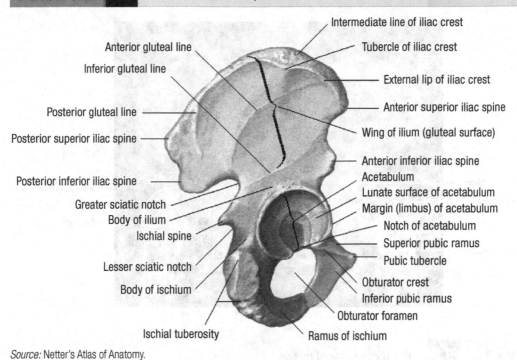

- Intermediate line of iliac crest
- Anterior gluteal line
- Inferior gluteal line
- Tubercle of iliac crest
- External lip of iliac crest
- Posterior gluteal line
- Anterior superior iliac spine
- Posterior superior iliac spine
- Wing of ilium (gluteal surface)
- Anterior inferior iliac spine
- Acetabulum
- Posterior inferior iliac spine
- Lunate surface of acetabulum
- Greater sciatic notch
- Margin (limbus) of acetabulum
- Body of ilium
- Notch of acetabulum
- Ischial spine
- Superior pubic ramus
- Pubic tubercle
- Lesser sciatic notch
- Obturator crest
- Body of ischium
- Inferior pubic ramus
- Obturator foramen
- Ischial tuberosity
- Ramus of ischium

Source: Netter's Atlas of Anatomy.

TABLE **9.1** **Differences between male and female pelvises.[3]**

	MALE	FEMALE
Overall pelvic bones	Thicker and heavier	Thinner and lighter
Lesser pelvis	Deep and narrow, oval	Wide and shallow, circular
Greater pelvis	Deep	Shallow
Pubic arch	Narrow and deep	Wide and shallow
Acetabulum	Large	Small
Obturator foramen	Round	Oval
Ischial tuberosity	Further apart	Closer together

Art courtesy FCIT, http://etc.usf.edu

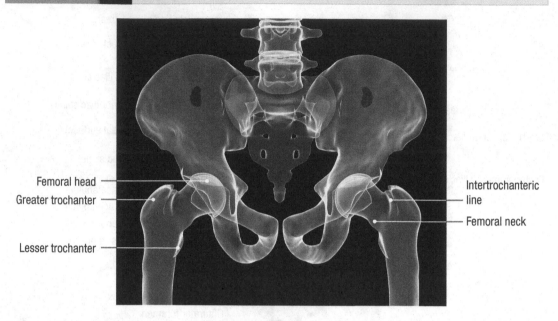

FIGURE **9.3**   Hip joint.

TABLE **9.2**   Hip active range of motion.[2]

MOVEMENT	NORMAL MOVEMENT	PLANE	AXIS
Flexion	0°–120°	Sagittal	Frontal
Extension	0°–30°	Sagittal	Frontal
Abduction	0°–45°	Frontal	Sagittal
Adduction	0°–30°	Frontal	Sagittal
Internal rotation	0°–45°	Transverse	Vertical
External rotation	0°–45°	Transverse	Vertical

Pelvic and Hip Joints

Lumbosacral joint

The lumbosacral joint consists of the articulation between the L5 and S1 vertebrae and is supported by the iliolumbar ligaments[6,8] (Figure 9.4). The facets located on S1 are faced posteriorly and medially and prevent the L5 vertebrae from moving in the anterior direction.

Sacrococcygeal joint

Mostly a cartilaginous joint, the sacrococcygeal joint consists of the articulation of the sacrum apex to the coccyx with support from the sacrococcygeal ligaments (anterior, posterior, lateral) (Figure 9.5) and intercornual ligaments.[8]

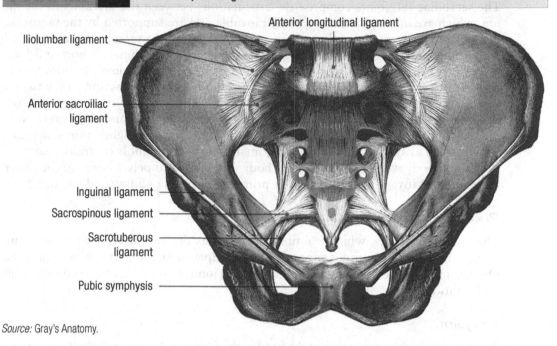

FIGURE 9.4   Anterior pelvic ligaments.

- Anterior longitudinal ligament
- Iliolumbar ligament
- Anterior sacroiliac ligament
- Inguinal ligament
- Sacrospinous ligament
- Sacrotuberous ligament
- Pubic symphysis

Source: Gray's Anatomy.

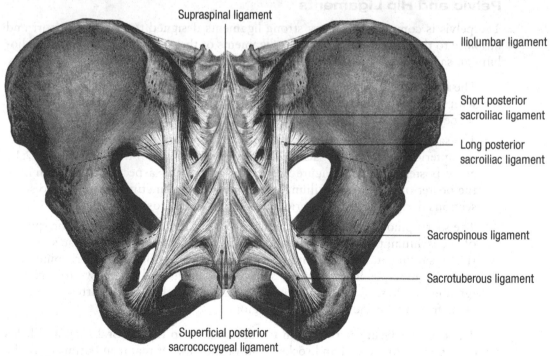

FIGURE 9.5   Posterior pelvic ligaments.

- Supraspinal ligament
- Iliolumbar ligament
- Short posterior sacroiliac ligament
- Long posterior sacroiliac ligament
- Sacrospinous ligament
- Sacrotuberous ligament
- Superficial posterior sacrococcygeal ligament

Source: Gray's Anatomy.

Sacroiliac joints

The sacroiliac (SI) joints comprise the articulations between the sacrum and the ilium, which are interlocking and slightly movable and are supported by the sacroiliac ligaments. The ligaments of the sacroiliac joint span from the sacrum to the ilium and include the anterior SI ligament (Figure 9.4), posterior SI ligament (short and long portion) (Figure 9.5), and sacroiliac interosseous ligaments.[8] Indirect stabilization is provided to the sacroiliac joint via the sacrospinous ligament (sacrum to the ischial spine) and sacrotuberous ligament (attaches from the sacrum to the ischial tuberosity) (Figures 9.4 and 9.5, respectively). These will be discussed later in this review.

The interlocking joints form a syndesmosis joint, and the slightly movable joints are classified as synovial, although the primary role of this joint is for transmission of forces and body weight from the axial body to the hip and pelvic bones of the lower extremity.[4,6] Movements of the SI joint primarily occur via gliding and rotating.[4,6]

Pubic symphysis

The pubic symphysis, which is a fibrocartilaginous disc, connects the two separate pubic bones anteriorly and is supported by the superior and arcuate pubic ligaments. Only a small degree of movement occurs at this joint, limited mainly to compression and rotation.

Hip joint

The hip joint is the articulation of the head of the femur and the acetabulum, which creates a ball and socket joint. Surrounding the articulating ends of the surfaces is cartilage that reduces the friction during movement. A fibrous capsule surrounds the hip joint.

Pelvic and Hip Ligaments

The pelvis is comprised of many strong ligaments designed to provide support and mobility to the region (Table 9.3). The ligaments of the sacral region include the iliolumbar, sacroiliac, sacrospinous, and sacrotuberous ligaments:[4,6,8]

- The iliolumbar ligament lies between the fifth lumbar and first sacral vertebrae, with strands to the iliac crest and iliac fossa just below the crest in a triangular shape (Figure 9.4).

- The sacroiliac ligament has two portions: an anterior portion that runs between the anterior surface of the sacrum to the anterior surface of the ilium (Figure 9.4) and a posterior portion (Figure 9.5) from the posterior aspect of the sacrum into the posterior aspect of the ilium. The portions are sometimes divided into subsections: long and short posterior sacroiliac and interosseous ligaments.

- The sacrospinous ligament runs between the sacrum and coccyx and the spine of the ischium; the sacrotuberous connects the posterior inferior iliac spine (PIIS), sacrum and coccyx, and the ischial tuberosity. Both the sacrospinous and sacrotuberous ligaments help stabilize the pelvis and create two foramina (greater and lesser sciatic) that are conduits for muscles, nerves, arteries, and veins from the pelvic to the gluteal region.

The capsular ligament runs from the acetabulum to the femoral neck and helps provide stability to the ball and socket joint of the hip. Of major importance are the iliofemoral, ischiofemoral, and pubofemoral ligaments because they provide major

TABLE 9.3	Pelvic and hip ligaments and their major functions.[4,8]
LIGAMENT	**FUNCTION**
SI Joint	
Iliolumbar	Prevents anterior displacement of the fifth lumbar vertebra
Sacroiliac (anterior, posterior, interosseous)	Connection between sacrum and ilium; limits sacral counternutation
Sacrospinous	Limits sacral nutation
Sacrotuberous	Limits sacral nutation
Hip Joint	
Capitis femoris ligament	Limits hip adduction
Inguinal ligament	Maintains continuity of soft tissue running from the abdomen to the lower leg
Iliofemoral	Limits hip hyperexetension
Ischiofemoral	Limits hip extension
Pubofemoral	Limits hip abduction and extension

The inguinal ligament runs between the anterior superior iliac spine (ASIS) to the pubic tubercle and functions as a site for muscle attachment.

support to the joint. The iliofemoral ligament (Figure 9.6) connects the ilium and the neck of the femur with two separate bands that form a "Y," often referred to as the "Y ligament of Bigelow."[8] The pubofemoral ligament extends from the anterior pubis to the neck of the femur, covered partially by the "Y" ligament. Posteriorly, the ischiofemoral ligament runs between the ischium and the neck of the femur (Figure 9.7). The transverse acetabular ligament runs along the inferior glenoid lip of the acetabulum and forms a foramen that acts like a conduit for the blood supply. The capitis femoris ligament (also known as ligamentum teres) runs from the femoral fovea (the hole in the head of the femur) to the transverse acetabular ligament, helping to attach the femur head to the acetabulum and assisting with blood supply to that region.

The head and neck of the femur are angled to facilitate articulation with the acetabulum. The angle of inclination is found between the

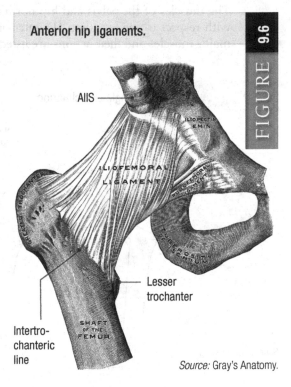

Anterior hip ligaments.

FIGURE 9.6

AIIS

Lesser trochanter

Intertrochanteric line

Source: Gray's Anatomy.

FIGURE   9.7

Posterior hip ligaments.

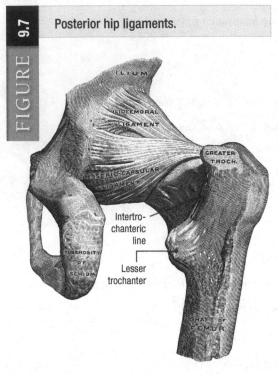

Source: Gray's Anatomy.

axes of the femoral neck and the femoral shaft in the frontal plane. This angle varies in degrees but begins at about 150° in infants and decreases to about 125° in adults. Women tend to have a slightly smaller inclination than men because of the width of the pelvis. Inclination that is increased beyond a normal range is called coxa valga, and smaller than normal inclination is called coxa vara (Figure 9.8). The angle of torsion (also known as the angle of anteversion) is found between the axes of the femoral head and the femoral condyles in the transverse plane.[6] Most often, this angle is viewed from above looking down the shaft of the femur. The angle of torsion is about 40° at birth and decreases over time. Adults have approximately a 15° angle; however, it is also dependent upon gender.[10] An increase in the angle is called "anteversion" and a decrease in the angle is called "retroversion." Anteversion causes the femur to medially rotate to help restore joint congruence at the hip. Conversely, retroversion causes external femoral rotation to help joint congruence at the hip.

Pelvic and Hip Muscles

The muscles of the pelvis and hip normally fall into four groups, according to location with respect to the hip joint: (1) anterior, (2) posterior, (3) medial, and (4) lateral. The major muscles and their actions are listed in Table 9.4.

FIGURE   9.8   **Angle of inclination.**

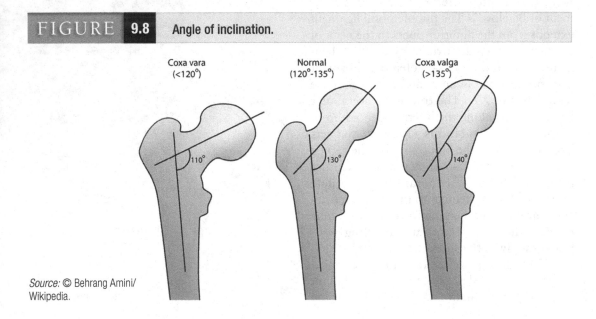

Source: © Behrang Amini/ Wikipedia.

TABLE 9.4	Hip/pelvis muscles and their major functions.[6,9]
MUSCLE	**ACTIONS**
Anterior	
Iliopsoas Psoas major and minor Iliacus	Hip flexion, lumbar spine flexion if the femur is stabilized
Sartorius	Hip flexion, abduction, external rotation, knee flexion
Quadriceps femoris Rectus femoris Vastus lateralis Vastus intermedius Vastus medialis	Hip flexion (rectus femoris), knee extension
Tensor fascia latae	Hip flexion, abduction, internal rotation
Posterior	
Hamstrings Biceps femoris Semitendinosus Semimembranosus	Knee flexion Internal rotation of the tibia with the flexed knee (semitendinosus and semimembranosus) External rotation of the tibia with the flexed knee (biceps femoris) Hip extension with the knee in extension
Gluteal maximus	Hip extension, external rotation Isolated with knee flexed 90°
Piriformis	External rotation of hip
Gemellus superior	External rotation of hip
Gemellus inferior	External rotation of hip
Obturator internus	External rotation of hip
Obturator externus	External rotation of hip
Quadratus femoris	External rotation of hip
Medial Muscles	
Adductor longus	Hip adduction
Adductor brevis	Hip adduction
Adductor magnus	Hip adduction
Gracilis	Hip adduction
Pectineus	Hip adduction
Lateral Muscles	
Gluteus medius	Hip abduction, internal rotation
Gluteus minimus	Hip abduction, internal rotation
Iliotibial band	Assists hip abduction, knee flexion and extension, depending on position of knee

FIGURE 9.9 Sacral plexus.

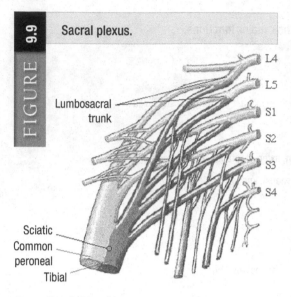

L4
L5
S1
S2
S3
S4

Lumbosacral trunk

Sciatic
Common peroneal
Tibial

Source: Netter's Atlas of Anatomy.

Neurovascular Structures

The hip and pelvis region is innervated by numerous nerves arising primarily from the lumbar plexis (T12–L4 or L5) sacral plexus[3,4,9] (Figure 9.9) (L4–S4), and coccygeal plexus (S4–S5).

The largest branch of the lumbar plexus is the femoral nerve, which supplies the skin and muscles of the anterior thigh region. The obturator nerve, also arising from the lumbar plexus, divides into an anterior and posterior portion that leave via the obturator foramen and supply the muscles of the medial thigh (adductors).

The sacral plexus has 12 nerve branches, of which the sciatic and pudendal are considered to be the two main branches. The major branches of the sacral plexus exit the pelvis via the greater sciatic foramen. The sciatic nerve is formed by ventral rami of L4 through S3 and converges on the anterior surface of the piriformis muscle. The L4 through S3 branches pass through the greater sciatic foramen inferior to the piriformis and into the gluteal region before innervating the hamstring and adductor magnus muscles. The sciatic nerve has two distant branches: the tibial nerve and the common peroneal nerve (common fibular). The pudendal nerve leaves the pelvis via the greater sciatic foramen between the piriformis and coccygeus muscles, and then hooks around the sacrospinous ligament and lesser sciatic foramen into the muscles of the perineum.

The coccygeal plexus is a small part of the plexus formed by the anterior rami of S4 and S5 and the coccygeal nerve. It supplies nerve innervations to the coccygeus, levator ani, and the sacroccygeal joint region.

LIGAMENTOUS AND SPECIAL TESTS

The case scenarios in this chapter will require you to select and utilize common and not-so-common special tests. Providing details on how to perform each special test is beyond the scope of this review, but Table 9.5 will briefly highlight various special tests that will be useful to review before beginning the case scenarios. Not all special tests are listed in the table; only the major or common specials tests are included. For a more thorough review, please refer to your favorite evaluation text or journal articles.

TABLE 9.5	Ligamentous and special tests for the hip, pelvis, and sacrum.[1,5,7,11]
SPECIAL TEST	**FUNCTION**
Ligamentous	
Anterior distraction (gapping test)	Assesses integrity of anterior sacroiliac ligaments
SI distraction (iliac compression test)	Assesses integrity of posterior sacroiliac ligaments
Gaenslen's	Assesses for SI dysfunction by placing a rotational force on the SIJ; also assesses for hip pathology or L4 nerve lesion

(continued)

TABLE 9.5	Continued.
SPECIAL TEST	**FUNCTION**
Hip	
Patrick's (FABER)	Assesses for pathology of the SI joint and hip joint
Hip scouring	Assesses for possible defects in the articular cartilage of the femur or acetabulum and for labral tears
Muscle Pathology	
Adductor contracture	Assesses adductor muscle group length and tightness
Abductor contracture	Assesses abductor muscle group length and tightness
Ely's	Assesses rectus femoris length and tightness
Noble's compression	Assesses the ITB while in non-weight-bearing position
Ober's	Assesses ITB and tensor fascia latae tightness
Piriformis	Assesses sciatic nerve impingement secondary to piriformis muscle tightness
Thomas	Assesses for hip flexion contractures, knee extension, and ITB tightness
Trendelenburg	Assesses hip stability and hip abduction (gluteus medius) weakness
Bony	
Allis' sign	Assesses femoral, tibial length, and hip dislocation
Anvil (hips)	Assesses femoral neck/head fracture
Fulcrum	Assesses for femoral shaft stress fracture
Neurological	
Femoral nerve traction	Assesses for femoral nerve pathology

REFERENCES

1. Anderson M, Parr G, Hall S. *Foundations of Athletic Training: Prevention, Assessment, and Management.* 4th ed. Baltimore: Lippincott Williams & Wilkins; 2008.

2. Clarkson H. *Joint Range of Motion and Function Assessment: A Research-Based Practical Guide.* 3rd ed. Baltimore: Lippincott Williams & Wilkins; 2006.

3. Clemente CD. *Anatomy: A Regional Atlas of the Human Body.* 4th ed. Baltimore MD: Lippincott Williams & Wilkins; 1997.

4. Cohen SP. Sacroiliac joint pain: a comprehensive review of anatomy, diagnosis, and treatment. *Anesth Analg.* 2005;101(5):1440–1453.

5. Konin JG, Wiksten D, Isear JA, Brader H. *Special Tests for Orthopedic Examination.* 3rd ed. Thorofare NJ: Slack; 2006.

6. Levangie PK, Norkin CC. *Joint Structure and Function: A Comprehensive Analysis.* Philadelphia PA: F. A. Davis; 2001.

7. Magee DJ. *Orthopedic Physical Assessment.* 5th ed. Philadelphia PA: WB Saunders; 2007.

8. Moore K, Dalley A. *Clinically Oriented Anatomy.* 5th ed. Baltimore MD: Lippincott Williams & Wilkins; 2005.

9. Moore KL, Agur AMR. *Essential Clinical Anatomy.* Baltimore MD: Lippincott Williams & Wilkins; 2005.

10. Radin EL. Biomechanics of the human hip. *Clin Orthop.* 1980:152;28–34.

11. Robinson H, Brox J, Robinson REB, Solem S, Telje T. The reliability of selected motion and pain provocation tests for the sacroiliac joint. *Man Ther.* 2007;12:72–79.

CASE

9.1

Shaun is a graduate athletic training student at a local university. She is responsible for team coverage of the dance department, including all shows and dress rehearsals, and daily treatment of injuries or conditions. During a dress rehearsal, one of the dancers, Tracey, missed her mark and landed with one foot on the floor and the other on a raised platform about one foot off the ground. Tracey continued to perform her routine but felt some slight discomfort in her low back region.

HISTORY

Tracey, being a dancer, is in great physical condition, especially her lower body. She does not approach Shaun when the incident occurs. Instead, Tracey just ices her lower back and does some extra stretching. After a week of self-treatment, Tracey approaches Shaun in the backstage area after a rehearsal. Tracey explains her incident and says that her low back is still not getting better. Tracey rates her pain about a 5/10, but her biggest complaint is pain upon movement, especially landing from jumps and turning when bearing weight on the left leg with the right leg stretched out.

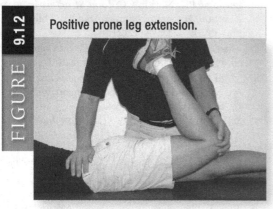

FIGURE 9.1.1 — Negative straight leg raise.

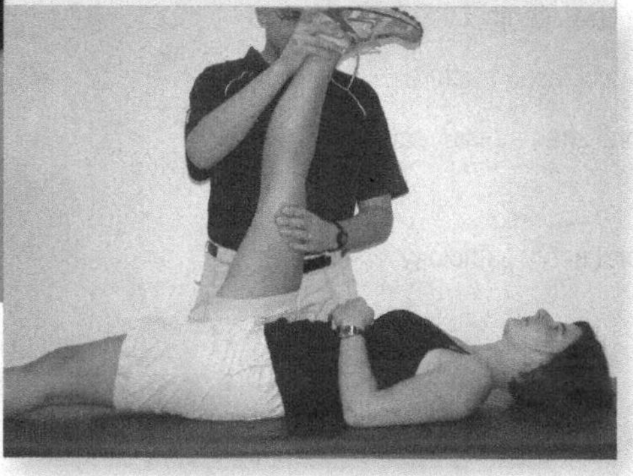

FIGURE 9.1.2 — Positive prone leg extension.

Increased area of pain is located between the sacrum and ilium.

PHYSICAL EXAMINATION

To inspect the area of the low back region, Shaun requests that Tracey remove her leotard. Shaun then examines for scoliosis or pelvic tilt abnormalities, looking for discoloration or abnormalities in the area, which are all absent. Palpation of the lumbar region from L1 to L5 is painless for Tracey. Palpation of the fascia of the lower lumbar area, especially at the intersection of the sacrum and ilium region on the left side, reveals tenderness. Examination of Tracey's ROM in her lumbar, hip, and pelvis areas reveals greater than normal ranges, most likely because she is a dancer. There is marked pain with leg extension on her affected side. The straight leg raise (Figure 9.1.1) does not reproduce pain, but prone hip extension on the affected side produces discomfort (Figure 9.1.2). Another special test also produces discomfort on her affected side (Figures 9.1.3, A and B). Reflexes of the lower extremity and sensation in her hips, lumbar, and pelvis are normal. Leg length is equal bilaterally.

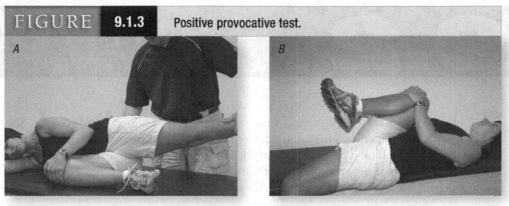

FIGURE **9.1.3** Positive provocative test.

A

B

A and B show the same test performed two different ways.

? QUESTIONS CASE 9.1

Please answer the following questions based on the above case information.

9.1 / **1.** Based on the information presented in the case, determine (a) the differential diagnoses and (b) the clinical diagnosis.

9.1 / **2.** The area in question has multiple ligamentous support structures. Please identify the major ligament structures and their function in the sacral region.

9.1 / **3.** What are the most common pain-referral sites for this injury?

9.1 / **4.** What are some of the provocative or diagnostic tests used to differentiate this pathology? Are these tests valid and reliable?

9.1 / **5.** Do you think Shaun should have removed Tracey's leotard for inspection of the area?

CASE

9.2

Sumpta is a 19-year-old starting defensive soccer player at a local junior college. She was kicking soccer balls in practice during team drills, performing the same drills she had performed for several days during the week as she prepared for a divisional semi-final soccer game. Today she began experiencing some discomfort, and when practice was over, she sought out care from Judy, the athletic trainer who visited the college twice a week.

HISTORY

Judy begins her evaluation by asking Sumpta to describe the problem. Sumpta states, "During today's practice I began experiencing pain in my right thigh after taking a shot on goal." Further questioning reveals that the involved leg was Sumpta's dominant limb and that she felt a twinge in that leg after the goal kick. She attributes her pain to fatigue from kicking many shots during the last couple of days in practice. Sumpta also says, "While I continued with practice, I noticed I didn't produce the same type of explosiveness off each kick I normally do and that the pain became worse as the practice continued. In fact, the ball speed got worse with each shot." Sumpta denies any history of lower leg trauma or pathology and reports a pain of 5/10. Sumpta has great lower leg muscular tone and overall general conditioning.

PHYSICAL EXAMINATION

Sumpta is alert and in moderate discomfort (5/10) without movement of the right leg. Judy observes a noticeable alteration in Sumpta's gait: decreased knee extension, particularly during the swing phase. Soft tissue palpation reveals localized tenderness over the upper middle myotendinous junction of the quadratus femoris and a slight palpable defect. There is no visible abnormality, swelling, or discoloration. Judy assesses active and passive ROM using a goniometer, followed by isometric muscle testing, the results of which are shown in Table 9.2.1. Ligamentous testing of the knee is unremarkable. Neurovascular testing is also unremarkable.

TABLE	9.2.1	Sumpta's range of motion results.

EXAM	JOINT MOTION	FINDINGS	
AROM	Knee flexion	Right 110°	Left 135°
	Knee extension*	Right 35°–short of full extension	Left 0°–full extension
PROM	Knee flexion*	Minor-to-moderate pain at mid-to-end ROM	
	Knee extension	Minimal-to-no discomfort	
RROM	Knee flexion (prone, mid-range)	4+/5 with pain	
	Knee extension (short sitting, mid-range)	2+/5	

*Increased pain is noted with these motions.

Judy discusses the results of her examination with Sumpta. They initially do not agree on an immediate course of action. After some persuasion, Sumpta does agree to follow Judy's plan, though Sumpta wants to know when she can play again.

❓ QUESTIONS   CASE 9.2

Please answer the following questions based on the above case information.

9.2 / **1.** Based on the information presented in the case, determine (a) the differential diagnoses and (b) the clinical diagnosis.

9.2 / **2.** Judy discussed some immediate treatment care for the injury. Based on the information provided, what immediate care do you think she recommended to Sumpta?

9.2 / **3.** Based on the clinical diagnosis, what section of muscle(s) does this type of injury usually affect and why?

9.2 / **4.** Based on the clinical diagnosis, what type of muscles and muscle actions are usually associated with this type of injury?

9.2 / **5.** Sumpta reluctantly agreed to the immediate course of action. When she asked about returning to play, what factors did Judy need to consider before allowing her to return to play?

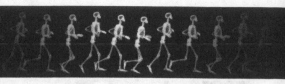

E merson, a recreational roller hockey player, was practicing with a group of friends during the weekend when he was hit in the upper leg by an opponent's knee. Emerson hobbled along until the pain subsided and continued to play the rest of the day. He did note limited knee motion and decided to take the rest of the week off from hockey because of slight discomfort. The following week, he played again and continued to experience pain in his right upper leg. Feeling concerned, Emerson went to a local college's free sports medicine clinic looking for some medical advice. He was seen by Lacretia, a new certified athletic trainer at the clinic.

HISTORY

Lacretia begins her examination by gathering a medical history and ascertaining the MOI. Emerson, a licensed electrician by trade, tells her that he was "kneed" in the upper thigh (Figure 9.3.1) about seven days ago playing roller hockey. Emerson explains, "The pain has gotten a little worse, but I managed to play again this weekend and scored a couple of goals."

FIGURE 9.3.1

Emerson's location of pain.

Area of pain is in the circle on the anterior thigh.

PHYSICAL EXAMINATION

Emerson is alert, oriented, and in minor discomfort when at rest. Further evaluation reveals some palpable tenderness, but no significant loss of motion (90% compared with the uninvolved limb) or strength (95% compared with the uninvolved limb). Believing this is a relatively simple case, and after the radiographs she ordered were negative for a fracture, Lacretia's diagnosis is a thigh bruise. She prescribes RICE and schedules a follow-up visit with Emerson in a couple of weeks if needed.

FOLLOW-UP PHYSICAL EXAMINATION

Three weeks later, Emerson returns to the free sports medicine clinic. Even though he followed the prescribed plan and limited his recreational activities, his pain is worse and he has lost more motion at his knee. In fact, he states to Lacretia, "Now I can't even kneel real well to do my job." Palpation over the affected area of the quadriceps produces slight discomfort and demonstrates an unusual hardness in the center of the muscle. His active ROM is now at 70 percent of the uninvolved leg, and the strength of his quadriceps is approximately 80 to 85 percent. Ligamentous testing is WNL. Neurologically, Emerson is intact. Lacretia again orders radiographs. A standard antero-posterior and lateral view reveals a significant finding (Figure 9.3.2).

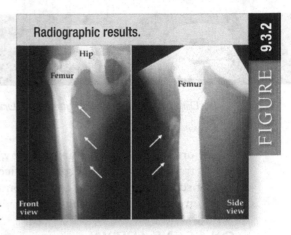

Radiographic results.

Source: Sloan, R. (1998). Hughston Health Alert, with permission.

? Q U E S T I O N S   CASE 9.3

Please answer the following questions based on the above case information.

9.3 / **1.** Based on the information presented in the case, determine and define the clinical diagnosis.

9.3 / **2.** Based on the information presented in the case, do you believe Lacretia took an adequate history? If not, what if any additional questions would you ask as the evaluating clinician?

9.3 / **3.** Based on the information presented in the case, the initial radiographs were unrevealing, yet the follow-up radiographs three weeks later were positive. Why do you suppose that was the case?

9.3 / **4.** During the initial history and physical examination, Lacretia could have provided some basic rehabilitation to help decrease the likelihood of developing this condition. If you were the evaluating clinician, what basic rehabilitation would you have recommended?

9.3 / **5.** Overall, do you believe Lacretia adequately evaluated Emerson's condition? Do you believe that Lacretia ever overstepped her boundaries as a certified athletic trainer? Why?

9.4

by Dilip Patel, M.D., Michigan State University, Kalamazoo Center for Medical Studies

During an early morning fall day, Stephanie and Joseph, the certified athletic trainers covering football practice at a Division II college, are called over to the line of scrimmage after the completion of a play. They find one of the players, Juan, lying on his back supporting his hip.

ON-SCENE ARRIVAL

Juan appears to have a patent airway but is in obvious discomfort. Joseph is trying to determine exactly what happened, while Stephanie immediately observes that Juan's left hip is flexed, adducted, and internally rotated. Stephanie immediately turns to one of the athletic training students and informs her to initiate the emergency action plan and call 9-1-1.

HISTORY

Juan, who is calm but clearly in discomfort, states, "As I cut to the left I got knocked down to the ground and landed on another player. A second player landed on my flexed hip from the front, and it felt weird. After that I couldn't move my leg."

PHYSICAL EXAMINATION

Joseph further questions Juan about his pain level. Juan is alert and in severe discomfort (9/10) but very calm considering the current situation. Palpation to the left hip reveals tenderness and apparent displacement of the femoral head, posteriorly. Reflex testing reveals hyporeflexia on the involved side only. Juan's vital signs appear in Table 9.4.1, A and B. Stephanie and Joseph decide it is best

TABLE	9.4.1	Juan's vital signs.

A. On-field vital signs.

VITAL SIGNS	FINDINGS
Pulse	98, regular, and bounding
Respiration	22 and labored
Blood pressure	138/82
Pupils	PEARRL
Mental status	Alert

B. Off-field vital signs.

VITAL SIGNS	FINDINGS
Pulse	78 and regular
Respiration	12 and normal
Blood pressure	120/76
Pupils	PEARRL
Mental status	Alert

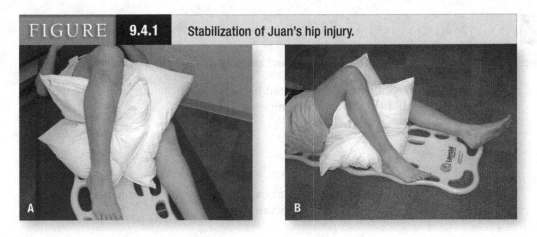

FIGURE 9.4.1 Stabilization of Juan's hip injury.

to remove Juan from the field while waiting for EMS so the team can continue to practice. They prepare to move him by stabilizing the limb with a soft splint (Figure 9.4.1, A and B).

Having arrived on the sideline, they continue to monitor Juan's vital signs and neurological status while waiting for EMS. When EMS arrives, Juan is packaged and transported to the local hospital for further evaluation.

Please answer the following questions based on the above case information.

9.4 / **1.** Based on the information presented in the case, determine (a) the differential diagnoses and (b) the clinical diagnosis.

9.4 / **2.** Based on the clinical diagnosis above, identify two or three history questions you as the evaluating clinician may have asked.

9.4 / **3.** (a) Do you believe Joseph and Stephanie performed a complete neurovascular exam? (b) What is the clinical significance of a neurovascular exam in this case? (c) What should the exam assess?

9.4 / **4.** There is one common MOI for this injury that typically does not relate to athletics. Identify this MOI and the pathomechanics involved.

9.4 / **5.** As the evaluating clinician, what if anything would you have done differently in managing the case, particularly on the field?

9.4 / **6.** If there are no complications, that is, no concomitant injuries, how long will it take before Juan can return to full sports participation?

Twenty-one-year-old Jenny is a cross-country athlete at a local university. She presented to Sarah, a member of the athletic training staff. Jenny complained of right upper leg pain into the pelvic region and has an extensive history of lower leg pathology.

HISTORY

Sarah asks about when the pain started, and Jenny responds, "I don't remember doing anything specific to my leg, but it has progressively gotten worse over the last three weeks. I tried running through the pain because this is my senior year and I didn't want to miss any meets." Jenny describes pain that begins as a dull ache in the anterior area in her groin region and then radiates to her right lateral hip (Figure 9.5.1). Jenny states that initially the pain would go away after track practice. Now the pain is getting worse during her long-distance training. There is some resolution at night after she rests, although lately she says the pain has been waking her at night. When Sarah questions Jenny about any training changes she has made, Jenny states that she had increased her weekly mileage over the last month from 20 miles a week to 35 miles a week and has been running a lot more on the road and other concrete surfaces, rather than around the track at the university. Jenny also had low iron levels at the beginning of the season and has not been taking her prescribed iron supplements. Jenny rates her pain at 7/10 during her workouts and at 4/10 during ADLs.

PHYSICAL EXAMINATION

Jenny is alert, oriented, and in moderate discomfort. An observation of Jenny's gait reveals obvious gait abnormality with compensation when stepping with her right foot. Sarah notes no significant swelling, ecchymosis, or deformity in the groin or upper right thigh. However, she does note palpable tenderness in the groin area just inferior to the right ASIS and a diffuse pain that did not increase upon palpation over the lateral hip. Active ROM is limited by comparison with the uninvolved limb in the direction of hip flexion and extension. Resisted ROM is also decreased, 4/5, in flexion and extension when compared bilaterally. Circulation and dermatomes were all WNL. A leg length discrepancy was also noted, with the affected leg being shorter by approximately 1/4 inch than the contralateral leg.

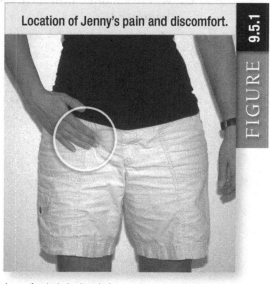

Location of Jenny's pain and discomfort.

FIGURE 9.5.1

Area of pain is in the circle.

Please answer the following questions based on the above case information.

9.5 / **1.** Based on the information presented in the case, determine (a) the differential diagnoses and (b) the clinical diagnosis.

9.5 / **2.** Based on the information presented in the history portion of the case, what is one of the hallmark signs indicating this clinical diagnosis?

9.5 / **3.** What significance does the low iron play in this case?

9.5 / **4.** What, if any, special tests could a clinician perform to aid in the physical examination and clinical diagnosis?

9.5 / **5.** Where should Sarah have referred Jenny in order to confirm the clinical diagnosis?

by Dilip Patel, M.D., Michigan State University, Kalamazoo Center for Medical Studies

J J, a 16-year-old long distance runner was training for his district cross-country meet. He was up to 30 miles per week until about four weeks ago, when he started having pain over his left hip bone. Not wanting his condition to get worse, his parents scheduled an appointment with his family doctor, Dr. Loughton. When JJ and his mother arrived at the clinic, they were asked to complete several documents, including the pain profile document shown in Figure 9.6.1. Once completed, they were escorted to an examination room, where Eric, a licensed PA, ATC, began his evaluation.

HISTORY

Eric initiates the evaluation by asking JJ several questions about the injury. He is able to determine that while training for an upcoming race, JJ's pain has gradually increased in intensity since its onset. JJ states, "The pain is worse during running; however, I have this achy pain all the time over the hip bone (Figure 9.6.2). Eric also learns that JJ's mile time has slowly been deteriorating from a 5-minute mile to an 8-minute mile. For the past week or so, JJ has had to stop running after about half an hour. JJ appears to be in otherwise excellent health. He has no history of direct trauma to the left hip area and denies any previous history.

PHYSICAL EXAMINATION

JJ is alert and in minor-to-moderate discomfort while sitting on the table. JJ appears to be a normally developed adolescent male. Observation of JJ's gait pattern appears unremarkable. Eric notes mild redness and poorly demarcated soft tissue swelling over the anterior third of the left iliac crest. Palpation reveals localized tenderness over the anterior third of the iliac crest. JJ also notes that although he is not in acute pain right now over the iliac crest, a dull aching pain intensifies on the site during activity, particularly running. The abdomen is soft and

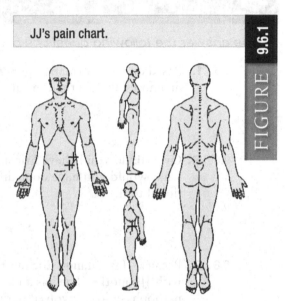

JJ's pain chart.

FIGURE 9.6.1

Crosses equal location of general pain.

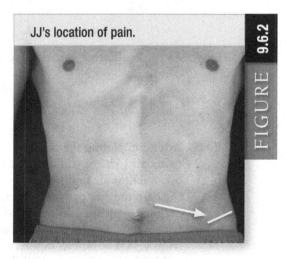

JJ's location of pain.

FIGURE 9.6.2

Pain is located by the arrow and the line.

non-tender. Left hip PROM is pain free, but there is pain with active hip abduction and flexion. Resisted muscle testing reveals 3+/5 for hip abduction and 3/5 for trunk flexion.

DIAGNOSTIC IMAGING

After some discussion with JJ's mom, Eric orders a set of plain film radiographs, including lateral and A/P views of both iliums for comparison. The radiographs identify widening of the physis and new bone growth along the left iliac crest.

Based on these results, Eric outlines a treatment plan for JJ that includes the use of crutches for a period of time. He documents his findings into the laptop computer he brought into the exam room.

? QUESTIONS   CASE 9.6

Please answer the following questions based on the above case information.

9.6 / **1.** Based on the information presented in the case, determine (a) the differential diagnoses and (b) the clinical diagnosis.

9.6 / **2.** Overall, do you believe Eric adequately evaluated JJ's condition? If not, what would you have done differently? Would you have added any additional tests?

9.6 / **3.** Because JJ is a minor, Eric must share the results of the physical examination with JJ's mother. She has a medical background and asks Eric to explain the pathophysiology involved in this condition. If you were the evaluating clinician, how would you describe the condition?

9.6 / **4.** As the evaluating clinician, describe how you would consider treating JJ's condition.

9.6 / **5.** After completing the physical examination, Eric documented his findings electronically. Using your athletic training room's computer tracking software, document your findings electronically as if you were the treating clinician. If the case did not provide information you believe is pertinent to the clinical diagnosis, please add this information to your documentation. If you do not have access to injury-tracking software, consider downloading a trial version from CSMI Solutions (Sportsware) by going to www.csmisolutions.com/cmt/publish/service_software_dl.shtml and following the on-screen directions.

CASE 9.7

by Joel Beam, Ed.D., ATC, University of North Florida, Jacksonville

S ara, an 18-year-old midfielder and co-captain of her high school soccer team, started noticeably limping after kicking the ball toward the goal during an early season soccer match. She continued to play for several minutes, but she was not running or playing to her full potential. The coach substituted her, and Al, the certified athletic trainer, approached her on the sideline to determine the extent of the problem.

HISTORY

Sara states that she had felt a twinge in her left groin area after she kicked the ball into the net. Al questions Sara further and learns that her groin had been bothering her for some time. Sara says, "My groin has been a little tender for a while, and honestly, I just thought I had been overdoing it recently, you know, getting ready for the season and everything." She denies suffering any significant trauma, and although Al does not notice any abnormalities during practices, Sara claims to be performing less than 100 percent and that this is starting to worry her. Her chief complaints are slight discomfort in the adductor/groin area, pain in the lower abdominal area, and increased pain when she pushes off to change direction. She rates her pain as 5/10 at rest and 8/10 with activity.

PHYSICAL EXAMINATION

Sara is alert and in moderate-to-severe discomfort and appears to be very upset. Al receives permission to palpate Sara's groin and lower abdominal area. Palpation reveals no palpable defects or abnormalities. He does note tenderness near the pubic symphysis and adductor muscle origins. Sara's pain is aggravated with active hip flexion, pivoting on her leg, and kicking a ball. Quadricep and hamstring resistive ROM is WNL. Al does note some weakness on the involved limb when he performs a resistive muscle test (Figure 9.7.1). Ligamentous testing of the SI joint and an Ober's test are unremarkable. Neurologically, Sara is intact.

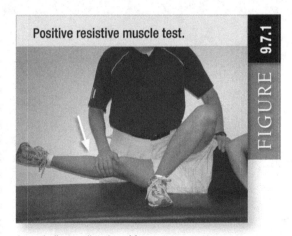

Positive resistive muscle test.

FIGURE 9.7.1

Arrow indicates direction of force.

Al's initial diagnosis is a muscle strain, and he prescribes an appropriate course of action, which includes rest, muscle strengthening, various therapeutic modalities to control pain, and limited activities.

FIGURE 9.7.2

Positive radiographic findings.

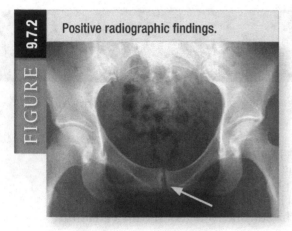

Note the abnormal widening of the pubic symphysis.

Source: Image reprinted with permission from eMedicine.com, 2009. Available at http://emedicine.medscape.com/article/87420-media.

DIAGNOSTIC IMAGING

Over the course of two weeks, Sara's pain during her activities has not lessened. Al consults with his team's physician, and after consultation, Al and the physician decide Sara should be seen by an orthopedic surgeon. Her parents send her to their orthopedic surgeon, who orders radiographs as part of the physical examination. The images suggests that, based on her age, activity level, and sport participation, there appears to be an abnormal widening of the pubic symphysis on the anteroposterior (AP) films (Figure 9.7.2).

? QUESTIONS   CASE 9.7

Please answer the following questions based on the above case information.

9.7 / 1. Based on the information presented in the case, determine (a) the differential diagnoses and (b) the clinical diagnosis.

9.7 / 2. This injury/condition can be exacerbated by repetitive stresses for athletes in which sports?

9.7 / 3. According to research by Mandelbaum and Mora, there are four primary clinical types of this condition. Please identify them.

9.7 / 4. It has been suggested that the major etiology of this condition is muscle imbalance. Please describe the muscle imbalance relationship and possible rationale behind it.

9.7 / 5. Overall, do you believe Al adequately evaluated Sara's condition? Are there any another special tests a clinician could perform to help guide the physical examination?

9.7 / 6. The signs and symptoms of this condition often mimic other common injuries in this region. Do you therefore think all athletes who present with the above scenario should be immediately referred for diagnostic imaging?

9.8

Over the course of a four-month club hockey season, Montclair, a 20-year-old goalie, has been playing despite pain in his lower right groin area. He attributed the pain to a mild groin injury that occurred earlier in the season. But because the groin pain has increased during the season, Montclair's coach suggested visiting the local sports medicine clinic in order to prevent any recurrence next season. When Montclair arrived at the clinic, he completed the paperwork provided by the office staff, which included a medical history, pain profile, and pain activity indicator, before he was to be seen by Joel, a staff athletic trainer.

FIGURE   9.8.1

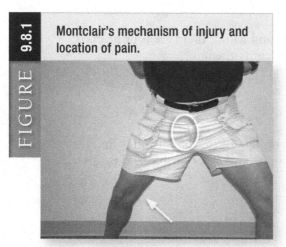

Montclair's mechanism of injury and location of pain.

The arrow demonstrates movement of the right leg laterally and back as if simulating a goalie pad save. Montclair has a difficult time pin-pointing the exact location, but area of pain is in the circle.

HISTORY

After a few minutes of small talk and introductions, Joel begins his examination by reviewing Montclair's past medical history and gathering additional information. He then proceeds by asking, "So tell me what is going on?" Montclair responds, "The pain comes and goes, but it is normally more noticeable during the hockey season and less during the off season." He continues, "Most of my pain occurs when I kick my right leg out to block the puck, especially when I go to the side and back (Figure 9.8.1). Occasionally, the pain is so bad during practice and games that I can't get the right leg completely out to the side; however, the deep groin pain seems to get better with rest." Further questioning reveals pain with increased intra-abdominal pressure (i.e., sneezing or coughing). Montclair also describes pain radiating to his testes and frequently experiencing low-back pain. He denies suffering any specific trauma. Pain is rated as 3/10 at rest and 8/10 with increased activity.

PHYSICAL EXAMINATION

Montclair is alert, oriented, and in minor discomfort at rest. Palpation reveals point tenderness near the pubic tubercle and superficial inguinal ring with no palpable mass. AROM is limited in hip extension and abduction, while hip adduction and trunk flexion RROM produces increased pain and a deficit (3/5) on the involved side. Ligamentous testing is WNL; however, one special test is positive (Figure 9.8.2). Joel notes no abnormal neurological findings of the lower extremities and no testicular abnormalities as well.

After completing the physical examination, Joel discusses Montclair's options, including referral to a physician for further evaluation. Joel tells Montclair the condition he thinks Montclair is suffering from. He bases his diagnosis on the length of time Montclair has been experiencing problems and the fact that the location of the pain appeared more lateral and proximal than normally seen with a groin strain or avulsion. However, Joel says that diagnostic imaging such as an MRI can help confirm whether his diagnosis is accurate.

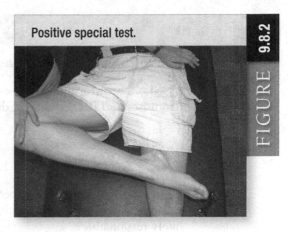

Positive special test.

FIGURE 9.8.2

DIAGNOSTIC IMAGING

The physician's evaluation reveals dilation of the superficial inguinal ring on the affected side, which was palpable when the scrotum was inverted with the little finger. An MRI of the pelvis demonstrates marrow signal changes on the right side (where he complained of pain) and appeared to be primarily involving the rectus abdominis insertion.

Please answer the following questions based on the above case information.

9.8 / **1.** Based on the information presented in the case, determine (a) the differential diagnoses and (b) the clinical diagnosis.

9.8 / **2.** (a) In most cases, the pain experienced by Montclair in and around the pubic tubercle suggests injury to which structure(s)? (b) What mechanism is most likely responsible?

9.8 / **3.** What is the name of the special test performed in Figure 9.8.2? What is considered a positive finding? Was it appropriate to perform in this case?

9.8 / **4.** If you were the treating clinician, what treatment or rehabilitation protocols would you suggest to treat the injury/condition?

9.8 / **5.** Why is this type of injury/condition difficult to diagnose?

L isa, an 18-year-old collegiate freshman field hockey player, initially reports pain in her anterior and medial left hip during pre-season camp. She presented to Jill, the athletic trainer who was covering field hockey. Lisa had an apparent deviation in gait and was unable to flex her hip or lift her left leg onto the plinth during the initial evaluation.

HISTORY

Jill begins her evaluation of Lisa by determining Lisa's MOI. Lisa states that she began experiencing soreness in her groin region the day before, while running, but that the pain became worse with backpedaling and change in direction movements. Upon waking the next morning, Lisa felt increased discomfort and pain while ambulating and when trying to lift her leg. Lisa denies any previous history of injury to her left hip/groin, though she did report a previous history of left lateral knee pain and ITBFS. Pain was rated at 8/10.

PHYSICAL EXAMINATION

Lisa is alert and very anxious because this is only the third day of pre-season camp and her coach is upset with her already for seeing the athletic trainer. Jill's initial evaluation reveals point tenderness over the iliopsoas and adductor muscle group. Range of motion testing reveals deficits in AROM and RROM (Table 9.9.1).

TABLE	9.9.1	Lisa's range of motion results.	
		FINDINGS	
EXAM	**JOINT MOTION**	**RIGHT**	**LEFT**
AROM	Hip flexion (short-sitting)*	120°	90°
	Hip extension (prone)	30°	20°
	Hip abduction (side-lying)	45°	40°
	Hip adduction (supine)*	30°	15°
PROM	Hip flexion	Minimal-to-no discomfort	
	Hip extension*	Minor-to-moderate pain at mid-to-end ROM	
	Hip abduction*	Minor-to-moderate pain at mid-to-end ROM	
	Hip adduction	Minimal-to-no discomfort	
RROM	Hip flexion (short-sitting)*	3+/5 with pain	
	Hip extension (prone)	4+/5	
	Hip abduction (side-lying)	5/5	
	Hip adduction (supine)*	3+/5 with pain	

*Increased pain is noted with this motion.

Ligamentous testing and neurological testing is unremarkable. Jill makes a clinical diagnosis. She and an athletic training student then treat Lisa over the next week, using a regimen of rest, ultrasound, cryotherapy, wrapping (for support), and therapeutic exercises (stationary biking and progressive resistive exercises with cuff weights and Thera-Band®).

After a week of treatment, Lisa's strength and ROM improve, and she is permitted to return to limited practice with prophylactic wrapping. However, three days later, she beings to complain of hip pain.

FOLLOW-UP PHYSICAL EXAMINATION

Lisa now describes a snapping sensation in her left lateral hip while lowering her leg from a flexed hip position; however, Jill is unable to reproduce the problem. Lisa's left hip ROM is equal bilaterally, and effusion is noted in the inguinal area. Lisa resumes her initial treatment program.

Lisa's soreness persists over the next several weeks, and her pain begins to radiate from the left anterior medial hip into the lateral hip. She is placed on crutches and progresses to a normal weight-bearing status. Significant point tenderness over the left greater trochanter and palpable snapping ITB are now noted, despite conservative treatment. Her coach is getting very annoyed at both Jill—for not doing her job—and Lisa—for not trying to play through the pain.

FIGURE 9.9.1

Positive special test.

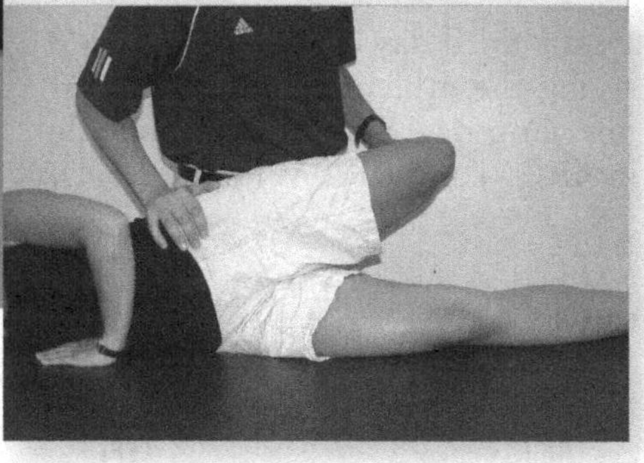

An orthopedic evaluation finds a positive special test (Figure 9.9.1) and negative radiographs. No significant clinical improvement was noted after three months of rest, ultrasound, cryotherapy, prophylactic wrapping, therapeutic exercises, oral medications, and cortisone injections. The special test is still positive, and the snapping sensation is now worse.

| ? | QUESTIONS | CASE 9.9 |

Please answer the following questions based on the above case information.

9.9 / 1. Based on the information presented in the case, determine (a) the differential diagnoses, and (b) identify the final clinical diagnosis made by the orthopedic surgeon.

9.9 / 2. Based on the physical examination, what was Jill's initial clinical diagnosis? How do you think this initial condition resulted in the final condition?

9.9 / 3. (a) What is the purpose of the special test in Figure 9.9.1? (b) Is there a modification to this special test? (c) If so, what is the reliability of this modified test?

9.9 / 4. What caused Lisa's snapping sensation to occur?

9.9 / 5. In this case, the coach became very upset at both Lisa and Jill. If you were the evaluating athletic trainer, how would you respond to a coach's comments that you are not doing your job? If another athlete told you that Lisa was out dancing at a club during the time when she was supposedly suffering from the lateral hip pain, would you use this information to defend yourself against the coach?

Dewalt, a middle-aged recreational runner, spent four months training for a marathon by following a prescribed running program that included adequate rest and recovery. The training regimen went smoothly, and Dewalt finished the marathon with a respectable time for his age group. Two days after the race, he abruptly began experiencing pain in his knee. After about a week, Dewalt sought medical advice from Jonas, a family physician.

HISTORY

Dewalt tells Jonas that he went for a short run a couple days after the marathon. After about 15 minutes, he suddenly felt a sharp pain in his right knee. He decided to stop running immediately and walked back to his house. He tried running again two days later, with the same result.

PHYSICAL EXAMINATION

Dewalt presents with right lateral knee pain around the joint line with point tenderness on the lateral aspect of the distal femur. His strength is equal bilaterally, and flexibility of the hip, thigh, and hamstring musculature are equal bilaterally and above average for his age. Because Dewalt insists on running for an upcoming event, Jonas injects him with cortisone in the area of tenderness.

Dewalt continues to run after the injection with no pain for about a month. Then, during a run, the pain starts abruptly again.

FOLLOW-UP PHYSICAL EXAMINATION

Dewalt visits an orthopedic physician who prescribes orthotics, massage, and rest. Approximately a month later, Dewalt begins running but has to stop after two weeks. Dewalt then follows the same treatment protocol off and on for several months to no avail. After approximately a year and a half after the initial event, surgery is performed with no subsequent bouts of pain or discomfort.

Please answer the following questions based on the above case information.

9.10 / **1.** Based on the information presented in the case, determine (a) the differential diagnoses and (b) the clinical diagnosis.

9.10 / **2.** What are some common causative factors for the development of this condition?

9.10 / **3.** What two common special tests are used to assist in determining the clinical diagnosis? How would you perform them on Dewalt?

9.10 / **4.** What is the usual course of conservative therapy for this condition?

9.10 / **5.** What is the common procedure to alleviate the tension/stress of the ITB if surgery is indicated?

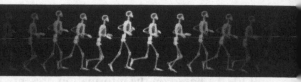

Danielle, an 18-year-old gymnast, has been competing since she was five years old. She reported for her pre-participation physical on the first day of practice at the college level. She passed her general medical screening, which looked at areas such as the heart, lungs, and eyes, and she also passed her orthopedic screenings. However, she tells the athletic trainer, Kathy, that her left gluteal and leg region has been bothering her for quite some time.

HISTORY

When asked, Danielle does not report any specific trauma that caused sudden pain in the area, but she does mention that she has fallen on her buttocks a number of times over the years, explaining, "It's just part of being a gymnast." The pain is described as somewhat radiating, as it goes down her leg sometimes but is mostly confined to her gluteal region. Danielle says that when she works out during practice, the pain lessens, but then the pain increases about two hours after practice. She says that she is uncomfortable when sitting in chairs and when driving for extended periods of time.

PHYSICAL EXAMINATION

Kathy examines Danielle's legs bilaterally and notices that the foot of the affected leg is rotated more externally. All lumbar spine ROM is normal. Her hip ROM and strength measurements are listed in Table 9.11.1. Palpation reveals some discomfort

TABLE 9.11.1   Danielle's range of motion results.

EXAM	JOINT MOTION	FINDINGS	
		RIGHT	LEFT
AROM	Hip flexion (short-sitting)	120°	120°
	Hip extension (prone)*	30°	25°
	Hip abduction (side-lying)	45°	45°
	Hip adduction (supine)*	30°	30°
	Hip external rotation (sitting)*	45°	40°
	Hip internal rotation (sitting)	45°	30°
RROM	Hip flexion (short-sitting)	5/5	4+/5
	Hip extension (prone)*	5/5	3+/5
	Hip abduction (side-lying)	5/5	4/5
	Hip adduction (supine)	5/5	5/5
	Hip external rotation (sitting)*	5/5	3+/5
	Hip internal rotation (sitting)	5/5	4/5

*Increased pain is noted with this motion.

in the lateral central gluteal region. A straight leg raise test reveals some pain and discomfort on her affected side, and Trendelenburg's test is normal. Leg length tests are equal. She does have discomfort side-lying with hip flexion at 60° and knee flexed with pressure applied downward (Figure 9.11.1).

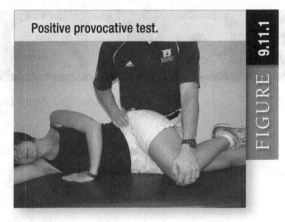

Positive provocative test.

FIGURE 9.11.1

? QUESTIONS   CASE 9.11

Please answer the following questions based on the above case information.

9.11 / **1.** Based on the information presented in the case, determine (a) the differential diagnoses and (b) the clinical diagnosis.

9.11 / **2.** What other observations or special tests could be used to help diagnose this injury? Please explain what indicates a positive finding and what information you would gain from performing the test.

9.11 / **3.** (a) What population seems more likely to suffer from this condition? (b) Why is this condition likely to cause sciatic nerve symptoms?

9.11 / **4.** As the treating clinician, (a) how would you treat this condition? (b) What methods, including those used by other health care professionals, can be implemented to relieve this condition if conventional therapy does not work?

by Dilip Patel, M.D., Michigan State University, Kalamazoo Center for Medical Studies

A lbert, an athletic trainer, is volunteering to help provide medical coverage for a field day event at a local middle school. After a short running event AJ, a 6th grader, reports to the medical tent with his father, Paul. AJ is complaining of mild left hip pain and has a limp.

HISTORY

Albert asks AJ to describe his pain. AJ says the pain is mild, aching, and feels like it is deep in his left hip area. His father reports that he has noticed AJ limping after playing outside, particularly toward the end of the day. This has been the case off and on over the past several weeks. AJ has never complained of pain and has not stopped or restricted his play activities. Today is the first time AJ has complained of hip pain. AJ is in excellent general health. He has not had any recent history of fever or other symptoms, according to his father.

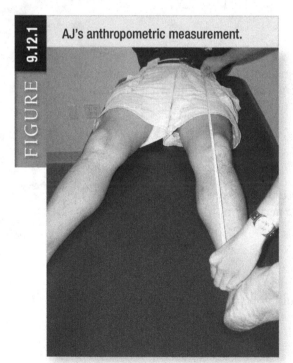

FIGURE 9.12.1

AJ's anthropometric measurement.

Left leg appears to be 1 inch shorter than right leg.

PHYSICAL EXAMINATION

Upon examination, AJ appears to be a healthy-looking young man who is not in any acute pain or distress. He walks with an antalgic gait favoring the left leg. His spine is straight without scoliosis. While standing, he has full, pain-free flexion and extension at the hips and knees. He has relatively decreased abduction of the left hip in the extended position, compared with that of the right side. In the prone position, he has a noticeable decrease in internal rotation and extension of the left hip.

Albert performs an anthropometric measurement (Figure 9.12.1) and notes a 1-inch difference between the right and left leg. There is no muscle atrophy in the lower limbs. Patellar and Achilles deep-tendon reflexes are 2+ bilaterally. Sensitivity to light touch is intact. Examination of AJ's knees, ankles, and feet is unremarkable.

Please answer the following questions based on the above case information.

9.12 / 1. Based on the information presented in the case, determine (a) the differential diagnoses and (b) the clinical diagnosis.

9.12 / 2. (a) Please explain why you ruled out at least two of your differential diagnoses. (b) Explain the clinical diagnosis.

9.12 / 3. (a) How can the clinical diagnosis be confirmed? (b) What will you advise the athlete and his parents to do at this time?

9.12 / 4. What is the etiology of this condition?

9.12 / 5. Describe the treatment, course, and prognosis of this condition.

9.12 / 6. (a) Who is most affected by this condition? (b) What are the potential complications of the condition?

Joshua is working in a sports medicine clinic that provides free injury screenings to the community. Adalyn, age 11, reports to the clinic to have her hip evaluated. Her parents are present for the initial evaluation, and they help explain the situation.

HISTORY

Adalyn describes localized pain to her left hip/groin area that has been progressively getting worse, which is why her parents brought her to the clinic. Adalyn actively participates in volleyball with her church league, and Adalyn reports that her hip pain began several weeks ago, although she cannot specifically remember suffering any traumatic events. She also reports pain in her left knee. She rates her pain as 5/10 at rest and 8/10 with activity.

TABLE 9.13.1 Adalyn's manual muscle testing results.

MOTION	RIGHT SIDE	LEFT SIDE
Hip flexion	5/5	3+/5
Hip extension	5/5	3/5
Hip abduction	5/5	4/5
Hip adduction	5/5	3/5
Hip internal rotation	5/5	3/5
Hip external rotation	5/5	4/5

PHYSICAL EXAMINATION

Joshua notes that Adalyn is able to bear weight but has a noticeable gait abnormality when walking, with the toes facing externally on the affected side. Joshua also notes that Adalyn is slightly overweight. Joshua notes no apparent abnormalities, swelling, or discoloration at the hip joint. Adalyn sits on a table in the examination room, and Joshua notices more external rotation and abduction of the hip during flexion. Results of Adalyn's manual muscle testing are located in Table 9.13.1. Because of her young age and his physical findings, Joshua knows he needs to refer Adalyn to a specialist.

Please answer the following questions based on the above case information.

9.13 / **1.** Based on the physical findings, determine (a) the differential diagnoses and (b) the clinical diagnosis.

9.13 / **2.** Diagnostic imaging can help confirm and classify the severity of the condition. Please identify the three classifications and the amount of movement that may occur with each classification.

9.13 / **3.** Why is the pain associated with this condition often felt elsewhere than the specific place of injury?

9.13 / **4.** (a) Where do you think Joshua should refer Adalyn for a further diagnostic workup? (b) If you were the evaluating clinician, what do you think the best course of treatment for this condition might include?

9.13 / **5.** What population and risk factors are most commonly associated with this condition?

9.13 / **6.** Overall, do you believe Joshua adequately evaluated Adalyn's condition? If you were the evaluating clinician, what would you have done differently?

CONCLUSION

The case scenarios presented in this chapter are some of the most common injuries seen by athletic trainers. When conducting an assessment for the thigh, hip, groin, and pelvis, it is important to think about related structures surrounding these areas. Consider that injuries to areas such as the knee can cause pain in the thigh and that injuries to internal organs can refer pain to the groin area. In addition, the anatomical complexity of these areas requires the athletic trainer to review the plethora of special tests and know when and how to apply them. As presented, the case scenarios in this chapter should assist the athletic trainer to become competent and confident in her skills and provide situations in which she must think "outside the box" when evaluating and treating an athlete with a thigh, hip, groin, or pelvis injury.

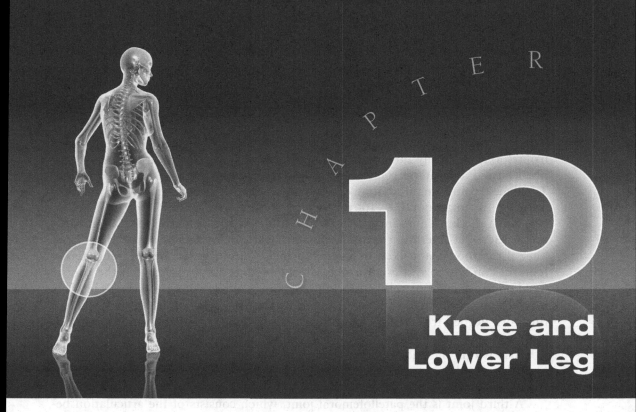

10

Knee and Lower Leg

INTRODUCTION

T his chapter will examine the clinical evaluation and management of 16 different knee and lower-leg pathologies, using a combination of on-field and off-field scenarios presented in a variety of settings with a diverse patient population. The traumatic and overuse injuries presented in this chapter are a mixture of acute and chronic pathologies as well as bony and ligamentous conditions. As in each chapter, we attempted to identify many of the common conditions frequently encountered in clinical practice by athletic trainers. As a reminder, some of the cases presented in this and other chapters have intentionally been written with inappropriate actions, procedures, or treatments in order to allow you to critically analyze the cases and identify the inappropriate decision(s). The following introduction is a cursory overview of the anatomical arrangement and basic functioning of the knee complex. For further review, we suggest reading texts and journal articles that specifically examine the structure and function of the knee complex.

Trauma to the knee complex results in a variety of injuries such as sprains, strains, contusions, fractures, dislocations, and subluxations. Injuries to the knee complex are common in both competitive and recreational sports. More than 50 percent of all reported collegiate sports injuries occur at the lower extremity, with knee and ankle injuries accounting for most of the lower-extremity injuries.[3] Injury to the anterior cruciate ligament (ACL) accounts for 3 to 5 percent of all collegiate injuries, with the highest incidences occurring in women's gymnastics, women's basketball, and men's spring football.[3] Over 50 percent of all high school athletic injuries reported by certified athletic trainers were injuries sustained to the knee complex.

ANATOMICAL REVIEW

T
he main joint of the knee complex is the tibiofemoral joint, a hinge joint that consists of the convex femur joined with the concave tibia. It is at this joint that flexion and extension of the knee occur in the sagittal plane around a frontal axis, normally ranging from 0° to 135° or more. The joint also allows for tibial medial and lateral rotation—but only when the joint is in a flexed position. Tibial medial and lateral rotation occur in the transverse plane around a vertical axis, normally ranging from 0° to 10° for each motion.

When the knee goes into full extension during an open kinematic chain situation, the tibia laterally rotates within the last 30° of extension to "lock" the knee if the foot is not fixed to a solid surface. This allows for the larger medial femoral condyle to rest comfortably on the medial tibial plateau.[5] If the foot is fixed on the ground or solid surface, the femur medially rotates on the tibia. This mechanism is known as the "screw home mechanism." This mechanism decreases the work needed from the quadriceps to maintain an extended knee in the standing position.[5]

Also within the knee is the proximal tibiofibular joint, consisting of the convex fibula head and the concave lateral condyle of the tibia. This joint is a synovial joint that allows for slight movement while dorsiflexion occurs at the ankle joint.

A third joint is the patellofemoral joint, which consists of the articulation between the intercondylar groove of the femur and the patella. The patella is considered to be a sesamoid bone and provides increased leverage for the quadriceps musculature. During flexion of the tibiofemoral joint, the patella glides distally on the femoral condyles. During extension of the tibiofemoral joint, the patella glides in a cranial direction. As the patella moves within the femoral condyles, or tracks, there is a slight rotation that occurs, otherwise known as the patellar tilt.[5] This patellar tilt accommodates for the irregularity between the medial and lateral femoral condyles. The patella tilts medially during 0° and 30° of flexion and over 100° of flexion. Lateral patella tilt occurs between 20° and 100° of flexion.[5] The mediolateral movement that the patella undergoes during knee motion is known as a patellar shift. The patella shifts medially with medial tibial rotation at all angles of knee flexion. The patella shifts laterally during knee extension.[5]

Tibiofemoral Joint and Ligaments

To provide stability of the knee, there are several ligaments that cross the tibiofemoral joint. The ACL attaches at the anteromedial intercondylar eminence of the tibia and the posterior aspect of the lateral condyle of the femur[7] (Figure 10.1). This ligament prevents anterior translation of the tibia on the femur. The posterior cruciate ligament attaches along the posterior portion of the intercondylar area of the tibia and the anterior lateral surface of the medial condyle of the femur. It prevents posterior translation of the tibia on the femur. The medial collateral ligament attaches at the medial epicondyle of the femur and continues down to the medial condyle and medial surface of the tibia (Figure 10.2). The deep fibers of this ligament are attached to the medial meniscus and to the thick fibrous capsule, increasing the incidence of injury to all three structures when the medial collateral ligament is stressed to its breaking point.[7] The lateral collateral ligament is attached at the lateral femoral epicondyle and continues to attach at the lateral surface of the fibula head.

FIGURE **10.1**   Anterolateral aspect of the knee complex.

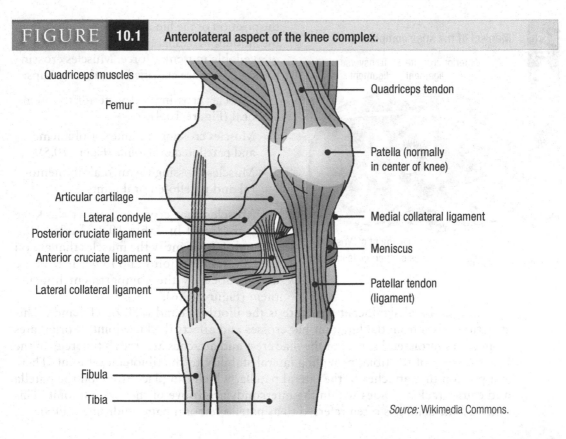

Quadriceps muscles

Femur

Quadriceps tendon

Patella (normally in center of knee)

Articular cartilage

Lateral condyle

Posterior cruciate ligament

Anterior cruciate ligament

Lateral collateral ligament

Medial collateral ligament

Meniscus

Patellar tendon (ligament)

Fibula

Tibia

Source: Wikimedia Commons.

Menisci

Menisci are fibrocartilage structures in the knee. The medial and lateral menisci deepen the articular surface of the tibia to allow for improved stability. These structures also act as shock absorbers. The medial meniscus is "C" shaped, whereas the lateral meniscus is shaped like the letter "O" and is more mobile than the medial menisci (Figure 10.3). Both menisci are thicker along the outer periphery and thinner in the central part. The menisci do not have a good arterial blood supply; therefore, the healing time of an injured menisci is prolonged and occurs primarily on the outer third of the structure.

Muscles

Dynamically, the muscles crossing the tibiofemoral and patellofemoral joints are a combination of single- and two-joint muscles acting on the knee, the patella, and the hip joint. Therefore,

Anteromedial aspect of the knee complex.

FIGURE 10.2

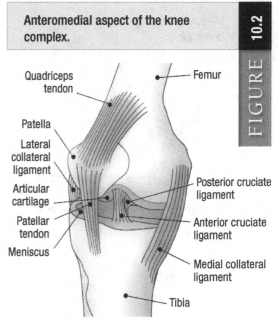

Quadriceps tendon

Patella

Lateral collateral ligament

Articular cartilage

Patellar tendon

Meniscus

Femur

Posterior cruciate ligament

Anterior cruciate ligament

Medial collateral ligament

Tibia

Source: National Institute of Arthritis and Musculoskeletal and Skin Diseases (NIAMS).

FIGURE 10.3

Menisci of the knee complex.

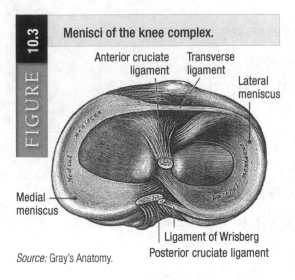

Anterior cruciate ligament

Transverse ligament

Lateral meniscus

Medial meniscus

Ligament of Wrisberg

Posterior cruciate ligament

Source: Gray's Anatomy.

the position of the hip and knee will affect both the amount of available ROM and the amount of available muscular force. Muscles crossing the knee joint are classified into three groups:

- Muscles crossing the posterior tibiofemoral (Figure 10.4).
- Muscles crossing the anterior tibiofemoral and patellofemoral joints (Figure 10.5).
- Muscles crossing the medial tibiofemoral and patellofemoral joints.

Muscles that cross and affect the knee joint are listed in Table 10.1. Tables 10.2 through 10.5 identify the muscles that act on the tibiofemoral joint and lower leg. These are grouped by the compartment housing them (Figure 10.6).

An additional significant structure is the iliotibial band (ITB or IT band). This structure arises from the hip joint but crosses and affects the knee joint. It originates from the anterolateral aspect of the iliac crest and attaches at Gerdy's tubercle on the lateral aspect of the tibia, providing lateral stability to the tibiofemoral joint. There is a portion that attaches to the lateral patella, which can place stress on the patella and cause tracking issues within the intercondylar groove of the femoral joint. This patella maltracking is often referred to as patello femoral pain syndrome (PFPS).

FIGURE 10.4

Muscles crossing the posterior knee complex.

FIGURE 10.5

Muscles crossing the anterior knee complex.

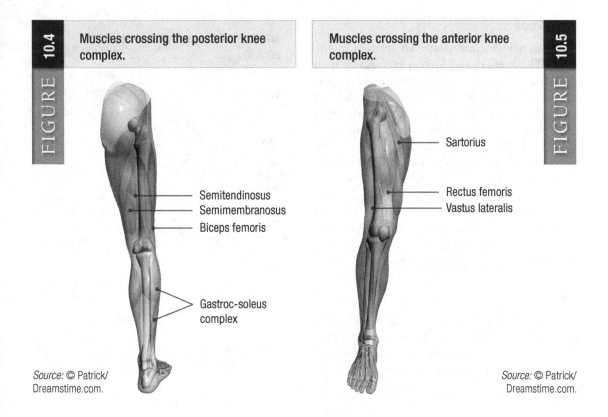

Semitendinosus
Semimembranosus
Biceps femoris

Gastroc-soleus complex

Sartorius

Rectus femoris
Vastus lateralis

Source: © Patrick/ Dreamstime.com.

Source: © Patrick/ Dreamstime.com.

| TABLE | 10.1 | Muscles acting on tibiofemoral and patellofemoral joints.[1,7] |

MUSCLE	ORIGIN ATTACHMENT	INSERTION ATTACHMENT	ACTIONS
Anterior			
Vastus medialis	Linea aspera of the femur	Tibial tuberosity via the patella ligament	Knee extension
Vastus lateralis	Linea aspera of the femur	Tibial tuberosity via the patella ligament	Knee extension
Vastus intermedius	Anterior shaft and linea aspera of the femur	Tibial tuberosity via the patella ligament	Knee extension
Rectus femoris	Anterior inferior iliac spine (AIIS)	Tibial tuberosity via the patella ligament	Knee extension, hip flexion
Posterior			
Biceps femoris	Long head: Ischial tuberosity Short head: Linea aspera and the lateral supracondylar line of the femur	Head of fibula and lateral tibial condyle	Knee flexion, hip extension, posterior pelvic rotation, lateral tibial rotation
Semimembranosus	Ischial tuberosity	Posterior medial condyle of the tibia	Knee flexion, hip extension, posterior pelvic rotation, medial tibial rotation
Semitendinosus	Ischial tuberosity	Pes anserine tendon	Knee flexion, hip extension, posterior pelvic rotation, medial tibial rotation
Medial			
Gracilis	Anterior body of pubis, inferior ramus of pubis	Pes anserine tendon	Hip adduction, hip flexion, knee flexion, anterior rotation of pelvis, tibial medial rotation
Sartorius	Anterior superior iliac spine (ASIS)	Pes anserine tendon	Hip flexion, abduction, and lateral rotation simultaneously; knee flexion, tibial medial rotation

| TABLE | 10.2 | Muscles of the anterior compartment of the lower leg.[1,8] |

MUSCLE	ORIGIN ATTACHMENT	INSERTION ATTACHMENT	ACTIONS
Tibialis anterior	Lateral tibial condyle, proximal 2/3 of the anterior tibia, proximal 2/3 of the interosseous membrane	First cuneiform and first metatarsal	Dorsiflexes the foot at the ankle joint, inverts foot at the tarsal joints
Extensor digitorum longus	Proximal 3/4 of fibula, proximal interosseous membrane, lateral tibial condyle	Dorsal surface of toes 2–5 on the middle and distal phalanges	Extends toes 2–5 at MTPJ and IPJs, dorsiflexes foot at ankle joint
Extensor hallucis longus	Middle of anterior fibula, middle of interosseous membrane	Distal phalanx of great toe	Great toe extension, at the MTP and IPJs, dorsiflexion of foot at the ankle joint
Peroneus tertius	Distal 1/3 of anterior fibula, distal 1/3 of interosseous membrane	Dorsal surface of base of the fifth metatarsal	Dorsiflexion of foot, aids in eversion of foot

TABLE	10.3	Muscles of the lateral compartment of the lower leg.[1,8]

MUSCLE	ORIGIN ATTACHMENT	INSERTION ATTACHMENT	ACTIONS
Peroneal longus	Head of the fibula and proximal 2/3 of lateral fibula	First cuneiform and first metatarsal	Eversion of foot and a weak plantarflexor
Peroneus brevis	Distal 2/3 of lateral fibula	Lateral side of base of the fifth metatarsal	Eversion of foot and a weak plantarflexor

TABLE	10.4	Muscles of the superficial posterior compartment of the lower leg.[1,8]

MUSCLE	ORIGIN ATTACHMENT	INSERTION ATTACHMENT	ACTIONS
Gastrocnemius	Medial and lateral femoral condyles	Posterior surface of calcaneus via Achilles tendon	Ankle plantarflexion, knee flexion
Soleus	Soleal line of tibia and head of proximal 1/4 of fibula	Posterior surface of calcaneus via Achilles tendon	Ankle plantarflexion, steadies leg on foot
Plantaris	Lateral condyle and distal lateral supracondylar line of femur	Posterior surface of calcaneus via Achilles tendon	Ankle plantarflexion, knee flexion

TABLE	10.5	Muscles of the deep posterior compartment of the lower leg.[1,8]

MUSCLE	ORIGIN ATTACHMENT	INSERTION ATTACHMENT	ACTIONS
Popliteus	Distal posterolateral femur	Proximal posterior tibia medial side	Tibial medial rotation, knee flexion
Tibialis posterior	Proximal 2/3 of posterior tibia, fibula, and interosseous membrane	Metatarsals 2–4 and all tarsal bones except talus	Ankle plantarflexion, inversion of foot
Flexor digitorum longus	Middle 1/3 of posterior tibia	Plantar surface of distal phalanges 2–5	Flexion of toes 2–5 at MTP and IP joints, ankle plantarflexion, supports longitudinal arch
Flexor hallucis longus	Distal 2/3 of the posterior fibula and distal 2/3 of interosseous membrane	Plantar surface of distal phalanx of the great toe	Great toe flexion at the MTPJ and IPJ, ankle plantarflexion, supports longitudinal arch

| FIGURE | 10.6 | Anterior, lateral, and superficial posterior compartment muscles. |

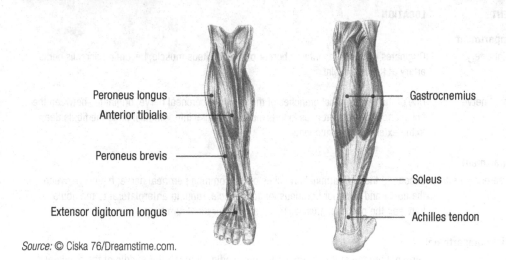

Peroneus longus

Anterior tibialis

Peroneus brevis

Extensor digitorum longus

Gastrocnemius

Soleus

Achilles tendon

Source: © Ciska 76/Dreamstime.com.

Neurovascular Structures

In this chapter, we will be examining a variety of tibiofemoral, patella, and lower-leg injuries. Some of those injuries may include traumatic injuries such as tibiofemoral joint dislocations or ruptures of collateral ligaments. These types of injuries can compromise the neurovascular structures in the area of the knee complex. Two important structures to keep in mind are the popliteal artery and the sciatic nerve.

The popliteal artery is an extension of the femoral artery and passes through the popliteal fossa. The popliteal artery then branches into the anterior and posterior tibial arteries at the inferior border of the popliteus muscle.[8] The anterior tibial artery passes through the anterior compartment of the lower leg and supplies the muscles in this same compartment. The anterior tibial artery then becomes the dorsalis pedis artery at the ankle joint. The posterior tibial artery runs in the deep posterior compartment of the lower leg and supplies the muscles of this compartment. The peroneal artery branches from the posterior tibial artery at the distal border of the popliteus to supply the lateral aspect of the lower leg. Finally, the posterior tibial artery ends at the origin of the abductor hallucis muscle by dividing into the medial and lateral plantar arteries. Reports have suggested that trauma occurs to the popliteal artery in 20 to 40 percent of knee dislocations.[4,6]

The sciatic nerve is the largest nerve in the body, running posteriorly down the lower extremity. It divides at the popliteal fossa into the tibial nerve—the medial portion—and the common peroneal nerve—the lateral portion. The tibial nerve (L4–S3) innervates the gastrocnemius and soleus and runs the length of the lower leg. The common peroneal nerve (L4–S2) initially wraps around the fibula head, which can be significant in trauma to the lateral aspect of the knee and can cause peroneal nerve palsy.[8] This nerve then divides into the deep peroneal nerve—which innervates the anterior tibialis muscle—and the superficial peroneal nerve—which innervates the peroneus longus. The three nerves, the tibial, the deep peroneal, and the superficial peroneal, run through the deep posterior, lateral, and anterior lower leg compartments, respectively (Table 10.6).[8]

TABLE	10.6	Lower leg neurovascular structures organized by compartment.

COMPARTMENT	LOCATION
Anterior compartment	
Anterior tibial artery	Originates opposite the inferior border of the popliteus muscle, becoming dorsalis pedis artery at the ankle joint
Deep peroneal nerve	One of the two terminal branches of the common peroneal nerve; originates between the fibula and superior peroneus longus muscle, running inferiomedial on to the fibula deep to the extensor digitorum longus
Lateral compartment	
Superficial peroneal nerve	Second of the two terminal branches of the common peroneal nerve; begins between the fibula and superior peroneus longus muscle, running anterolateral to the fibula between the peroneal muscles and the extensor digitorum longus
Deep posterior compartment	
Tibial nerve	Terminal branch of the sciatic nerve, descending through the middle of the popliteal fossa, posterior to the popliteal artery and vein, descending deep to the soleus and inferiorly on the tibialis posterior; terminates forming the medial and lateral plantar nerves
Posterior tibial artery	Terminal branch of the popliteal artery, passing deep to the origin of the soleus, passing inferomedially on the posterior surface of the tibialis posterior muscle running posterior to the medial malleolus where it is separated by the tendons of the tibialis posterior and flexor digitorum longus

Common Injuries

Injuries to the knee complex occur as a result of either a unidirectional force or two or more forces applied to the knee over a flexed or extended joint (i.e., multidirectional)[2] during both contact (player vs. player or player vs. equipment) and non-contact (pivoting) situations.[3] Individually, these forces include isolated hyperextension, hyperflexion, varus, valgus, anterior displacement, posterior displacement, and axial loading. However, certain combinations of forces applied to the knee complex are known to cause specific injury patterns and normally include a rotational force (i.e., external or internal rotation).[2] During a hyperextension force, the primary restraint against injury is the posterior cruciate ligament (PCL); the ACL and posterior capsule act as secondary restraints. A varus stress results in trauma to the lateral collateral ligament (LCL) and possibly the ACL and PCL. A unidirectional valgus force can cause isolated damage to the medial collateral ligament (MCL). A valgus and rotational force (e.g., pivoting in basketball) can result in trauma to the MCL, the ACL, and the menisci. Anterior translation, which displaces the tibia anteriorly, results in trauma to the ACL, the MCL, and/or the LCL.[2] Other anatomical structures such as the menisci, joint capsule, iliotibial band, and neurovascular tissue are also susceptible to and result in concomitant ligament damage.

LIGAMENTOUS AND SPECIAL TESTS

The case scenarios in this chapter may have you select and use a variety of ligamentous and special tests in order to adequately evaluate the injury. The details on how to perform each special test are beyond the scope of this section; however, Table 10.7 provides a general list of tests that may be required and useful for you to review before beginning the case scenarios. For a more thorough review, please refer to your favorite evaluation text or journal article(s).

TABLE 10.7	Ligamentous and special tests of the knee complex.
LIGAMENTOUS TESTS	**FUNCTIONS**
Uniplanar Instability	
Valgus stress	Assesses integrity of MCL and joint capsule
Varus stress	Assesses integrity of LCL
Anterior drawer	Assesses integrity of ACL (anteromedial bundle)
Lachman's stress	Assesses integrity of ACL (posterolateral bundle, tight in extension) and posterior oblique ligament
Posterior drawer	Assesses integrity of PCL, acruate-popliteus complex, and posterior oblique ligament
Godfrey's	Assesses Integrity of PCL
Rotary Instability	
Slocum drawer	Assesses anterior rotational knee instability
Lateral pivot shift	Assesses anterolateral knee instability (ACL, posterolateral capsule, arcuate ligament complex, or ITB)
Hughston drawer	Assesses posterior rotational knee instability
SPECIAL TESTS	**FUNCTIONS**
McMurray	Assesses for meniscal lesions
Apley's compression	Assesses for meniscal lesions
Sweep	Assesses accumulation of joint fluid
Patellar tap test or ballotable patella	Assesses moderate-to-severe joint effusion
Patella	
Clarke's sign	Assesses for chondromalacia patella
Apprehension	Assesses for a subluxating or dislocated patella, suggesting laxity of the medial patellar retinaculum
Patellar glide	Assesses mobility of the patella

(continued)

TABLE 10.7	Continued.
SPECIAL TESTS	**FUNCTIONS**
ITB	
Ober's	Assesses for ITB tightness
Noble's compression	Assesses ITB while non-weightbearing
Renne's	Assesses ITB while weightbearing

List of ligamentous and special tests is not exhaustive, and reliability of some tests may be questionable.

REFERENCES

1. Clarkson H. *Musculoskeletal Assessment: Joint Range of Motion and Manual Muscle Strength.* Philadelphia PA: Lippincott Williams & Wilkins; 2000.

2. Hayes CW, Brigido MK, Jamadar DA, Propeck T. Mechanism-based pattern approach to classification of complex injuries of the knee depicted at MR imaging. *Radiographics.* 2000;20:S121–S134.

3. Hootman JM, Dick R, Agel J. Epidemiology of collegiate injuries for 15 sports: summary and recommendations for injury prevention initiatives. *J Athl Train.* 2007;42(2):311–319.

4. Kaufman SL, Martin LG. Arterial injuries associated with complete dislocation of the knee. *Radiology.* 1992;184:153–155.

5. Levangie PK, Norkin CC. *Joint Structure and Function: A Comprehensive Analysis.* 3rd ed. Philadelphia PA: F. A. Davis; 2001.

6. Merrill KD. Knee dislocations with vascular injuries. *Orthop Clin N Am.* 1994;25:707–713.

7. Moore K, Dalley A. *Clinically Oriented Anatomy.* 5th ed. Baltimore MD: Lippincott Williams & Wilkins; 2005.

8. Moore KL. *Clinically Oriented Anatomy.* 3rd ed. Baltimore MD: Lippincott Williams & Wilkins; 1992.

I t was a rainy and muddy Friday night, and Tyler was covering a collegiate football game as a certified athletic trainer. Jim, a junior defensive back, was attempting to block a pass when he felt a pop in his left knee as he was jumping vertically. Jim instantly fell to the ground grabbing his knee. Tyler ran out onto the field, and as he arrived at Jim's side, Tyler noted that Jim was breathing heavily and rolling around on the ground holding his knee. After 20 seconds, Tyler calmed Jim down enough to get a history.

HISTORY

Tyler begins to question Jim about the injury. Jim states, "As I was trying to block the pass, my foot got stuck in the mud. As I jumped up, I tried to rotate and felt a pop in my knee." Jim's chief complaint is pain and tenderness along the medial joint line of the left knee. Tyler and another player assist Jim off the field. While walking over to the sideline, Jim complains that his knee feels like it is giving out.

PHYSICAL EXAMINATION

On the bench, Jim is very alert and in moderate-to-severe discomfort (7/10 on a numerical pain scale). Tyler begins evaluating Jim, noting some left-knee joint effusion. A flexed carrying position of the knee was noted sometime later. Active ROM is limited and produces pain with knee flexion. Passive ROM with overpressure produces pain (flexion). A locking sensation is noted with knee extension. Knee flexion and extension strength is reduced: 3+/5 and 3/5, respectively. Stress testing produces pain and laxity in multiple planes. Tyler tells Jim that he cannot return to the game and needs to be seen in the office tomorrow morning for a further evaluation and possible MRI. Tyler believes the best course of action would be immediate management for an acute knee injury.

? | Q U E S T I O N S | **CASE 10.1**

Please answer the following questions based on the above case information.

10.1 / **1.** Based on the information presented in the case, determine (a) the clinical diagnosis and (b) the common name for this condition.

10.1 / **2.** (a) Identify the bony and soft tissue structures that should have been palpated as part of the physical examination. Then (b) identify two or three other observations Tyler could have made during the initial assessment. (c) Why was the flexed carrying position noted sometime later during the evaluation and not initially?

10.1 / **3.** Based on Jim's MOI and his signs and symptoms, identify at least three ligamentous tests that could have been performed to assist in determining the clinical diagnosis. Describe how to perform each test.

10.1 / **4.** According to the evidence-based literature, which ligamentous tests used by clinicians are the most accurate in diagnosing this condition?

10.1 / **5.** Jim questions you as to why the doctor wants to see him tomorrow and why he needs an MRI. How do you answer him?

Sam, a 38-year-old construction worker and avid mountain biker, arrived at David's rehabilitation clinic five days after suffering a basketball accident. Sam was out playing basketball with his daughter when he landed awkwardly on his right leg. When Sam arrived at the clinic, his right knee was in an immobilizer, and he was on crutches. He appeared to be in moderate discomfort.

HISTORY

Sam reports that he was running down for a lay-up and misjudged the distance to the net. As he planted his right leg, he internally rotated just at the moment when his daughter came in from the side, knocking Sam off balance. He tried to catch his balance and immediately began to experience lateral knee pain. He recalls that he then limped into the house and explained to his wife what had just occurred. They put some ice on the knee to control swelling, and Sam says he took it easy for the rest of the night. The next morning, his knee was swollen, and he was having difficulty walking because of the pain and a funny sensation in his foot. He then went to a walk-in clinic, where the physician placed him in the knee immobilizer, gave him crutches, and referred him to an orthopedic specialist.

PHYSICAL EXAMINATION

Upon examination, five days after the injury, Sam presents with moderate discomfort (5/10–6/10) and an abnormal gait cycle. An observation of Sam's right knee reveals 2+ swelling and ecchymosis over the lateral joint line. A closer observation reveals some minor swelling into the popliteal fossa. David notes some tenderness over and around the lateral collateral ligament. Active ROM is decreased (15°–100°). Pain is also noted with passive tibial internal rotation. Strength testing reveals 3+/5 for knee flexion and extension. A closer look at Sam also reveals a decrease in ankle dorsiflexion and eversion active ROM and 1+/5 for ankle dorsiflexion and eversion strength. Knee ligamentous testing reveals instability at 0° and 20° of knee flexion (Figure 10.2.1). Tests for fractures are unremarkable. Neurologically, Sam presents with decreased peripheral sensation as shown in Figure 10.2.2.

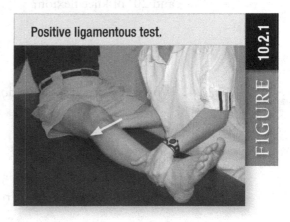

Positive ligamentous test.

FIGURE 10.2.1

Arrow indicates direction of force being applied to the medial knee.

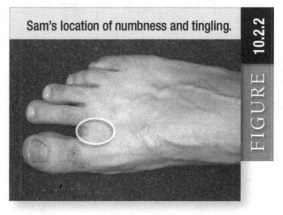

Sam's location of numbness and tingling.

FIGURE 10.2.2

Numbness and tingling are located within the circle.

Please answer the following questions based on the above case information.

10.2 / **1.** Based on the information presented in the case, determine (a) the differential diagnoses and (b) the clinical diagnosis.

10.2 / **2.** Figure 10.2.1 demonstrated a positive knee ligamentous test. The test revealed instability at 0° and 20° of knee flexion. What is the name of the test performed, and what is the diagnostic accuracy of this test?

10.2 / **3.** What is the clinical significance of varus ligamentous instability at both 0° and 20° of knee flexion?

10.2 / **4.** Why was a deficit in ankle dorsiflexion and eversion noted?

10.2 / **5.** How would you respond to Sam if he asks, "How is the doctor going to determine exactly what is wrong with me?"

CASE **10.3**

Mike, a 33-year-old male recreational triathlete, was training for a triathlon event. One day he began experiencing severe pain along the medial aspect of the left tibiofemoral joint line approximately 20 minutes into an easy run. Mike decided it would be best to stop running and walk back home because of the pain. The pain continued to increase during the day and was especially noticeable while he descended his stairs at home. Mike decided to stop by the university's sports medicine clinic several days later to pay a visit to Deb, one of the graduate assistant athletic trainers.

HISTORY

Deb has been working in the sports medicine clinic for several months and is happy to see Mike. She begins questioning him about his current situation. He explains what occurred earlier in the week and that he has been running 35 mi/wk and recently stepped it up to 50 mi/wk. He states, "After several days of complete rest, the initial pain went away, so I tried to return to running. However, after 5 minutes of jogging, the pain returned. I have a triathlon in five weeks and need to be ready."

PHYSICAL EXAMINATION

After Deb completes her physical examination of Mike, she determines that he is suffering from pes anserine bursitis. His initial treatment includes cryotherapy, anti-inflammatory medications, stretching, and therapeutic ultrasound (3 MHz at 1.2–1.5 w/cm²). During the second ultrasound treatment two days later, Mike begins complaining of intense bone pain along the medial aspect of the proximal tibia, forcing the termination of the ultrasound treatment. Deb refers Mike to an orthopedic surgeon, who orders radiographs of the left knee. The physician also provides Mike with a prescription of Tylenol® 800 mg every six hours to help alleviate pain.

DIAGNOSTIC IMAGING

The radiographs do not reveal any bony pathology. The physician decides to order a magnetic resonance imaging scan. The MRI is unremarkable for soft tissue trauma, but T1-weighted images demonstrate a small linear area of low signal intensity at the proximal aspect of the tibia, parallel to the tibial plateau medially and laterally, but more pronounced along the medial aspect (Figure 10.3.1).

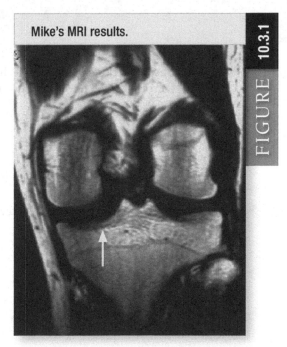

Mike's MRI results.

FIGURE 10.3.1

Arrow indicates area of increased signal intensity.

Please answer the following questions based on the above case information.

10.3 / **1.** Based on the information presented in the case, determine (a) the differential diagnoses and (b) the clinical diagnosis.

10.3 / **2.** (a) Overall, do you feel Deb performed an adequate history in this case? (b) Identify three or four history questions you as the evaluating clinician may have asked about extrinsic risk factors involved in the development of this condition?

10.3 / **3.** The findings of Deb's physical examination in this case are not well identified, except for the statement that "After Deb completes her physical examination of Mike, she determines that he is suffering from pes anserine bursitis." As the evaluating clinician, identify the steps you would have to follow to arrive at the initial clinical diagnosis of per anserine bursitis. Would you have considered the diagnosis of pes anserine bursitis, given the location of Mike's pain?

10.3 / **4.** Based on the case's clinical diagnosis, identity the possible intrinsic risk factors for the development of this condition.

10.3 / **5.** (a) Do you believe that Deb made a bad decision regarding the use of the therapeutic ultrasound? (b) Why did the therapeutic ultrasound produce intense pain at the injury site?

by William Holcomb, Ph.D., ATC, CSCS-D, University of Nevada, Las Vegas

A university basketball team was in the middle of its competitive season when Dylan, a 19-year-old male basketball player, reported to the athletic training clinic before practice. He was complaining of medial knee pain. Dylan was seen by Sean, the athletic trainer in charge of men's basketball.

HISTORY

Sean begins his assessment by asking, "So what's going on?" Dylan explains his chief complaints to Sean and specifically reports medial right knee pain that increases while engaged in activity and lessens when he is allowed to rest. He states that he has tried to ignore the pain, but the symptoms are getting worse as the season progresses. When asked about a specific MOI, he does not recall any specific event(s) during which he injured the knee. Dylan further reports a clicking sensation and noise with active knee flexion and extension and that his knee sometimes catches before giving away when he forces it to bend.

PHYSICAL EXAMINATION

Dylan is alert and oriented. He complains of moderate pain (5/10) even at rest, specifically along the medial femoral condyle near the joint line and adjacent to the medial border of the patella. This area is point tender when palpated. Active ROM reveals no deficits in knee flexion or extension. Muscle testing also reveals no weakness (5/5 for both flexion and extension); however, Sean does note that resisted movements do cause Dylan pain on the medial side of the knee.

DIAGNOSTIC IMAGING

The location of point tenderness is near the joint line, so Sean believes he is dealing with a possible torn medial meniscus. He decides the best course of action is to refer Dylan to Dr. Hansen, the team physician, for further evaluation and diagnostic imaging. The results of an MRI reveal a healthy, uninjured meniscus, but minor erosion of the medial femoral condyle is noted.

Because injury to the medial meniscus is ruled out, Sean and Dr. Hansen expand their assessment. Further palpation over the medial femoral condyle reveals a fibrous band running in a longitudinal fashion just medial to the patella. The area is point tender when palpated during knee extension; in fact, Dr. Hansen performs a special test that produces a positive finding (Figure 10.4.1).

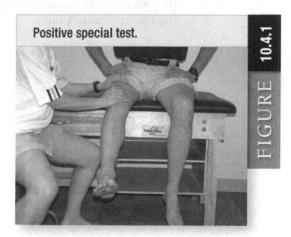

Positive special test.

FIGURE 10.4.1

Please answer the following questions based on the above case information.

10.4 / **1.**   Based on the information presented in the case, determine (a) the differential diagnoses and (b) the clinical diagnosis.

10.4 / **2.**   (a) What is the name of the special test shown in Figure 10.4.1? (b) As the evaluating clinician, how would you perform the test? (c) What is a positive finding?

10.4 / **3.**   What other special tests, if any, could be performed to assist in determining the clinical diagnosis?

10.4 / **4.**   Discuss the etiology of this condition. Include the following in your answer: (a) the definition of the condition, (b) the MOI, (c) a description of the asymptomatic condition, and (d) a description of the symptomatic condition.

10.4 / **5.**   (a) Describe the goals for management of this condition and the techniques that have been shown to be effective, including conservative methods. (b) Describe more aggressive treatments to be used should the conservative treatment methods fail.

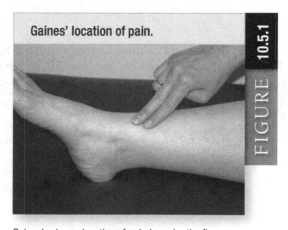

CASE

10.5

by William Holcomb, PhD, ATC, CSCS-D, University of Nevada, Las Vegas

G aines, a 21-year-old female, reported to her college's athletic training clinic after cross-country practice. She was complaining of recurring right lower leg pain and was worried because the team was in the final weeks of a four-month-long season. Shana, a certified athletic trainer, was glad to take a look at Gaines.

HISTORY

After some small talk about the upcoming meets, Shana begins to question Gaines about her problem. Gaines states, "I began experiencing pain after long training runs over the last several weeks, and it has been getting progressively worse. Normally the pain goes away with rest; but recently the pain has worsened, and now I have pain before exercise, during exercise, and after exercise." Gaines denies any previous history of lower leg trauma or chronic injuries. She rates her pain as 5/10 at rest and 8/10 during exercise.

PHYSICAL EXAMINATION

Gaines is alert and in moderate pain. Shana notes an area of increased palpable tenderness along the anterior medial border of the tibia, and she notes an area that is extremely tender (Figure 10.5.1). Knee AROM reveals no deficits. Shana does note a deficit in active ankle dorsiflexion. The remaining ankle ROM is unremarkable. Knee RROM reveals no muscular weakness. Ankle RROM is positive for pain and weakness in the inversion and plantarflexion directions. The remaining ankle movements are unremarkable.

> **Gaines' location of pain.**
>
> Gaines' primary location of pain is under the fingers.
>
> **FIGURE 10.5.1**

Shana believes she has a good idea of what is wrong and refers Gaines to the student health services for radiographs, which are negative for a stress fracture. Gaines is put on a conservative treatment consisting of cryotherapy and NSAIDs for pain and inflammation by the health center physician. After 10 days of this care, Shana realizes that Gaines has failed to have a resolution of her symptoms.

FOLLOW-UP PHYSICAL EXAMINATION

A follow-up neurological examination reveals no abnormalities with dermatomes or myotomes, and Tinel's sign over the superficial peroneal and saphenous nerves is negative. The dorsal pedal pulse is also found to be normal at rest and after exercise. The team physician orders a three-phase bone scan. Results are negative for a stress fracture, but a longitudinal uptake pattern along the distal third of the tibia is noted.

? | Q U E S T I O N S | **CASE 10.5**

Please answer the following questions based on the above case information.

10.5 / **1.** Based on the information presented in the case, determine (a) the differential diagnoses and (b) the clinical diagnosis.

10.5 / **2.** Explain how each of the differential diagnoses could be eliminated with confidence based on the physical examination and diagnostic tests.

10.5 / **3.** The clinical diagnosis is often graded based on the single criteria of pain. Describe what the four grades would be, based on the clinical diagnosis.

10.5 / **4.** (a) When Gaines reported to the athletic training clinic, what grade based on question 10.5/3. was she experiencing? (b) What does that mean for her participation in cross-country?

10.5 / **5.** If you were the treating clinician in this case, identify the possible interventions you may use to treat Gaines.

Jeannette is an 18-year-old female gymnast. While warming up with a tumbling pass on the floor during practice, she did not complete a full rotation when performing a back flip and landed on her right knee. At the time of the injury, she did not feel any substantial pain. When she went to complete another tumbling pass 10 minutes later she was unable to, and she was not able to complete the rest of the competition. She then sought the assistance of Sue, the university's new athletic trainer, who was covering the event.

HISTORY

Sue begins by questioning Jeannette about the MOI. Jeannette answers that she did not fully rotate during her back flip and landed straight down on her right knee (Figure 10.6.1). Jeannette says that she attempted another pass and was unable to complete the pass because "my knee felt unstable." Sue then proceeds to question Jeannette about her pain level on a 0 to 10 scale. Jeannette states that her pain level is 5/10 at rest.

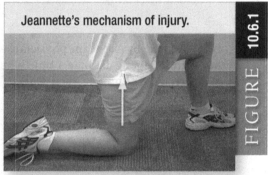

Jeannette's mechanism of injury.

Arrow indicates direction of force applied by the body to the flexed knee complex.

PHYSICAL EXAMINATION

Sue observes Jeannette's gait and notes an increase in right knee flexion during the stance phase of the right lower extremity (Figure 10.6.2). There is a slight antalgic gait pattern. Upon observation of the right knee, there is minimal-to-moderate general effusion noted of the right knee. Palpation reveals tenderness and guarding of the distal hamstrings. Jeannette's ROM results are in Table 10.6.1. Neurologically, there is no deficit. Ligamentous testing reveals a positive Godfrey's test, a positive posterior drawer, and a positive active quadriceps test. Sue also performs a Lachman's test, which is negative. A McMurry's test and Apley's compression and distraction tests are also negative.

Sue decides, based on her findings, to begin immediate care using RICE. Jeannette and Sue then discuss the options for the best course of action for competing in tomorrow's competition and decide it would be most appropriate to continue resting and to

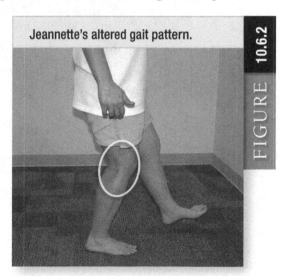

Jeannette's altered gait pattern.

Altered gait pattern indicated by circle.

TABLE	10.6.1	Jeannette's range of motion results.		
			FINDINGS	
MOTION	**JOINT MOTION**	**RIGHT**	**LEFT**
AROM	Knee flexion	115°	140°
	Knee extension	5°	5°–0°
PROM	Knee flexion	Minor-to-moderate discomfort at end range	
	Knee extension	Minor-to-moderate discomfort at end range	
RROM	Knee flexion	4–/5	
	Knee extension	4/5	

be evaluated by the team physician when possible. At the completion of treatment, Sue and Jeannette arrange a time when they can meet and perform further treatment the next day. Jeannette then walks out of the athletic training room to watch her teammates finish practice.

| ? | Q U E S T I O N S | CASE 10.6 |

Please answer the following questions based on the above case information.

10.6 / 1. Based on the information presented in the case, determine (a) the differential diagnoses and (b) the clinical diagnosis.

10.6 / 2. What other MOI(s) can cause this injury?

10.6 / 3. (a) In your opinion, and based on the information in the case, explain whether you think Sue took an appropriate history. (b) What other questions would you have asked as the evaluating clinician?

10.6 / 4. According to the case, it was reported that there was an antalgic gait pattern, but Jeannette's location of pain was not addressed. In what area do you think Jeannette would complain most about pain?

10.6 / 5. What could Sue have done to address the antalgic gait pattern?

10.6 / 6. The clinical diagnosis can be classified into one of three different grades. Describe the classification of each grade.

10.6 / 7. Overall, do you believe that Sue managed the condition appropriately? What else could have been done to assist with Jeannette's recovery?

10.7

Melissa, an 18-year-old female high school soccer player, was standing in as goalie during a soccer match. When an offender got past the last defender, Melissa decided to challenge the defender rather than wait for the offender to take a shot. In doing so, the two girls knocked knees. Instantly, Melissa fell to the ground, grabbing her left knee. She immediately knew that something was really wrong and started calling for Sara, the per diem athletic trainer on the sideline. The referee called time, and Sara rushed onto the scene to perform an on-field assessment.

HISTORY

Sara was paying close attention to the match, so she saw Melissa's MOI. However, she still starts the evaluation by asking Melissa what happened. Melissa is extremely upset at this point and is unable to maintain her composure enough to tell Sara exactly what happened. All Sara understood is, "I heard a pop, and now I can't move my knee." Sara proceeds to examine Melissa on the field based on what she had seen from the sidelines.

PHYSICAL EXAMINATION

As Sara begins her observation, she immediately notes an abnormality of the left knee with the patella riding toward the mid-thigh. Sara continues to attempt to calm Melissa in order to assess where she is feeling the most pain and to keep her from further injuring herself as she continues to move and writhe in pain. When Melissa is finally calm, about 6 minutes later, and Sara asks her to attempt to straighten her leg, she is unable to do this without severe pain.

Sara decides it is best to leave Melissa in this position and attempt to immobilize her as best as possible. She also decides to activate EMS and asks a coach to stay with Melissa to keep her calm so she can call 9-1-1. Melissa is left on the field because Sara did not want to attempt weight-bearing, in light of Melissa's pain level and inability to actively straighten the left knee. After activating EMS, Sara returns and attempts to splint the injury in Melissa's current position.

When the paramedics arrive, they also notice a defect of the left anterior thigh, with moderate swelling of the knee joint. Melissa is stabilized by the paramedics, with the knee left in flexion, and transported to the hospital via ambulance.

DIAGNOSTIC IMAGING

At the hospital, radiographs are immediately performed to rule out a fracture and/or dislocation of the knee. The radiographs show the patella floating in the middle of the femur, with a portion of the patella located distal to the femoral condyles. Melissa is immediately brought to the operating room.

FOLLOW-UP EXAMINATION

Twelve weeks after the initial insult, Melissa receives a prescription to start rehabilitation. Melissa spends 12 weeks immobilized, 6 weeks in a straight leg cast, and then 6 weeks in a hinge brace locked at 0° to 90°. She has just been released to full ROM within the brace during daily activities. She returns to the athletic training room and conveys the instructions to start rehab. Sara evaluates Melissa to start the rehab process. Sara finds that Melissa has limited knee flexion ROM to 105°, and extension ROM is WNL. Melissa is unable to actively contract the left quadriceps; her hamstring strength is 2+/5, gastrocnemius strength is 3/5, and dorsiflexion strength is 3/5.

❓ QUESTIONS   CASE 10.7

Please answer the following questions based on the above case information.

10.7 / 1. Based on the information presented in the case, determine (a) the differential diagnoses and (b) the clinical diagnosis.

10.7 / 2. Why do you believe that Melissa was unable to actively extend her knee?

10.7 / 3. (a) Overall, do you believe that Sara managed the situation appropriately? (b) What if anything could she have done better to manage the situation?

10.7 / 4. What are some possible consequences of Sara's on-scene actions?

10.7 / 5. After Melissa arrived at the hospital, how do you think this case was managed medically?

10.7 / 6. Now that Melissa is cleared to begin rehabilitation, what should be the first thing Sara should concentrate on in Melissa's rehabilitation? Please explain your reasoning.

CASE 10.8

andy is a 27-year-old female training to be a police officer. While running the obstacle course at the police academy she came across some uneven ground. As she transitioned from one obstacle to another, her knee twisted, causing her to fall to the ground. She landed on her right knee and immediately experienced anterior knee pain, an inability to bear weight through the right lower extremity, and an inability to move the knee into extension or flexion. Samantha, the certified athletic trainer assisting in medical coverage for the cadets, was then called to the scene to evaluate Sandy's condition.

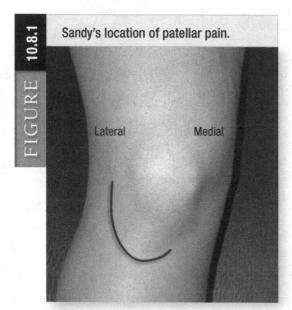

FIGURE 10.8.1

Sandy's location of patellar pain.

Lateral   Medial

Sandy's primary location of pain is along the line.

HISTORY

Before Samantha begins her SAMPLE history, she makes an initial assessment, making sure there is no immediate threat to Sandy's life. Samantha then asks Sandy what happened and what her chief complaints are. Sandy explains that while she was running from one obstacle to another, her right foot got stuck on the ground while her upper leg and torso continued to move, causing a rotational force at the knee. Sandy also states, "When I looked at my knee, I noticed a bump on the outside of my knee that disappeared when I attempted to move my knee." Samantha asks about the location of pain, to which Sandy responds, "It's in the front of my knee and around my kneecap" (Figure 10.8.1). Sandy's chief complaints are pain and the inability to move her knee without excessive pain.

PHYSICAL EXAMINATION

Sandy is in obvious discomfort. Samantha begins her physical examination by completing a more thorough assessment of the involved knee. She notes an increase in swelling of the right knee but no other obvious deformity. Sandy is unable to perform active or passive knee flexion without severe pain. Samantha determines that Sandy is stable medically but requires transport to the hospital for medical management of her right knee pain, according to Academy regulations. While waiting for EMS to arrive, Samantha applies ice to Sandy's right knee and remains with Sandy, ensuring that she remains medically stable.

After radiographs are completed and it is concluded that Sandy did not suffer any bony trauma, she is placed in a knee immobilizer and told to continue the use of the knee immobilizer for one week. She is given crutches because she was having difficulty bearing weight and walking with the immobilizer. She is also instructed to apply ice for the next 24 hours and then to switch to heat after that. She can take a NSAID twice a day for pain. Finally, she is given a prescription for rehabilitation, with pain being her only restriction, and told to follow up with an orthopedic physician if necessary.

FOLLOW-UP EXAMINATION

Sandy returns to see Samantha the next day in order to apprise her of the outcome of the ER visit. Samantha proceeds to perform a follow-up evaluation of Sandy's knee. Sandy's ROM and girth measurements can be found in Tables 10.8.1 and 10.8.2, respectively. An isolated vastus medialis contraction is fair on the right, good on the left. Sandy demonstrates a positive special test on the right and negative on the left (Figure 10.8.2). Patella location appears to be more lateral on the right than the left, and there is an observable patella alta on the right when compared with the left. There is positive point tenderness along the medial side of the patella.

TABLE 10.8.1 Sandy's range of motion results.

| MOTION | JOINT MOTION | FINDINGS | |
		RIGHT	LEFT
AROM	Knee flexion	120°	140°
	Knee extension	−5° (lacks full extension)	5°–0°
RROM	Knee flexion	4/5	5/5
	Knee extension	3–/5	5/5

TABLE 10.8.2 Sandy's girth measurements.

	RIGHT	LEFT
6 inches above superior patella	60 cm	64 cm
4 inches above superior patella	52 cm	54 cm
Knee joint	35 cm	32 cm
2 inches below inferior patella	33 cm	30 cm

FIGURE 10.8.2 Positive special test.

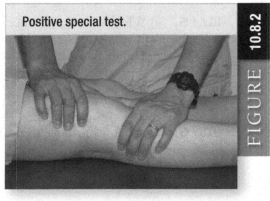

Force is applied along the medial patella pushing laterally.

Please answer the following questions based on the above case information.

10.8 / **1.** Based on the information presented in the case, determine (a) the differential diagnoses and (b) the clinical diagnosis.

10.8 / **2.** Based on the information presented above, do you think Samantha took a thorough history and physical examination? What else could Samantha have asked or performed to help make the diagnosis?

10.8 / **3.** Do you believe that Samantha performed the necessary immediate care steps? Explain your answer.

10.8 / **4.** At the emergency room, Sandy underwent several radiographs to rule out bony trauma. The radiographs were negative for fractures, but an Insall-Salvati ratio of 1.4 did show up, along with proper alignment of the patella in the femoral groove. What is an Insall-Salvati ratio, and why is it significant?

10.8 / **5.** (a) What is the significance of knowing that the patella is in proper alignment within the femoral groove? (b) What are some other factors that may contribute to a patella dislocation?

10.8 / **6.** (a) What is the name of the test in Figure 10.8.2? (b) What does it assess?

10.8 / **7.** After completing each physical examination, Samantha documented her findings. Please document your findings from both examinations as if you were the treating clinician. If the case did not provide information you believe is pertinent to the clinical diagnosis, please feel free to add this information to your documentation.

CASE 10.9

Jessica is an athletic trainer who was covering a professional power weight-lifting event. She was nearby when Antonio, a 28-year-old male, started to perform a power clean maneuver with 350 lbs. Antonio collapsed while attempting to throw the weight in the upward direction from the floor to the chest. As he was collapsing, he attempted to throw the weight away from his body but was unsuccessful.

HISTORY

Upon arrival at the scene, Jessica determines that Antonio is alert and demonstrates signs of life. She quickly determines that there is no obvious injury from the weight falling on Antonio, though he is writhing in pain and complaining of right knee and thigh pain. An initial assessment of the cervical, thoracic, and lumbar spine and neurological screening are unremarkable. Jessica asks Antonio what happened, and he responds, "My knee just gave out and was no longer able to support me. My knee really hurts now!" While he is explaining to Jessica what happened, he is holding on to his leg rocking back and forth in an attempt to manage his pain. Jessica proceeds to ask Antonio if he could point to his pain. Antonio points to his superior patella and distal anterior thigh area.

PHYSICAL EXAMINATION

Upon observation of the knee, Jessica notices Antonio's right knee is in a flexed position. She also notes immediate formation of edema of the right knee by comparison with the left. When Jessica asks Antonio to attempt to actively extend the right knee, he is unable. He grimaces in pain in the attempt. Jessica then passively moves the right knee into extension without complaints of pain from Antonio. Jessica realizes Antonio is going to be unable to walk on his own and proceeds to immobilize the knee. With assistance from two competitors she gets Antonio to the side so she can further evaluate his injury.

SIDELINE PHYSICAL EXAMINATION

After immobilizing him and safely getting him to the side so that the event could continue, Jessica further evaluates Antonio's injury. Upon observation, the right-knee edema is worsening. Upon palpation, Jessica finds a defect in the right quadriceps area above the superior pole of the patella. Jessica determines that Antonio requires further medical evaluation. Antonio is transported by EMS to the hospital.

Please answer the following questions based on the above case information.

10.9 / **1.** Based on the information presented in the case, determine (a) the differential diagnoses and (b) the clinical diagnosis.

10.9 / **2.** What questions might Jessica have asked in this particular situation to help establish the proper clinical diagnosis?

10.9 / **3.** Describe how you think Jessica should have immobilized Antonio's knee.

10.9 / **4.** What medical studies or diagnostic imaging may be ordered for this injury upon evaluation at the emergency room?

10.9 / **5.** Based on the information presented in the case, what if anything should have been done differently?

10.9 / **6.** What medical management do you think is required for the above injury?

E va is a 23-year-old who has recently started to experience an increase in right anterior knee pain, primarily while running. Her knee pain has become progressively worse over the last month, leading Eva to seek a medical examination from her primary-care physician. The physician referred her to a local physical medicine clinic, where she was to be evaluated by Jonathan, an athletic trainer and physical therapist.

HISTORY

While interviewing Eva and obtaining a history, Jonathan learns that Eva has been training for the Saginaw City Marathon for about three weeks and that this is her first time training for such an event. During their continued discussion about her marathon training, Eva reveals that her marathon is four months away. She reports pain in the area depicted in Figure 10.10.1 that gets worse with running, especially during the first mile and after activity. Eva reports that the pain has progressively gotten more intense while running and that the pain is lasting longer throughout her running. At approximately mile two, the pain subsides but then increases after continued running. Jonathan asks Eva to describe her pain. Eva describes it as, "sharp when I am running and a dull ache when I am resting." Pain is rated as 8/10 during activity.

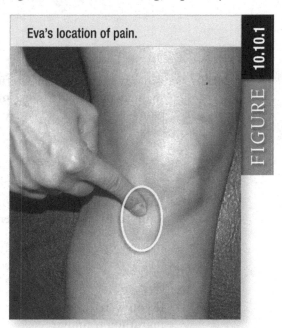

Eva's location of pain.

FIGURE 10.10.1

Eva's location of pain is under the finger and within the circle.

PHYSICAL EXAMINATION

Eva presents with normal knee AROM and PROM. Manual muscle testing reveals normal hamstring strength bilaterally. Right quadriceps strength is 4/5 with pain elicited. Left quad strength is 5/5. Palpation reveals positive point tenderness along the patella tendon and inferior pole of the patella. There is mild effusion noted along the inferior aspect of the patella tendon. Ligamentous stress tests are negative. A Clarke's sign is negative.

Please answer the following questions based on the above case information.

10.10 / **1.** Based on the information presented in the case, determine (a) the differential diagnoses and (b) the clinical diagnosis.

10.10 / **2.** What other history questions could Jonathan have asked to help with his differential diagnoses and to assist him in determining which special tests to perform?

10.10 / **3.** What, if any, other special tests could you as the evaluating clinician perform to assist in determining the differential diagnoses?

10.10 / **4.** What would be the most effective rehabilitation program for Eva so that she may participate in her marathon training with the least amount of pain?

10.10 / **5.** Based on the history that Jonathan acquired from Eva, what stage of the injury is Eva presently experiencing?

10.10 / **6.** If you were Jonathan, what would you advise Eva to do regarding her marathon training?

Sandra, an 18-year-old freshman for a Division I volleyball team, reports to Kerri, the athletic trainer responsible for women's volleyball. Sandra's chief complaint is of anterior right knee pain. The volleyball team has been in two-a-days for the past five days.

HISTORY

After some small talk, Kerri begins questioning Sandra about her current chief complaint. Kerri learns that Sandra's pain just started within the last two days and has progressively worsened during this day. Sandra reports pain in the anterior aspect of the knee but is unable to pinpoint the location (Figure 10.11.1). She points to a diffuse area of the anterior knee, patella tendon, and inferior pole of the patella. Sandra states that her pain is most severe with jumping when attempting to spike the ball. She also reported increased pain when performing her squatting exercises and climbing up stairs. She denies pain at rest; however, she does admit that this preseason is the most challenging she has ever experienced and that not training this summer was a really bad idea.

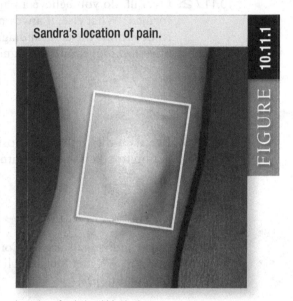

Sandra's location of pain.

FIGURE 10.11.1

Location of pain is within the box.

PHYSICAL EXAMINATION

Upon Sandra's arrival to the athletic training room, Kerri notes a normal gait pattern. Evaluation of the right knee reveals normal quad strength, hamstring strength at 4/5, and VMO contraction delayed compared with the contralateral VMO. The right VMO bulk is also diminished when compared with the left. Sandra exhibits normal bilateral ROM of the knee, hip, and ankle. Patella motion is limited with a medial glide. Lateral, superior, and inferior glides are normal. Kerri also notes a patella alta and squinting patella. Sandra exhibits a positive patellar tilt test and a positive patellar grind test. Ligamentous and meniscal tests are negative. Point tenderness is present along the lateral and medial aspects of the patella. Standing posture reveals positive foot pronation and positive genu valgus.

After completing the evaluation, Kerri decides it is necessary to begin a rehabilitation program to improve Sandra's current state. She informs Sandra's coach that Sandra can practice but with modifications. The coach is very upset with this decision and tells the 18-year-old to "suck it up." This does not sit well with Kerri.

? | Q U E S T I O N S | CASE 10.11

Please answer the following questions based on the above case information.

10.11 / **1.** Based on the information presented in the case, determine (a) the differential diagnoses, and (b) the likely clinical diagnosis.

10.11 / **2.** Overall, do you believe an appropriate physical examination was performed? What else, if anything, would you do as the evaluating clinician to determine the clinical diagnosis? Describe how to perform these evaluative techniques and the significance they would have on your findings.

10.11 / **3.** Based on the clinical diagnosis, what do you think is the best course of action to take as far as treatment?

10.11 / **4.** Many individuals use McConnell taping to assist in managing this condition. (a) What is McConnell taping? (b) What is its efficacy in treating the condition?

J ohn is a 25-year-old industrial worker for a Fortune 500 company. He was walking within the warehouse where pallets were being moved, when he was struck below the anterior knee by a forklift. The driver of the forklift realized what had happened and immediately put the emergency action plan into effect. Doug, a certified athletic trainer and emergency medical technician, was the first person to respond to the incident.

ON-SCENE ARRIVAL

When Doug arrives on the scene, he sees John lying on the ground, exhibiting grimaces and writhing from severe pain. Doug observes John's knee and immediately notices that the left knee is severely deformed. Doug performs a rapid assessment and confirms a painful, swollen, deformed knee. He also quickly gathers a history of the MOI, determines that medical evaluation is necessary, and asks Stan (another worker) to activate EMS. Baseline vital signs are: blood pressure, 118/70; radial pulse, 90 and strong; and respiration, 14 and regular.

PHYSICAL EXAMINATION

Closer observation of the left knee and foot reveals discoloration of the left foot. The left foot appears to be a grayish-bluish color. He also notices moderate effusion of the knee joint. Doug then proceeds to splint the injury. As Doug is splinting the injury, the EMS staff arrives, helps Doug splint the injury, and then transports John to the local emergency department.

DIAGNOSTIC IMAGING

At the hospital, John is evaluated by the ER physician. Radiographs are taken and reveal a noticeable deformity of the tibiofemoral joint.

? Q U E S T I O N S   **CASE 10.12**

Please answer the following questions based on the above case information.

10.12 / **1.** Based on the information presented in the case, determine (a) the differential diagnoses and (b) the clinical diagnosis.

10.12 / **2.** Based on the information provided in the case, is there anything else that Doug should have assessed further?

10.12 / **3.** In what position was the knee when Doug splinted the injury? What materials do you think were used?

10.12 / **4.** (a) What other types of injuries does Doug need to be concerned with in addition to vascular damage? (b) How might he assess the problems?

10.12 / **5.** (a) Based on the clinical diagnosis, what if any ligamentous structures could be affected? (b) What is the most likely treatment?

10.13

J ennifer, an athletic trainer, was completing paperwork in the general athletic training room when Susie, a track runner, came to the athletic training room limping, barely weight-bearing on her left lower extremity.

HISTORY

Jennifer immediately places Susie on the table and starts taking a history. She asks Susie how the injury occurred. Susie reports that she was bouldering on the university recreation center's climbing wall and that while she was on the wall she fell from approximately six feet, landing on her left leg. Susie thinks that her left ankle turned inward (inverted) and that her knee was flexed (Figure 10.13.1). She says that she felt and heard an audible pop when she attempted to rise to her feet after the fall. Jennifer then asks Susie about her pain level and the location of her pain (Figure 10.13.2). Susie describes her pain as 8/10.

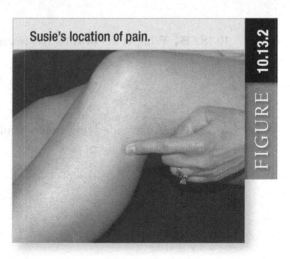

Susie's mechanism of injury.

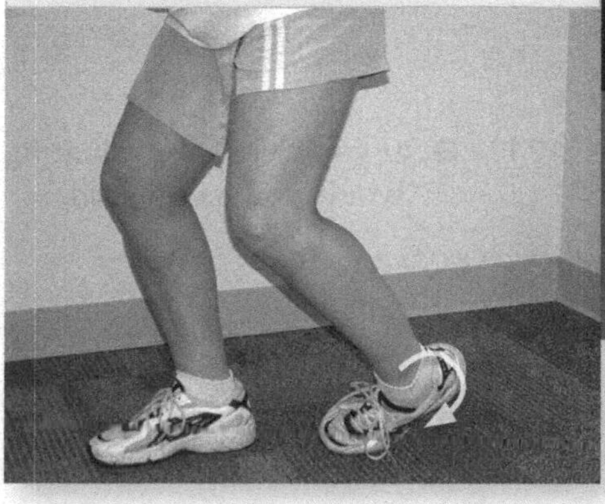

FIGURE 10.13.1

Ankle is rolling inward.

PHYSICAL EXAMINATION

Susie appears alert and cooperative but is experiencing severe discomfort. During the physical examination, Jennifer notes that Susie is point tender along the fibular head, with minimal effusion noted in the left knee area. Jennifer also notes that knee flexion ROM is 100° and extension lacks 8° (left knee ROM 8°–100°). Strength measurements are not made because of increased pain and limited ROM. A valgus stress test is negative bilaterally while varas testing produces pain. Tests of the ACL and PCL are negative.

Jennifer decides that, in order to properly manage the condition, she needs to refer Susie to the team physician to rule out secondary injury.

Susie's location of pain.

FIGURE 10.13.2

Location of pain is under the finger.

Please answer the following questions based on the above case information.

10.13 / **1.** Based on the information presented in the case, determine (a) the differential diagnoses and (b) the clinical diagnosis.

10.13 / **2.** Identify (a) the four classifications of this injury and (b) the most common MOI.

10.13 / **3.** If you were the evaluating athletic trainer, what other questions, if any, would you have asked?

10.13 / **4.** If you were evaluating this injury, which anatomical structures would you have palpated/tested, and why?

10.13 / **5.** What is the normal treatment for this condition?

10.13 / **6.** What underlying causes could have influenced this injury?

10.14

Kirk, a 24-year-old hurdler for an NCAA Division II Track and Field team, reports to the athletic training room complaining of medial left knee pain. Latisha, the head athletic trainer for track and field, takes Kirk over to a treatment table and starts taking a history.

HISTORY

Latisha begins by asking Kirk when and how the injury occurred. Kirk states that his pain started approximately three weeks ago for no apparent reason. He reports that he has had several incidents of medial knee pain intermittently over the last year. Latisha asks what makes his pain better and what makes his pain worse. Kirk replies that his pain is better with rest and the use of ice and anti-inflammatory drugs and worse with activity, specifically running and hurdling. Latisha asks him to describe his pain. He states, "It hurts in the middle part of my knee, like an ache that worsens when I hurdle." Kirk then points to the area of pain shown in Figure 10.14.1.

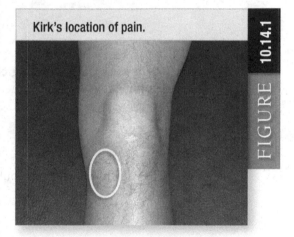

Kirk's location of pain.

FIGURE 10.14.1

Location of pain is within the circle, on the medial aspect of the tibia.

PHYSICAL EXAMINATION

Observation reveals no significant ecchymosis of the left knee when compared with the right. There is a slight increase in effusion along the medial aspect of the proximal tibia by comparison with the right. Kirk is also point tender at the insertion of the gracilis, sartorius, and semimembranosus. No other point tenderness is revealed. Ligamentous tests are within normal limits for the left knee. Manual muscle testing reveals 4/5 for the sartorius muscle and produces pain; 5/5 for quadriceps; lateral hamstrings are 5/5; medial hamstrings are 4/5 and produce pain. Hip abduction is 5/5; hip adduction is 4/5 and produces pain. Meniscal testing is negative, as are patella tests. Neurologically Kirk is intact.

Latisha discusses her findings with Kirk, and together they devise a modified training plan. Latisha also informs Kirk that if the overuse condition has not improved within seven days, she is going to refer him to the team's physician.

Please answer the following questions based on the above case information.

10.14 / **1.** Based on the information presented in the case, determine (a) the differential diagnoses and (b) the clinical diagnosis.

10.14 / **2.** What, if anything, did you recognize in the case that was inaccurate?

10.14 / **3.** What is the most appropriate way to manually test the muscles involved in this injury?

10.14 / **4.** If you were the evaluating clinician, what would be your treatment recommendations?

10.14 / **5.** What diagnostic imaging could be performed to help determine the clinical diagnosis?

H ugh is an athletic training graduate assistant for a Division I university. His primary responsibility is to evaluate, treat, and prevent athletic injuries for the women's field hockey team. The team has just started three-a-day practices for pre-season. At the first practice, the coach had the team go through what they have termed the "Gauntlet." Hugh quickly learns that the Gauntlet consists of several timed running tests, including the following: a 3-mile run, a 1-mile run, two 800-yard runs, two 400-yard runs, four 200-yard runs, and ten 50-yard runs. By the end of the week, Hugh starts to see an increase in injuries from poor conditioning over the summer. Lisa is the first of three players who report to the athletic training room complaining of anterior lower leg pain, especially with running.

HISTORY

Hugh asks Lisa to sit on the treatment table so he may ask her some questions regarding her symptoms. Lisa reports that she has anterior lower leg pain and numbness in the dorsal aspect of the foot. Lisa states that her pain started at the third practice on the first day of three-a-days. Initially, the pain and numbness occurred only while she was running and ceased when she completed the activity. Now, the pain is becoming more constant. She says, "My pain gets worse when I'm moving around or working out, and it gets better if I stop; but it never really goes away." She adds that her numbness is also getting more pronounced when she runs but does stop after she rests for 10 minutes. In fact, the numbness is most noticeable between the first two toes. Lisa reports that she has been icing after practice, but it has not helped. Hugh asks Lisa what her pain level is currently, on a 0 to 10 scale. Lisa states, "5/10."

PHYSICAL EXAMINATION

Hugh measures Lisa's knee and ankle ROM and finds no significant difference bilaterally. She does complain of some pain with active dorsiflexion, but no other motions are painful. All knee and ankle ligamentous tests are within normal limits. Strength testing is unremarkable except for DF, which is decreased on the involved side. Hugh palpates the anterior, medial, and lateral lower leg without report of pain. There is no obvious deformity or swelling present.

Hugh tells the coach that he is withholding Lisa from three-a-days because of her increased symptoms. The coach is clearly not happy about the decision and asks Hugh how long she has to sit out.

FOLLOW-UP EXAMINATION

Lisa remains on the sideline and sees little-to-no improvement in her symptoms. Meanwhile, Candice and Sandy report to the athletic training room a week later after the first practice of the day. Each athlete is also complaining of the same symptoms as Lisa. Candice states she started having minimal discomfort after performing the Gauntlet. She too has pain during activity that has progressively worsened with no paresthesia as this time. Initially, her pain appeared only during activity and subsided with rest. Now the pain is constant, increasing in intensity during running and decreasing with cessation of the activity. Sandy's pain is very similar, but she does complain of paresthesia in the dorsal aspect of the foot that increases with activity and does not fully cease with rest. She reports that her pain also started the day after performing the Gauntlet. She too complains that her pain and paresthesia are worsening. Candice reports her pain level at 6/10, and Sandy reports a pain level at 4/10.

The physical examination of Candice is normal as far as ROM, palpation, strength, and ligamentous tests, with some point tenderness noted in the anterior tibialis muscle belly. Sandy demonstrates increased pain with dorsiflexion, and her strength measurements are 4/5. All other strength and ROM measurements are within normal limits.

Hugh starts conservative treatment with both Candice and Sandy and also puts them on the injured list for the rest of three-a-days. Hugh suspects these injuries have a commonality of poor conditioning during the summer. He also suspects the Gauntlet is the triggering factor for these three individuals.

? **QUESTIONS**   **CASE 10.15**

Please answer the following questions based on the above case information.

10.15 / **1.** Based on the information presented in the case, determine (a) the differential diagnoses and (b) the clinical diagnosis.

10.15 / **2.** Was everything performed during the physical examination that could or should have been performed?

10.15 / **3.** (a) What diagnostic test can be done to confirm the clinical diagnosis?
(b) What are the normal ranges of pressure in the area of the injury?
(c) What is the treatment for the abnormal ranges?

10.15 / **4.** (a) What do you believe would be the most appropriate treatment in Lisa's case after she presented to Hugh? (b) What are some alternative activities that could be performed to allow for proper cardiovascular training but not worsen the condition?

10.15 / **5.** (a) Why do you think Hugh pulled Lisa out of practice? (b) What are the risks if she continues to play? (c) How long would you keep Lisa out of three-a-days? What would be your response to the coach if she told you she was not happy with the decision presented in this case?

10.15 / **6.** (a) How would you approach the coach and suggest that the training regime be changed? (b) If the coach were not receptive to Hugh's suggestions, what other course of action could he take?

CASE 10.16

Jayden, a 15-year-old boy and an active basketball player, has sought medical attention for right anterior knee pain. He has received a referral for physical therapy services from his primary-care physician and is now seeing Nate, a physical therapist/athletic trainer at a local sports medicine clinic.

HISTORY

Nate starts the evaluation by reviewing the physician's referral. It states that Jayden's CC is anterior knee pain. Nate then reviews the health questionnaire Jayden filled out in order to learn the location, severity, and description of Jayden's pain (Figure 10.16.1). He notices that Jayden described his pain as "a dull ache with some sharp pain." Nate examines the questionnaire for any other pertinent information on past medical history, but nothing else is noted. Nate asks Jayden how he injured his knee. Jayden responds that he could not remember a specific injury. He reports that the pain started approximately two weeks ago for no apparent reason. After talking a little more with Jayden, Nate finds out that the pain has been ongoing for several weeks, even months at a lower degree. Nate then asks about what activities Jayden performs regularly. Jayden states that he plays basketball and just started playing on two different league teams within the last few weeks. Nate finally asks Jayden if there are any specific activities that increase his pain or anything that relieves his pain. Jayden states that his pain is worse when he plays basketball and increases with jumping and that rest helps the most. Jayden also reports that he has tried some ice with some relief.

PHYSICAL EXAMINATION

Upon physical examination, Nate immediately notices an enlarged right tibial tuberosity, with no enlargement noted on the left. He has tenderness along the right tibial tuberosity. Range of motion measurements are equal bilaterally for both active and passive motion, with slight pain at end range of right knee flexion. The

FIGURE 10.16.1

Jayden's pain profiles.

1. Please rate your current level of pain at rest on the following scale (circle one):

   0 1 ② 3 4 5 6 7 8 9 10
   (no pain)   *(worst imaginable pain)*

2. Please rate your level of pain during activity on the following scale (circle one):

   0 1 2 3 4 5 ⑥ 7 8 9 10
   (no pain)   *(worst imaginable pain)*

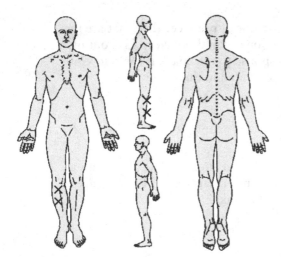

✕✕ = dull ache with some sharp pain.

position of the patella is alta on the right when compared with the left patella position. Ligamentous tests are negative. Manual muscle testing for the quadriceps is normal but causes pain on the right. All other strength measurements are within normal limits.

Nate has a pretty good idea of the clinical diagnosis and retreats to the back room to acquire a specialized patella tendon strap.

? QUESTIONS   **CASE 10.16**

Please answer the following questions based on the above case information.

10.16 / **1.** Based on the information presented in the case, determine (a) the differential diagnoses and (b) the clinical diagnosis.

10.16 / **2.** Identify the etiology for this clinical diagnosis.

10.16 / **3.** What are the three classifications for this clinical diagnosis?

10.16 / **4.** (a) What else, if anything, could Nate have asked in his history to assist with determining the differential diagnosis? (b) Is there anything else Nate should have evaluated?

10.16 / **5.** What would be an appropriate treatment?

10.16 / **6.** Jayden and his parents ask Nate if Jayden is able to continue playing basketball, because he has a tournament this weekend that he wants to compete in. What would be your response to this question? Would you allow Jayden to continue playing? Why or why not? When would you allow Jayden to return to playing if you feel he should not play?

10.16 / **7.** If conservative treatment does not work, what would be an alternative treatment?

CONCLUSION

A s seen in these case scenarios, there are a considerable number of structures that pass around the knee and down to the lower leg that can be involved in a variety of knee and lower leg injuries. Because the knee is involved in many lower extremity overuse injuries, it is extremely important to take a full and detailed history. A detailed history assists in determining what further evaluation techniques are necessary to guide the clinical diagnosis. It is also important to evaluate and treat knee injuries quickly and as effectively as possible because, as we have learned, the blood supply and nerve supply for the lower leg passes through the knee. In acute trauma situations if treatment is not timely, irreversible damage to the knee and lower leg may occur. For example, in the instance of the tibiofemoral dislocation, if this injury is not properly managed, there can be permanent damage to the lower leg if the popliteal artery has been compromised and is no longer supplying blood to the lower leg. Amputation can be a real possibility if immediate medical management is delayed.

The injuries presented in the chapter were detected and treated appropriately for the most part. There were some instances in which the athletic trainer forgot to perform an evaluation technique or ask an important history question. This allows you to think of what you might do in the particular situation. After all, it easier to think clearly when there is no stress involved than it is to think in a stressful situation. We hope that with these case scenarios, you may be able to work through these situations in a safe environment to prepare you for the real thing.

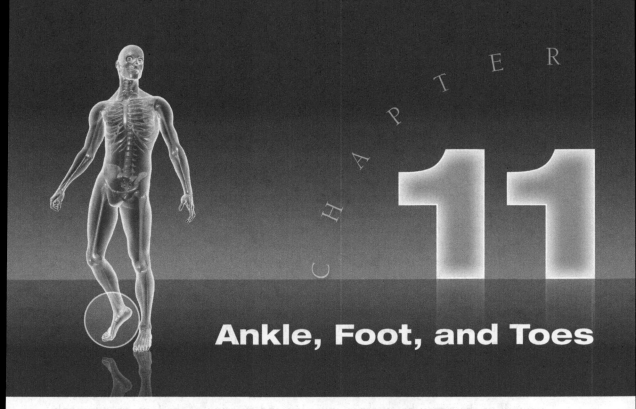

CHAPTER

Ankle, Foot, and Toes

INTRODUCTION

I n this chapter, we will examine the clinical evaluation and management of
18 different talocrural (ankle), tarsal (foot), and phalangal (toes) pathologies
using both on-field and off-field scenarios. These are presented in a variety of
settings with a diverse patient population, including collegiate, high school, performance arts, and the military. The ankle, foot, and toe pathologies presented in this
chapter include acute and chronic injuries, such as sprains, strains, and the bony and
neurovascular conditions typically encountered during the practice of athletic training. Several of the cases are actual situations that have occurred in our own clinical
practices. As a reminder, some of the cases presented in this chapter have intentionally been written with inappropriate actions, procedures, treatments, and general
mismanagement of the case by the clinician. This allows you to critically analyze the
cases in order to identify the inappropriate decision(s) and then be able to provide the
appropriate gold-standard treatment.

ANATOMICAL REVIEW

T he ankle-foot complex is comprised of the ankle, the foot, and the toes. It is
just as intricate as the wrist-hand complex, and so this overview of the anatomical structures will provide only a cursory review of the basic anatomical
arrangement and functioning of the joints. For further review, we suggest that you
read texts, original research, case reviews, and evidence-based practice reviews that
specially examine the structure and function of the ankle-foot complex and the most
appropriate methods of evaluating and managing the area. Biomechanics textbooks

will provide more detailed information about the joints, ligaments, and other structures that make up the complex, and volume 37(4) of the *Journal of Athletic Training* is dedicated to ankle pathology, clinical practice, and research.

The ankle-foot complex is made up of four distinct regions: the talocrural joint, the rearfoot (hindfoot), the midfoot, and the forefoot. Together, these four regions consist of 28 bones and numerous muscles originating from the lower leg and foot. The ankle-foot complex is responsible for a great deal of weight-bearing and responsible for bipedal stance and locomotion, both walking and running. Structurally similar to the wrist-hand complex, the ankle-foot complex receives much more attention from the medical community because there is a high rate of injury at the ankle-foot complex both athletically (competitively)[19,20,23,26,32,37,38,43] and recreationally.[11] This is because, as the distal end of the lower extremity, the ankle-foot complex provides a stable base of support for the body in a variety of positions that do not require great muscle activation or energy expenditure, and yet it acts as a rigid lever during the push-off phase of gait.[26]

Most acute trauma sustained to ankle-foot complex results either from direct compression, such as stepping on another player, falling from a height, or dropping sporting equipment on the foot or from a combination of direct compression and indirect or shearing force, with or without the foot being firmly planted.[3,15,23,27,30] For example, a player may be kicked from behind while his foot is firmly planted on the ground; or there may be excessive inversion and eversion of the foot, as commonly seen with a Jones fracture. When falling from a height, the force of the impact can be transmitted up the involved extremity, resulting in trauma to the knee, thigh, pelvis, or lumbar spine. Recurrent ankle injuries are also extremely common, and most patients suffer from a history of previous ankle sprains.[20] Chronic ankle instability is believed to be caused by mechanical instability, functional instability, and a combination of the two.[20] Table 11.1 is a brief summary of common ankle-foot complex injuries.

A thorough understanding of the injury mechanics and anatomy of the ankle-foot complex will assist in examining the extent of injuries.[3] The extent of an injury varies, depending on the MOI, foot position (i.e., pronated, dorsiflexed, everted), direction of the force applied, and type of protective equipment or shoe worn by the athlete. For example, the distal extension of the lateral malleolus limits the damage sustained to the deltoid ligament, but its position increases the risk of bony trauma when an excessive eversion force is applied to the ankle. Ligamentous sprains are more likely to occur when the ankle-foot complex is in a position in which the bony architecture conveys little stability.[3] The dome of the talus, which articulates with the tibia and fibula to form the ankle joint, is wider anteriorly than posteriorly, and when the foot is forced into dorsiflexion or rotated, it increases the risk of talus trauma. In cases of chronic ankle sprains, particularly those caused by functional instability, an athletic trainer would be prudent to assess the athlete for insufficiencies in proprioception and neuromuscular control.[20]

Ankle Complex

The ankle joint refers specifically to the talocrural joint. The talocrural is a uniaxial, modified-hinge joint formed by the talus, the medial malleolus of the tibia (tibiotalar), and the lateral malleolus of the fibula (talofibular). Together, these structures create what is often referred to as a mortise joint, because the rectangular cavity of the inferior ends of the tibia and fibula forms a deep socket or a boxlike mortise where the dome-shaped trochlea of the talus sits (Figure 11.1).[29] The distal ends of

TABLE 11.1	Ankle-foot complex injuries.	
NAME	**MECHANISM OF INJURY**	**SIGNS AND SYMPTOMS**
Phalange fracture	Axial load (e.g., jamming a toe) and direct compression (e.g., dropping a weight)	Pain, swelling, ecchymosis, difficulty wearing footwear Antalgic gait when a great toe fracture is suspected
Metatarsal fracture	Axial load (e.g., jamming a toe) and direct compression (e.g., dropping a weight)	Deep pain, swelling, ecchymosis, difficulty wearing footwear Antalgic gait
Acute Jones fracture	Inversion and plantarflexion force of the foot (e.g., tripping on a stair) and direct compression	Pain and tenderness within 1.5 cm distal to tuberosity of the fifth metatarsal; difficulty with weight bearing; swelling; ecchymosis
Talus fracture	Depends on the location of the fracture (i.e., lateral talar dome fractures occur with a severe inversion and dorsiflexion force; medial talar dome fractures occur with a severe inversion and plantarflexion force)	Tenderness and swelling over fracture site Pain upon bearing weight or inability to bear weight Antalgic gait
Calcaneus fracture	High-energy axial load such as falling from a height or inversion and compression when an anterior process fracture occurs	Severe heel pain and tenderness over the fracture site Pain with ankle dorsiflexion Inability to bear weight
Tarsal bone fracture (navicular, cuboid, cuneiforms)	Depends on location of fracture and direction of force	Pain, swelling, ecchymosis, difficulty wearing footwear Antalgic gait
Phalange dislocation	Direct trauma (e.g., kicking an object)	Severe pain, swelling, deformity, loss of function, open wounds
Ankle fracture, dislocation	Axial load and direct compression (e.g., falling from a height) with the foot inverted or everted	Severe pain, swelling, deformity, changes in neurovascular status, loss of function, open wounds

the tibia and fibula also create a distal tibio-fibular joint. The dome-shaped body of the trochlea is wider anteriorly than posteriorly and fits snugly into this concave undersurface of the distal surface of the tibia. This creates a very stable joint and contributes to a relatively simple hinge-like motion.[33]

As a uniaxial joint, the talocrural joint allows 1° of freedom. Dorsiflexion (ankle flexion) and plantarflexion (ankle extension) occur in an oblique sagittal plane around an oblique frontal axis and normally range from 0° to 20° and from 0° to 50°, respectively. The ROM de-

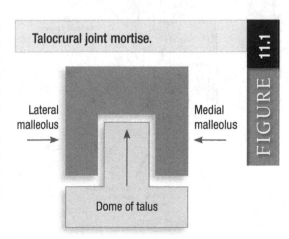

Talocrural joint mortise.

Lateral malleolus

Medial malleolus

Dome of talus

FIGURE 11.1

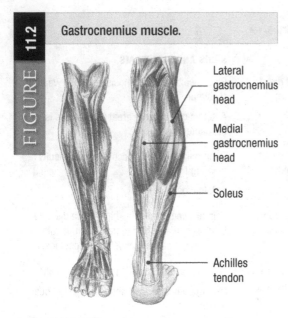

FIGURE 11.2

Gastrocnemius muscle.

Lateral gastrocnemius head

Medial gastrocnemius head

Soleus

Achilles tendon

Source: © Ciska 76/Dreamstime.com

pends on the position of the tibiofemoral joint. The gastrocnemius, a two-joint muscle, crosses the knee joint posteriorly, inserting on the distal ends of the femoral condyles and thereby influencing talocrural joint ROM (Figure 11.2). When the knee is extended, the gastrocnemius is taut, limiting dorsiflexion. When the knee is flexed, the muscle is allowed to slacken, and this increases the amount of available dorsiflexion.

During dorsiflexion, the wider anterior articular surface of the talus "wedges" itself between the medial and lateral malleoli, resulting in movement of the distal tibiofibular joint (syndesmosis) and an increase in the stability of the joint from the close packing of the bones and increased contact of the articular surfaces.[29,30] The dorsiflexed position is considered the safest position for the ankle against most ankle injuries, except for syndesmosis, also known as "high-ankle sprain." These sprains come about when external rotation and hyperdorsiflexion of the talus cause the widening of the mortise, resulting in disruption of syndesmosis and talar instability.[29,30,31] In a planterflexed and inverted position, the widened anterior articular surface of the talus moves out of the mortise, decreasing the ankle's bony stability and increasing the chances of lateral ankle sprains.[20,27,30,35]

Talocrural joint ligamentous structures

The stability of the ankle, particularly in dorsiflexion, is enhanced not only by the configuration of the ankle mortise but also by a fibrous joint capsule,

FIGURE 11.3

Lateral ankle ligaments.

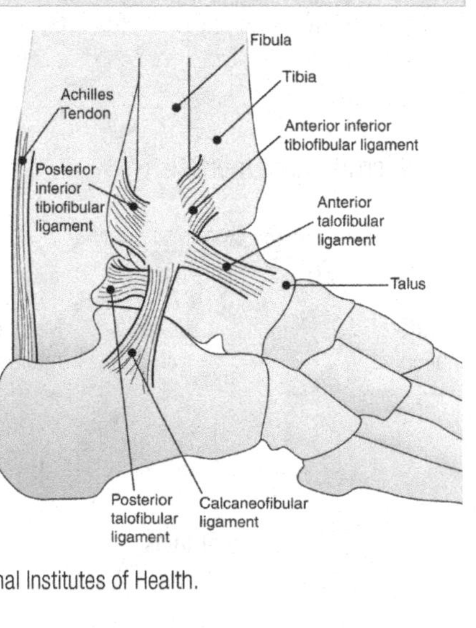

Fibula

Tibia

Achilles Tendon

Anterior inferior tibiofibular ligament

Posterior inferior tibiofibular ligament

Anterior talofibular ligament

Talus

Posterior talofibular ligament

Calcaneofibular ligament

Source: National Institutes of Health.

strong powerful ligaments, and several tendons crossing the joint. These tendons are bound by a thickening of the deep fascia called retinacula.[29] As the ankle moves into greater degrees of plantar flexion, there is a greater reliance on the ligaments, particularly the lateral ligaments, to provide ankle stability.[27] Many of the ligaments providing stability to the talocrural joint are in fact areas of increased density of the fibrous joint capsule. The exception is the calcaneofibular ligament, which is actually considered to be extracapsular.[35] The ligaments of the ankle (Table 11.2) are responsible for providing joint stability in different ankle positions and can be divided into the lateral group (the most commonly injured) (Figure 11.3), the medial group, and the ligaments of the syndesmosis.

	TABLE	11.2	Collateral ligaments of the ankle complex.[26, 29, 30, 33]

LIGAMENTS	LOCATION	FUNCTIONS
Lateral Collateral Ligaments[a]		
Anterior talofibular ligament (ATFL)	Flat band extending anteromedially from lateral malleolus to the talar neck	Prevents anterior displacement of the talus from the mortise and excessive inversion and internal rotation of the talus on the tibia
Calcaneofibular ligament (CFL)	Round cord passing posteroinferiorly from the tip of lateral malleolus to the lateral surface of the calcaneus	Restricts excessive supination of both the talocrural and subtalar joints and restricts excessive inversion and internal rotation of the rearfoot; tautest when the ankle is dorsiflexed
Posterior talofibular ligament (PTFL)	Thick, strong band running horizontally medially and slightly posteriorly from the malleolar fossa to the lateral tubercle of the posterior process of the talus	Provides restraint to both inversion and internal rotation of the loaded talocrural joint
Medial Collateral Ligaments[b]		
Anterior tibiotalar ligament (ATTL)	Extends from the anteromedial portion of the medial malleolus to the superior portion of the medial talus	Prevents excessive eversion of the talus at the subtalar joint; anterior portion also resist talar external rotation
Tibiocalcaneal ligament (TCL)	Apex of the medial malleolus to the calcaneus directly below the malleolus	
Posterior tibiotalar ligament (PTTL)	Posterior aspect of medial malleolus to the posterior portion of the talus	
Tibionavicular ligament (TNL)	Runs beneath and slightly posterior to the ATTL, inserting on the medial surface of the navicular	Limits lateral translation and external rotation of the tibia on the foot
Distal Tibiofibular Syndesmosis		
Anterior inferior tibiofibular	Flat, strong ligament originating from the longitudinal tubercle on the anterior aspect of the lateral malleolus, attaching on the anterolateral tubercle of the tibia	Maintains the fibula tight to the tibia and prevents excessive fibular movement and external talar rotation
Posterior inferior tibiofibular	Originates on the posterior tubercle of the tibia and runs obliquely, distally, and laterally to the posterior lateral malleolus	Works with the anterior inferior tibiofibular ligament to hold the fibula close in the fibular groove of the tibia
Transverse	Thick, strong structure with twisting fibers passing posterior to the tibial margin to the osteochondral junction on the posterior and medial margins of the distal fibula	Prevents posterior talar translation
Interosseous	Originates at the anteroinferior triangular segment of the medial aspect of the distal fibular shaft, then courses to insert on the lateral surface of the distal tibia	Believed to act as a "spring," allowing for slight separation between the medial and lateral malleolus during dorsiflexion at the talocrural joint

[a]Lateral ligaments placed in order of injury with ATFL first, CF second, and PTFL least likely to be injured.

[b]Medial collateral ligament is normally referred to as the deltoid ligament and is often described as a strong, flat, and triangularly shaped ligament on the medial aspect of the ankle.

Musculature structures of the ankle complex

The muscular tendons that cross the complex dynamically are responsible for providing a broad array of activities, including locomotion and balance. These muscle tendons are classified into three groups:

1. Muscles crossing anterior to the malleoli
2. Muscles crossing posterior to the malleoli
3. Muscles crossing lateral and medial to the talocrural joint

There are three muscles that have tendons that cross over the anterior aspect of the ankle. These muscle tendons have origins in the anterior compartment of the lower leg and travel distally to insert onto various locations in the foot complex. These three muscles include the tibialis anterior, the extensor digitorum longus (EDL), and the extensor hallucis longus (EHL). The tibialis anterior is responsible for ankle dorsiflexion and foot inversion (Figure 11.4). The EDL is the primary agonist for metatarsophalangeal and interphalangeal joint extension of the lesser four toes. The EHL is the primary agent of great toe extension.

The other muscles that have tendons crossing over either the posterior, medial, or lateral aspect of the ankle have origins in the lateral and posterior compartment of the lower leg and travel distally to insert onto various locations in the foot complex. The gastrocnemius and soleus merge distally to form the Achilles tendon, which inserts on the calcaneus and is responsible for ankle plantarflexion (Figure 11.3). Laterally, the peroneus longus and brevis are responsible for ankle eversion. The peroneus longus also assists in ankle plantarflexion as the muscle inserts onto the lateral side of the base of the first metatarsal and medial cuneiform. Medially, the "Tom, Dick and Harry" muscles act to invert and flex the toes. Tom, the tibialis posterior, is a foot inverter and weak plantar flexor. Dick, the flexor digitorum longus (FDL), is responsible for flexion of the second through fifth distal interphalangeal joints. Harry, the flexor hallucis longus, is responsible for great toe interphalangeal joint flexion.

FIGURE 11.4 Muscles crossing anterior to the malleoli.

Tibialis anterior

Extensor digitorum longus

Extensor hallucis longus

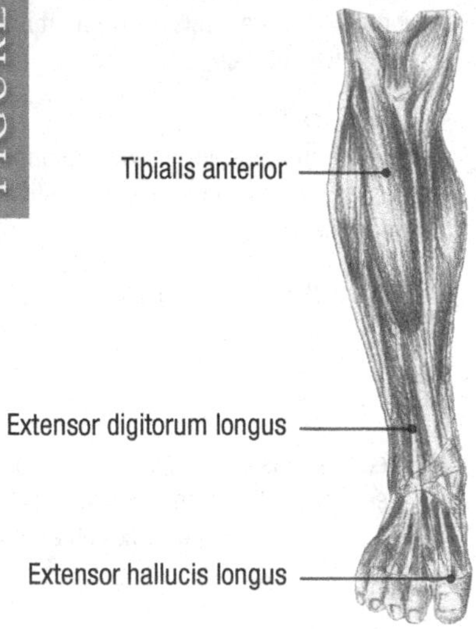

Source: © Ciska 76/Dreamstime.com

Foot Complex

The foot complex consists of three regions: the rearfoot (posterior segment), the midfoot (middle segment), and the forefoot (anterior segment). Each area consists of several tarsal joint articulations, which are supported by and work in tandem with a variety of structures, including: dorsal, plantar, and interosseous tarsal ligaments; intrinsic and extrinsic muscles; bursae; retinacula; arches (lateral, medial longitudinal, transverse); and the plantar fascia. Please note that not all of these articulations or structures will be discussed here.

Rearfoot

A main part of the rearfoot is the subtalar joint or talocalcaneal joint. The joint is formed by the articulations between the talus and calcaneus bones and is an intricate structure held together by an articular capsule and by anterior, posterior, lateral, medial, and interosseous talocalcaneal ligaments.[30] The subtalar joint is responsible for stability and shock absorption, and it serves as a lever arm for the Achilles tendon during plantarflexion (i.e., calcaneus). As a composite joint, the subtalar joint is formed by three separate plane articulations between the talus (superiorly) and the calcaneus (inferiorly).[26] Together, the three planes create a triplanar motion that allows the talus to rotate around a single oblique joint axis. This movement gives the subtalar joint 1° of freedom, allows for pronation and supination, and similar to the talocrural joint, converts torque between the lower leg (internal and external rotation) and the foot (supination and pronation).[20, 26]

The component triplanar motions that allow for supination and pronation include (1) abduction/adduction, (2) inversion/eversion, and (3) plantarflexion/dorsiflexion.[26] The extent that each component motion contributes to supination or pronation varies from person to person and is dependent on the location of the axis. Furthermore, supination, pronation, and movement of the talus and/or calcaneus are dependent on whether an individual is bearing weight or not (Table 11.3). If an individual is not bearing weight, it means that the distal end of the lower leg is not fixed to the ground. During weight-bearing, the distal end of the lower leg is fixed and the calcaneus is not free to move about the axis; therefore, the talus must move on the calcaneus. Supination and pronation are described by the motion of the calcaneus, a distal, non-weight-bearing segment.

Subtalar joint motion is often recorded based on the frontal plane component of motion, usually inversion (movement of the foot inward) and eversion (movement of the foot outward). Inversion and eversion ROM values vary significantly among researchers,[26,33] and the values depend on the starting position, whether one is in subtalar neutral,[26] and whether measurement is based on movement of the calcaneus or combined movement of the calcaneus and talus. Eversion (valgus) of the calcaneus has been measured at 5° to 10° and inversion (varus) at 20° to 30°.[26]

TABLE 11.3	Component movement of subtalar supination and pronation.[26]	
	NON–WEIGHT-BEARING	**WEIGHT-BEARING**
Supination	Calcaneal inversion (varus)	Calcaneal inversion (varus)
	Calcaneal adduction	Talar abduction (lateral or external rotation)
	Calcaneal plantarflexion	Talar dorsiflexion Tibiofibular lateral rotation
Pronation	Calcaneal eversion (valgus)	Calcaneal eversion (valgus)
	Calcaneal abduction	Talar adduction (medial or internal rotation)
	Calcaneal dorsiflexion	Talar plantarflexion Tibiofibular medial rotation

Midfoot

The talocalcaneonavicular joint (TCNJ) and calcaneocuboid joint (CCJ) are part of the midfoot and create a functional articulation between the rearfoot (talus and calcaneus) and the midfoot (navicular and cuboid).[42]

Talocalcaneonavicular joint. The TCNJ is formed by the articulations between the head of talus, with a socket formed by the posterior surface of the navicular, and the articular surface of the calcaneus.[29] As part of the transverse tarsal joint (Chopart's joint), the TCNJ is reinforced by the dorsal talonavicular and the plantar calcaneonavicular ligament, often known as the "spring ligament." The spring ligament consists of the superomedial calcaneonavicular ligament, the inferior calcaneonavicular ligament, and a ligament called "the third ligament" that is comprised of fibers running from the notch between the calcaneal facets to the navicular tuberosity.[40] The spring ligament's structural location is vital because its complex supports the talar head with assistance from the posterior tibial tendon located beneath it. In fact, dysfunction of the posterior tibial tendon can cause stretching of the spring ligament, resulting in collapse of the medial longitudinal arch and a less effective push-off during ambulation.[12] This increases the risk of biomechanical changes to the foot and lower extremity.

Calcaneocuboid joint. The CCJ is formed by the articulation between the anterior surface of the calcaneus and the posterior surface of the cuboid.[29] Also part of the transverse tarsal joint, the CCJ is reinforced by the dorsalcalcaneocuboid, long plantar, plantar calcaneocuboid (short), and bifurcate ligament. Together, the TCNJ and CCJ increase the ROM during inversion and eversion and permit the forefoot to remain evenly distributed on the ground while walking on uneven surfaces.[26,29,39]

Forefoot

The tarsometatarsal joint (TMTJ), intermetatarsal joint (IMTJ), metatarsophalangeal joint (MTPJ), and interphalangeal joint (IPJ) are all part of the forefoot. Each joint creates a continuous functional articulation between itself and the next midfoot.

Tarsometatarsal joints. The TMTJs consist of five articulations between the metatarsal (MT) and the distal row of the tarsal bones (Table 11.4). The articulations of the TMTJs are plane synovial joints that permit only gliding and sliding joint movements. The first TMTJ is the only joint possessing a well-developed joint capsule (joints 2–5 share a capsule) and is the most mobile. The second TMTJ is much stronger and more stable than the other joints because of its more posterior position.[26] The relative immobility of the second TMTJ makes it susceptible to acute and repetitive trauma, particularly stress fractures.[7,13,14,21,22]

The main function of the TMTJ is to help regulate the position of the metatarsals and phalanges during weight bearing and allow the foot to conform to the uneven surfaces during weight bearing. The TMTJs are supported by thin dorsal ligaments (second through fifth metatarsals), a strong plantar ligament, and the main stabilizing structure, a Y-shaped interosseous ligament often called Lisfranc's ligament.[34]

Intermetatarsal joints. The IMTJs are situated between the metatarsal bones, creating the proximal and distal IMTJs. They are functionally related to the TMTJs because the TMTJs require the metatarsal bones to move relative to the adjacent bone, therefore requiring an IMTJ to move when a TMTJ moves. The IMTJs are plane

TABLE 11.4	Tarsometatarsal joint articulations.
JOINT	**ARTICULATION**
First TMTJ	First (medial) cuneiform and base of first MT
Second TMTJ	Second (intermediate) cuneiform and base of second MT
Third TMTJ	Third (lateral) cuneiform and base of third MT
Fourth TMTJ	Cuboid and base of fourth MT
Fifth TMTJ	Cuboid and base of fifth MT

joints that permit slight gliding movement of one metatarsal relative to another.[29] The proximal IMTJ, which is closely entwined with the TMTJ joint, is supported by a fibrous joint capsule and intermetatarsal ligaments (dorsal, plantar, and interosseous). The intermetatarsal ligaments connect all of the metatarsals except for the first and second metatarsals. In this situation, the Lisfranc ligament extends from the first cuneiform to the base of the second metatarsal and helps to prevent separation of the first ray and the second metatarsal.[16] The distal IMTJ is also stabilized by a fibrous joint capsule and the deep transverse ligament, which connects the heads of the metatarsal bones. Together, the deep transverse ligament and interosseous ligament assist in maintaining the transverse arch of the foot.

Metatarsophalangeal joint. The MTPJ consists of five articulations between the heads of the metatarsals and the base of the proximal phalanges (Table 11.5). As a condyloid joint, the MTPJ allows for 2° of freedom, flexion and extension, limited abduction and adduction, and some rotation. The first MTPJ allows for a greater degree of flexion (0°–45° vs. 0°–40°) and extension (0°–70° or 80° vs. 0°–40°) than the second through fifth joints.[10] The MTPJs in general are responsible for allowing the foot to pivot at the toes in order to allow the heel to rise off the ground while still maintaining a base of support provided by the toes during walking, running, and balancing.[9,26]

The MTPJ is stabilized by a fibrous capsule, collateral ligaments (medial and lateral), and a plantar plate. The first MTPJ is the largest and most complex of the five articulations. It consists of four bones—two of which are sesamoid bones encap-

TABLE 11.5	Metatarsophalangeal joint articulations.
JOINT	**ARTICULATION**
First MTPJ	First MT (MT-I) and proximal phalanx of first toe
Second MTPJ	Second MT (MT-II) and proximal phalanx of second toe
Third MTPJ	Third MT (MT-III) and proximal phalanx of third toe
Fourth MTPJ	Fourth MT (MT-IV) and proximal phalanx of fourth toe
Fifth MTPJ	Fifth MT (MT-V) and proximal phalanx of fifth toe

sulated within the flexor hallucis brevis tendon—nine ligaments, and three points of muscle attachment.[9] Structurally, the first MTPJ is supported by the fan-shaped medial and lateral collateral ligaments, each consisting of two subparts—the metatarsophalangeal ligament and the metatarsosesamoid ligament—along with two bands of the plantar plate.[2] The first MTPJ is susceptible to damage to the soft tissue support structures of the joint, most notably, "turf toe."[2,4,6]

Interphalangeal joint. Nine IPJs are situated between the phalanges of the toes, creating two separate articulations: the proximal interphalangeal joint (PIPJ) and the distal interphalangeal joint (DIPJ). The PIPJ is located between the proximal and middle phalange bones of toes two through five. The proximal and distal phalanges of the great toe create a generic IPJ similar to the thumb. The DIPJ is located between the middle and distal phalange bones of toes two through five. The IPJs are plane synovial joints allowing for 1° of freedom, flexion, and extension (sagittal plane). The IPJs function to smooth the shifting of weight from foot to foot during gait and to help maintain stability during weight bearing by pressing the toes down against the ground.[26]

Muscular structures

Dynamically, the foot-complex musculature has its origins in both the lower leg and foot and its insertion on the tarsal, metatarsals, and/or phalanges. These muscles are divided into intrinsic and extrinsic muscles (Table 11.6).

Neurovascular Structures

The ankle and foot joints, similar to all joints, are susceptible to neurological and vascular dysfunctions. These dysfunctions can occur from acute trauma or repetitive trauma and result in entrapment of the nerve(s) or vessel(s). Conditions include peroneal nerve entrapment, tarsal tunnel syndrome, intermetatarsal neuroma, and anterior compartment syndrome (distribution of the deep peroneal nerve).

The peripheral nerves innervating the ankle and foot complex include the tibial nerve, the deep and superficial peroneal nerves, and the medial and lateral plantar nerves (Table 11.7). As the sciatic nerve originates from the lumbosacral plexus, it approaches the popliteal fossa of the knee and diverges to form the tibial nerve (medially) and the common peroneal nerve (laterally). The tibial nerve (L4–S3) runs the length of the lower leg and innervates structures such as the gastrocnemius and soleus, eventually dividing into medial and lateral plantar nerves. The common peroneal nerve (L4–S2) winds laterally just below the proximal head of the fibula and branches to form the deep peroneal nerve (tibialis anterior) and superficial peroneal nerve (peroneus longus). The deep peroneal nerve runs inferomedially on the fibula, deep to and piercing the extensor digitorum longus as it descends to the interosseous membrane. It continues to course deep to the extensor retinacula with the anterior tibial artery. Because the deep peroneal nerve is part of the anterior compartment, it can become compressed with increased compartmental swelling, resulting in a loss of or abnormal sensation in the skin, between the first and second digits and/or loss of motor control in dorsiflexion.

The superficial peroneal nerve descends posterolaterally, eventually lying anterolateral to the fibula, between the peroneal muscles and the extensor digitorum longus. The nerve innervates the lateral compartment, containing the peroneus longus and brevis, and supplies the skin on the distal part of the anterior surface of the leg, most of the dorsum of the foot, and most digits.

TABLE	11.6	Intrinsic and extrinsic muscles of the foot complex.[19, 29]

LAYER	MUSCLE	ACTIONS
Intrinsic muscles of the foot		
Superficial	Abductor hallucis	Abduction of the great toe
	Abductor digiti minimi	Abduction and flexion of fifth toe
	Flexor digitorum brevis (FDB)	Flexion of PIPJ of lateral 4 toes
Middle	Quadratus plantae	Modifies the flexor digitorum's angle of pull. Assists in flexion of MTPJs 2–5.
	Tendons of the flexor hallucis longus (FHL)	Flexion of the IPJ of great toe
	Tendons of the flexor digitorum longus (FDL)	Flexion of DIPJs of lateral 4 toes
	Lumbricals	Flexion of the MTPJs and extension of IPJs of toes
Deep	Flexor hallucis brevis (FHB)	Flexion of MTPJ of great toe
	Adductor hallucis	Adduction of great toe
	Flexor digiti minimi brevis	Flexion of the MTPJ of fifth toe
Interosseous	Plantar interossei	Adduction of toes 3–5 and flexion of MTPJ
	Dorsal interossei	Abduction of toes 2–4 and flexion of MTPJ
Extrinsic muscles acting on the foot		
	Extensor hallucis longus (EHL)	Extension of IPJ of great toe
	Extensor digitorum longus (EDL)	Extension of MTPJs and IPJs of lateral 4 toes
	Flexor hallucis longus	Flexion of the IPJ of great toe

TABLE	11.7	Peripheral nerves and muscle innervations of the ankle-foot complex.

NERVE	MUSCLES
Tibial	Gastrocnemius, soleus, tibialis posterior, FHL, FDL
Deep peroneal	Tibialis anterior, EHL, EDL, EDB
Superficial peroneal	Peroneus longus and brevis
Medial plantar	FHB, FDB, abductor hallucis, first lumbrical
Lateral plantar	Flexor digiti minimi brevis, abductor digiti minimi, dorsal interossei, plantar interossei, adductor hallucis, second to fourth lumbricals

Passing through the tarsal tunnel is the posterior tibial nerve and its branches, the medial and lateral plantar nerves; the posterior tibial artery and vein; the flexor digitorum longus; the flexor hallucis longus; and the tibialis posterior. Compression of the tunnel from trauma[36,41] (e.g., eversion ankle sprain, tarsal fracture), biomechanical deficiencies[1,41] (e.g., pes planus, unstable medial longitudinal arch), or space-occupying lesions[24,25,28] (e.g., soft tissue mass, accessory muscle, cysts) predisposes patients to the development of tarsal tunnel syndrome.

Morton's neuroma affects the third common digital nerve, located in the region of the third webspace,[5,18] and supplies cutaneous information on the adjacent sides of the third and fourth toes. This is also the area where the nerve is the thickest, receiving branches from the medial and lateral plantar nerves. The wider nerve is easily irritated from stretching and shearing stresses between the metatarsal heads and the transverse intermetatarsal ligament.[8] Because the third common digital nerve provides only sensory information, motor deficits to the intrinsic or extrinsic musculature should not be evident, and any noted weakness should raise concerns that another diagnosis may be indicated.[17]

The anterior tibial artery, a branch of the popliteal artery, passes through the anterior compartment and ends at the ankle midway between the malleoli, where it becomes the dorsalis pedis artery. The dorsalis pedis artery is commonly used to assess distal circulation in a trauma situation. The posterior tibial artery is the larger of the terminal branches of the popliteal artery, and it passes deep to the soleus beyond and posterior to the medial malleolus. It continues until it branches into the medial and lateral plantar arteries, supplying blood to the foot.

LIGAMENTOUS AND SPECIAL TESTS

T he case scenarios in this chapter may require you to select and utilize different types of ligamentous and special tests in order to adequately evaluate the injury. The details on how to perform each special test are beyond the scope of this section; however, Table 11.8 provides a general list of tests that may be required and useful for you to review before beginning the case scenarios. For a more thorough review and determination of the sensitivity and specificity of each test, please refer to your favorite evaluation text or journal article(s).

TABLE 11.8	Ligamentous and special tests of the foot and ankle complex.
LIGAMENTOUS TEST	**FUNCTION**
Anterior drawer	Assesses integrity of the anterior talofibular (ATF) ligament and joint capsule
Eversion stress	Assesses integrity of the deltoid ligament, particularly the tibiocalcaneal ligament
Kleiger's	Assesses rotatory damage to the deltoid ligament or the distal tibiofibular ligament
MTP and IP varus and valgus stress	Assesses integrity of the collateral ligaments and joint capsule of the MTP and IP joints
Talar tilt/inversion stress	Assesses integrity of the calcaneofibular ligament

(continued)

TABLE	11.8	Continued.

SPECIAL TEST	FUNCTION
Feiss line	Assesses the amount of hyperpronation of the foot
Homan's sign	Assesses for deep vein thrombosis (DVT)
Interdigital neuroma	Assesses for interdigital neuroma
Long bone compression	Assesses fractures of the metatarsals or phalanges
Navicular drop	Assesses the amount of hyperpronation of the foot by measuring the height of the navicular tuberosity while the foot is NWB
Squeeze or compression	Assesses fibular fractures or syndesmosis sprains
Test for supple pes planus feet	Assesses the presence of supple pes planus
Tinel's sign	Assesses for tarsal tunnel syndrome
Thompson (Simmonds')	Assesses the integrity of the Achilles tendon

REFERENCES

1. Aldridge T. Diagnosing heel pain in adults. *Am Fam Physician*. 2004;70(2):332–338.

2. Allen L, Flemming D, Sanders T. Turf toe: Ligamentous injury of the first metatarsophalangeal joint. *Mil Med*. 2004;169(11):xix–xxiv.

3. Anderson SJ, Harmon KG, Rubin A. Acute ankle sprains. *Physician Sportsmed*. 2002;30(12):29.

4. Ashman C, Klecker R, Yu J. Forefoot pain involving the metatarsal region: differential diagnosis with MR imaging. *Radiographics*. 2001;21:1425–1440.

5. Ayub A, Yale SH, Bibbo C. Common foot disorders. *Clin Med Res*. 2005;3(2):116–119.

6. Bowers K, Martin R. Turf-toe: a shoe-surface related football injury. *Med Sci Sports Exerc*. 1976;8(2):81–83.

7. Carmont MR, Patrick JH, Cassar-Pullicino VN, Postans NJ, Hay SM. Sequential metatarsal fatigue fractures secondary to abnormal foot biomechanics. *Mil Med*. 2006;171(4):292–297.

8. Childs S. Diagnosis and treatment of interdigital perineural fibroma (a.k.a. Morton's neuroma). *Orthop Nurs*. 2002;21(6):35.

9. Childs S. Pathophysiology: the pathogenesis and biomechanics of turf toe. *Orthop Nurs*. 2006;25(4):276–282.

10. Clarkson H. *Musculoskeletal Assessment: Joint Range of Motion and Manual Muscle Strength*. Philadelphia PA: Lippincott Williams & Wilkins; 2000.

11. Conn JM, Annest JL, Gilchrist J. Sports and recreation related injury episodes in the US population, 1997–99. *Inj Prev*. 2003;9:117–123.

12. Conti S. Posterior tibial tendon problems in athletes. *Orthop Clin N Am*. 1994;25:109–121.

13. Dhami S, Sheikh A. Metatarsal stress fracture. *Gen Pract*. 2002;76.

14. Dixon S, Creaby M, Allsopp A. Comparison of static and dynamic biomechanical measures in military recruits with and without a history of third metatarsal stress fracture. *Clin Biomech*. 2006;21(4):412–419.

15. Gallaspy JB, May JD. *Signs and Symptoms of Athletic Injuries*. St. Louis MO: Mosby; 1996.

16. Glasoe W, Yack H, Saltzman C. Anatomy and biomechanics of the first ray. *Phys Ther*. 1999; 79(9):854–859.

17. Gonzalez P, Bowman R. Morton neuroma. *eMedicine* [electronic version]. 2006. Available from: http://www.emedicine.com/pmr/topic81. htm. Accessed June 20, 2008.

18. Gulick DT, Charles TK. Differential diagnosis of Morton's neuroma. *Athl Ther Today.* 2002;7(1): 39–42.

19. Hagglund M, Walden M, Ekstrand J. Injury incidence and distribution in elite football: a prospective study of the Danish and the Swedish top divisions. *Scand J Med Sci Sports.* 2005;15(1):21–28.

20. Hertel J. Functional anatomy, pathomechanics, and pathophysiology of lateral ankle instability. *J Athl Train.* 2002;37(4):364–375.

21. Hinz P, Henningsen A, Matthes G, Jäger B, Ekkernkamp A, Rosenbaum D. Analysis of pressure distribution below the metatarsals with different insoles in combat boots of the German Army for prevention of March fractures. *Gait Posture.* 2008;27(3):535–538.

22. Hod N, Ashkenazi I, Levi Y, et al. Characteristics of skeletal stress fractures in female military recruits of the Israel defense forces on bone scintigraphy. *Clin Nucl Med.* 2006;31(12):742–749.

23. Hootman J, Dick R, Agel J. Epidemiology of collegiate injuries for 15 sports: summary and recommendations for injury prevention initiatives. *J Athl Train.* 2007;42(2):311–319.

24. Hu Liang L, Stephenson G. These boots weren't made for walking: tarsal tunnel syndrome. *CMAJ: Suppl.* 2007;176(10):1415–1416.

25. Kinoshita M, Okuda R, Morikawa J, Jotoku T, Abe M. The dorsiflexion-eversion test for diagnosis of tarsal tunnel syndrome. *J Bone Joint Surg Am.* 2001;83-A(12):1835.

26. Levangie PK, Norkin CC. *Joint Structure and Function: A Comprehensive Analysis.* Philadelphia PA: F.A. Davis; 2001.

27. Lynch S. Assessment of the injured ankle in the athlete. *J Athl Train.* 2002;37(4):406–412.

28. Mizel MS, Hecht PJ, Marymont JV, Temple HT. Evaluation and treatment of chronic ankle pain. *J Bone Joint Surg Am.* 2004;86-A(3):622–632.

29. Moore K, Dalley A. *Clinically Oriented Anatomy.* 5th ed. Baltimore MD: Lippincott Williams & Wilkins; 2005.

30. Norkus S, Floyd R. The anatomy and mechanisms of syndesmotic ankle sprains. *J Athl Train.* 2001;36(1):68–73.

31. Nussbaum E, Hosea T, Sieler S, Incremona B, Kessler D. Prospective evaluation of syndesmotic ankle sprains without diastasis. *Am J Sport Med.* 2001;29:31–35.

32. Ostojic SM. Comparing sports injuries in soccer: influence of a positional role. *Res Sports Med.* 2003;11(3):203–208.

33. Otis C. Structure and function of the bones and noncontractile elements of the ankle and foot complex. In: *Kinesiology: The Mechanics & Pathomechanics of Human Movement.* Baltimore MD: Lippincott Williams & Wilkins; 2004:775–802.

34. Peicha G, Labovitz J, Seibert F, et al. The anatomy of the joint as a risk factor for Lisfranc dislocation and fracture-dislocation. *J Bone Joint Surg Br.* 2002;84-B:981–985.

35. Renstrom P, Konradsen L. Ankle ligament injuries. *Br J Sports Med.* 1997;31:11–20.

36. Romani W, Perrin D. Tarsal tunnel syndrome: case study of a male collegiate athlete. *J Sport Rehabil.* 1997;6(4):364.

37. Sheppard C, Hodson A. Injury profiles in professional footballers. *SportEX Med* [electronic version]. 2006. Available from: www.sportex.net. Accessed June 18, 2007.

38. Silbergleit. Fracture, foot. *eMedicine* [electronic version]. 2009. Available from; http://emedicine. medscape.com/article/825060-overview. Accessed June 11, 2009.

39. Starkey C, Ryan J. *Evaluation of Orthopedic and Athletic Injuries.* 2nd ed. Philadelphia PA: F.A. Davis; 2002.

40. Taniguchi A, Tanaka Y, Takakura Y, Kadono K, Maeda M, Yamamoto H. Anatomy of the spring ligament. *J Bone Joint Surg Am.* 2003;85-A(11):2174–2178.

41. Toth C, McNeil S, Feasby T. Peripheral nervous system injuries in sport and recreation: a systematic review. *Sports Med.* 2005;35(8):717–738.

42. Tweed J, Campbell J, Thompson R, Curran M. The function of the midtarsal joint: a review of the literature. *Foot.* 2008;18:106–112.

43. Walden M, Hagglund M, Ekstrand J. Injuries in Swedish elite football: a prospective study on injury definitions, risk for injury and injury pattern during 2001. *Scand J Med Sci Sports.* 2005;15(2):118–125.

44. Ward PJ, Porter ML. Tarsal tunnel syndrome: a study of the clinical and neurophysiological results of decompression. *J R Coll Surg Edinb.* 1998;43(1):35–36.

11.1

t is Monday morning, early in the soccer season, and Josh, the certified athletic trainer working with a university's women's soccer team, is getting ready for another week of two-a-day practices. The team is already warming up out on the field when one of the players races in to get Josh from the athletic training room. She explains that her teammate Jasmine was running for a pass when she fell to the ground, twisting her ankle. Josh grabs his athletic training kit and heads out to the field.

ON-SCENE ARRIVAL

When Josh arrives, Jasmine, a 21-year-old forward, is in obvious discomfort. An initial assessment reveals no immediate threats to Jasmine's life. He does see trauma (swelling and tenderness) to her right ankle. Her vital signs are shown in Table 11.1.1. Further assessment reveals that Jasmine is unwilling to bear weight on the involved limb.

HISTORY

On the sideline, Josh begins to gather more information regarding the injury. Jasmine says, "I was running down the field and I fell into a hole, my right ankle got caught and twisted downward and inward. I tried to catch myself, but it felt like it just kept going." Further questioning reveals no unusual sounds or sensation. Her pain level is 8/10, with increased pain around the anterior and distal lateral malleolus. She has no previous history of foot or ankle trauma.

Jasmine's vital signs.		TABLE 11.1.1
VITAL SIGNS	**FINDING**	
Pulse	96 and strong	
Respiration	19, labored, but regular	
Blood pressure	132/92	
Mental status	Alert, but in discomfort	

PHYSICAL EXAMINATION

After removing Jasmine's cleat, Josh immediately notes lateral ankle joint effusion. Pain and palpable tenderness are noted (Figure 11.1.1), increasing when the ankle is inverted. Anterior inferior tibiofibular tenderness is unremarkable. Active ROM is decreased in plantarflexion, inversion, and eversion. Passive ROM results in an increase in pain during combined inversion and plantarflexion, and during subtalar inversion only, and there is an abnormal end-feel. Resisted ROM demonstrates a decrease in muscle strength, particularly in eversion (2+/5). A test for a calcaneus fracture is unremarkable. Dorsal pedis and posterior tibial pulses

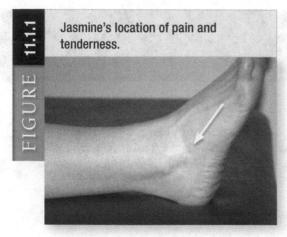

FIGURE 11.1.1

Jasmine's location of pain and tenderness.

Arrow indicates location of pain and tenderness.

are unremarkable. Dermatome, peripheral nerve, and deep-tendon reflex assessments are also unremarkable. Ligamentous testing reveals a positive anterior draw (Figure 11.1.2), and the test shown in Figure 11.1.3 is also positive. An external rotation test (Kleiger's test) is unremarkable.

Josh is fairly certain of the clinical diagnosis and discusses the results of his physical examination with Jasmine. He places an ice bag directly on Jasmine's right ankle and applies a wet compression wrap to secure the ice. The leg is elevated, and Josh molds a posterior splint and fits Jasmine for crutches.

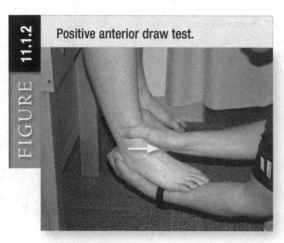

FIGURE 11.1.2

Positive anterior draw test.

Ankle is in a neutral position. Arrow indicates movement of the rearfoot.

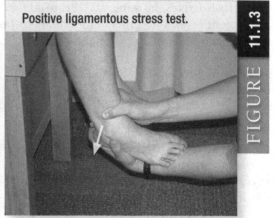

FIGURE 11.1.3

Positive ligamentous stress test.

Clinician's thumb is over the CFL with movement of the subtalar joint toward the midline.

Please answer the following questions based on the above case information.

11.1 / **1.** Based on the information presented in the case, determine (a) the differential diagnoses and (b) the clinical diagnosis.

11.1 / **2.** Based on the information presented in the case, do you believe Josh took an adequate history? If not, what, if any, additional questions would you ask as the evaluating clinician?

11.1 / **3.** Overall, do you believe Josh adequately evaluated Jasmine's condition given the clinical presentation? If not, what would you have done differently as the evaluating clinician?

11.1 / **4.** (a) What is the name of the ligamentous stress test performed in Figure 11.1.3? (b) Why is it used, and what is considered a positive finding?

11.1 / **5.** Josh assessed active and passive ROM as part of the on-field assessment; however, his clinical findings do not list any specific ROM limitations. (a) Why do you believe this is the case? (b) If you were doing the evaluation, how could you quantify AROM, particularly ankle dorsiflexion? (c) How much active dorsiflexion is considered normal during a walking gait?

While covering a pee-wee ice hockey tournament, Nichole, a graduate assistant athletic trainer from the local university, was summoned from the bench to the ice. A 12-year-old ice hockey forward named Mary had been tied up with an opposing player when another player fell into the two, landing on the lateral side of Mary's left ankle. Mary immediately fell to the ice, grabbing her ankle in pain. The referees stopped play, triggering Nichole into action. She arrived on the scene to observe Mary supporting her right ankle.

ON-SCENE ARRIVAL

Nichole shuffles to Mary to find her scared and in obvious discomfort. She is conscious and alert, with no immediate threats to life, and a rating of 14 on the GCS. A rapid assessment reveals trauma (tenderness) to her right ankle and lower leg. Vital signs are provided in Table 11.2.1. Nichole determines that Mary can skate off with assistance but will require an immediate assessment in the locker room. Mary's mother follows right behind when Mary gets off the ice.

TABLE 11.2.1	Mary's vital signs.	
VITAL SIGNS	**FINDING**	
Pulse	124, rapid and weak	
Respiration	21, shallow and labored	
Blood pressure	126/90	
Mental status	Alert and conscious	

FIGURE 11.2.1 Mary's mechanism of injury.

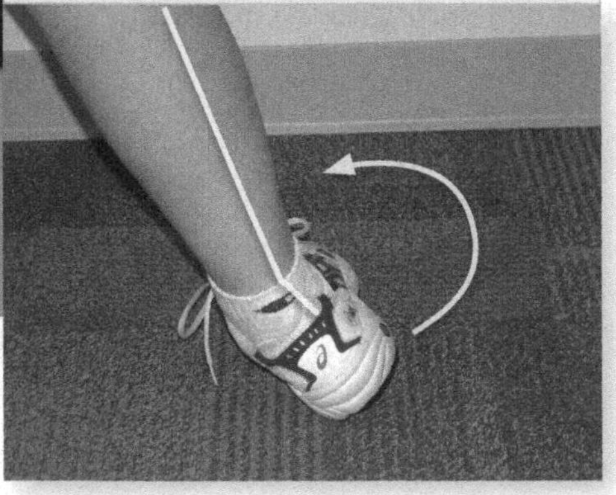

HISTORY

In the locker room, Nichole begins questioning Mary about the injury. Mary states, "The girl fell right on to my ankle and it rolled out" (Figure 11.2.1). Further questioning reveals that Mary felt a pop on the inside of her ankle. Mary's chief complaint is of pain and tenderness along the medial and lateral lower leg and difficulty with ankle inversion, eversion, and weight bearing. She denies any neurovascular deficits. Her pain level is 9/10, with increased pain around the anteroinferior and posteroinferior medial malleolus. Her mother reports no previous foot or ankle trauma.

PHYSICAL EXAMINATION

Nichole cuts Mary's skate lace and removes the skate to expose the ankle. There is immediate swelling around the medial and lateral malleolus. Mary is point tender over the distal end of the fibula and inferior to the distal medial malleolus. Nichole asks

Mary to actively dorsiflex, plantarflex, invert, and evert her right ankle. Mary refuses to do so because of the intense pain. Any attempt to bear weight on her right ankle increases Mary's pain on the medial side. Strength testing is deferred because of the pain. A Kleiger's test and eversion stress test are positive for pain and instability when compared with the uninvolved side. Neurovascularly, she is intact.

Nichole discusses her findings with Mary's mother and recommends an immediate medical referral, preferably to an orthopedic surgeon. Nichole stabilizes Mary's ankle and lower leg using a splint. Her CSM (circulation, sensation, movement) is unremarkable before and after application of the splint. As Nichole is providing home-instruction to Mary and her mother, the assistant coach approaches and wants to know the status of Mary and when she will return, because without her the team will probably lose the game. Nichole is at a loss for words.

Please answer the following questions based on the above case information.

11.2 / **1.** Based on the information presented in the case, determine (a) the differential diagnoses and (b) the clinical diagnosis.

11.2 / **2.** Mary presented with tenderness over and inferior to the distal medial malleolus. Identify the structures responsible for providing medial ankle joint stability.

11.2 / **3.** Based on the clinical presentation and the MOI, what is one pertinent history question Nichole could have asked to guide the physical examination?

11.2 / **4.** As the evaluating clinician, in addition to the obvious anatomical landmarks (e.g., malleoli), what other bony anatomical landmarks would you have assessed to guide the physical examination?

11.2 / **5.** Overall, do you believe Nichole made the correct decision by removing Mary from the ice after completing her on-ice evaluation? If not, why? What would you have done differently?

11.2 / **6.** As a new certified athletic trainer, how would you respond to the assistant coach's request for playing status? If a difference of opinion occurred, how and when should the situation be handled?

arcy, a 32-year-old ballroom dancer, and her partner Steve were practicing for a regional dance competition when Steve lost his footing and landed on the back of Marcy's ankle. She reported experiencing immediate pain and went straight to a local urgent care center. The on-duty PA provided an ICD-9 CM diagnosis of code 845.00. The recommended treatment from the nurse consisted of rest, heat, compression with an elastic wrap, and no dancing for three or four days but some walking on the foot within two days to prevent any stiffness. After five days, her ankle was no better, so Marcy sought out further medical care at a local sports medicine facility. After completing the necessary paperwork and supplying the nurse with her insurance information, Marcy was escorted to a treatment room where she was to be evaluated by Dr. Angus, MD, PhD, ATC.

HISTORY

Dr. Angus begins the evaluation by gathering some general information. Marcy describes the events that took place five days earlier and her symptoms since. After some discussion, Dr. Angus determines the exact MOI (Figure 11.3.1). Marcy states, "I used a heat pack like I was told, but it seemed to make the ankle worse." She continues, "The pain is the worst right here (Figure 11.3.2). When I do try to move my ankle, the pain is the greatest at the same spot, especially when I try to point my ankle upward." Further questioning by Dr. Angus reveals that Marcy is not only a ballroom dancer but is also a college professor teaching physics and has not been able to stand during class. Marcy's record indicates no previous history of lower leg, foot, or ankle trauma. Current pain is rated at 6/10 at rest and 8/10 with activity.

PHYSICAL EXAMINATION

Marcy is a 32-year-old female who is alert and in moderate-to-severe discomfort. A general observation of Marcy's right ankle and lower leg reveals swelling and ecchymosis over the anterior distal tibia-fibula joint. Marcy is point tender over this same area; however, no tenderness is elicited over the

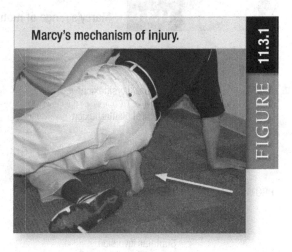

Marcy's mechanism of injury.

FIGURE 11.3.1

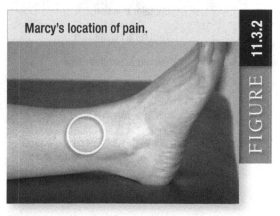

Marcy's location of pain.

FIGURE 11.3.2

Circle indicates location of pain and tenderness superomedial to the lateral malleolus.

length of the fibula. Active, passive, and resistive ROM are limited because of pain and swelling (Table 11.3.1). Dr. Angus performs an external rotation test, which is positive for pain and increased joint laxity in the involved limb. A squeeze test also increases Marcy's pain. Assessment of the lower leg dermatomes, myotomes, peripheral nerves, and deep tendon reflexes is unremarkable.

DIAGNOSTIC IMAGING

Based on the results of the physical examination, Dr. Angus orders A/P, lateral, and mortise views of the ankle and AP and lateral views of the entire length of the tibia and fibula. Results of the AP and mortise views suggest a tibiofibular clear space greater than 6.5 mm.

Dr. Angus discusses his findings with Marcy and provides her with a new ICD-9 CM code. He prescribes continued rest but recommends replacing the heat with ice (at least until the swelling and pain are under control). He places her in an NWB cast for two weeks. He tells her that this will be followed by progressive weight bearing in a cam walker. Recovery time he informs her could be six to eight weeks or longer.

TABLE	11.3.1	Marcy's range of motion results.		
			FINDINGS	
MOTION	**JOINT MOTION**	**LEFT**	**RIGHT**	
AROM	Talocrural dorsiflexion*	21°	11°	
	Talocrural plantarflexion	48°	18°	
	Forefoot inversion	35°	18°	
	Forefoot eversion*	15°	13°	
PROM	Talocrural dorsiflexion	Moderate-to-severe discomfort		
	Talocrural plantarflexion	Increased pain end-range motion		
	Subtalar inversion	Increased pain end-range motion		
	Subtalar eversion	Moderate-to-severe discomfort		
RROM	Talocrural dorsiflexion	3+/5 with pain		
	Talocrural plantarflexion	4/5		
	Subtalar inversion	3+/5 with pain		
	Subtalar eversion	3+/5		

*Pain increases to 8/10 with active dorsiflexion and eversion.

Please answer the following questions based on the above case information.

11.3 / 1. Based on the information presented in the case, determine (a) the differential diagnoses and (b) the likely clinical diagnosis.

11.3 / 2. What is the typical MOI for this injury?

11.3 / 3. Obviously, the ICD-9 CM code provided by the PA was incorrect. (a) What is an ICD-9 CM code, and based on the clinical diagnosis, (b) what is the correct ICD-9 code for this injury?

11.3 / 4. During the physical examination, Dr. Angus performed a neurological assessment including dermatomes, myotomes, peripheral nerves, and deep tendon reflexes. What are the two main deep tendon reflexes in the lower extremity?

11.3 / 5. Dr. Angus performed several provocative tests to determine the stability of the ankle. If the patient asked you to explain these tests and the purpose behind them, what would be your response?

11.3 / 6. If this dancer had been a football player and you were attempting to stabilize the ankle for further medical referral, describe how you could properly stabilize the joint.

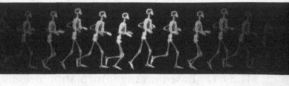

Ika'aka, a 19-year-old sophomore running back, reported to pre-season football in what he considered to be good shape. He believed this was his year to become a starter. He had been running four to five miles a day and was lifting every other day. He was excited to be at training camp. However, after three weeks of two-a-days, he began experiencing significant forefoot problems, so much that he was unable to give 100 percent when running. This forced him to seek out Al, the certified athletic trainer for the football team.

HISTORY

After some small talk about the summer and training camp, Al begins asking Ika'aka several history questions. Al learns that Ika'aka's problem has been progressively getting worse over the last five to six days. He explains, "My big toe is killing me. It was fine before camp, but once I got here and got on the field, all of the running, starting, and stopping, and jumping has made it difficult for me to run and jump. It really hurts when I do this [Figure 11.4.1]. I have been icing after practice, but nothing seems to be helping. It's so bad that even walking around has started to bother me." Al questions Ika'aka about his summer training, to which Ika'aka responds, "It went well. I learned from last year and got new shoes and gradually increased my training. In fact, when I got back I got a new pair of shoes for the new field." Further questioning reveals no previous ankle or foot injury. Ika'aka's pain at rest is 6/10 and 8/10 when running and jumping.

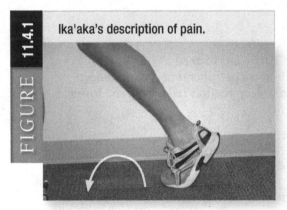

FIGURE 11.4.1

Ika'aka's description of pain.

Arrow indicates increase in pain to the first MTPJ during toe-off.

PHYSICAL EXAMINATION

Ika'aka is alert but anxious and in moderate discomfort without movement of the right hallux. Al's observation of the plantar surface of the right foot reveals an area of joint swelling at the first metatarsophalangeal joint (MTPJ) and evidence of friction blisters. Soft tissue and bony palpation reveals significant tenderness around the same area of swelling. Al assesses active and passive ROM using a goniometer and records his findings (Table 11.4.1) in his SOAP note. Resistive ROM testing reveals a deficit in first MTPJ flexion (4/5) and extension (3/5) when compared with the uninvolved side. Varus and valgus stress tests of the first MTPJ and DIPJ are unremarkable. Neurovascular testing is also unremarkable.

TABLE	11.4.1	Ika'aka's range of motion results.	

| MOTION | JOINT MOTION | FINDINGS | |
		RIGHT	LEFT
AROM	Flexion		
	First MTPJ	30°	45°
	First IPJ	80°	90°
	2–5 MTPJ	38°	40°
	2–5 PIPJ	34°	35°
	2–5 DIPJ	60°	58°
	Extension		
	First MTPJ	38°	70°
	First IPJ	–5°	0°
	2–5 MTPJ	40°	40°
	2–5 PIPJ	0°	0°
	2–5 DIPJ	0°	0°
PROM	First MTPJ flexion	Minimal discomfort, increased pain at end range of motion	
	First MTPJ extension*	Moderate to severe discomfort, limited to mid-range of motion	
	MTPJs, PIPJs, DIPJs 2–5	No discomfort or limit	

*Pain increases to 8/10 with passive extension.

Al discusses the results of his examination with Ika'aka. Al believes Ika'aka should be referred to the team's orthopedic surgeon for further evaluation and diagnostic testing. In the interim, Ika'aka is placed on the injured reserve list, is instructed to report to the athletic training room twice a day for treatment, and is placed in stiff-soled shoes until he sees the orthopedic surgeon. Ika'aka is displeased with the decision and walks out of the athletic training room, mumbling under this breath.

Two days pass, and Ika'aka does not return to the athletic training room for any follow-up treatment or physical examination.

? QUESTIONS   CASE 11.4

Please answer the following questions based on the above case information.

11.4 / 1. Based on the information presented in the case, determine (a) the differential diagnoses and (b) the clinical diagnosis and the common term used to describe the clinical diagnosis.

11.4 / 2. (a) In your opinion, was the MOI in this case typical for the injury? (b) What other mechanism, if any, may cause the injury?

11.4 / 3. If you were the evaluating clinician in this case, based on the clinical presentation, what one other item would you expect to observe during the inspection phase of the physical examination?

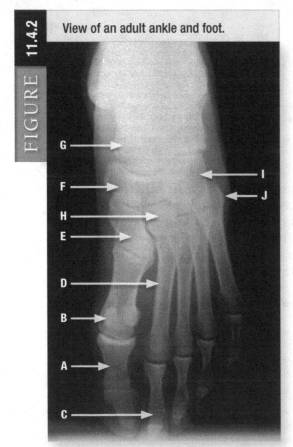

FIGURE 11.4.2

View of an adult ankle and foot.

11.4 / 4. (a) Identify the bony and soft tissue structures Al should have palpated as part of his evaluation specific to the foot. Then (b) identify the anatomical landmarks in Figure 11.4.2.

11.4 / 5. What is the purpose of the first MTPJ valgus stress test, and how is it performed? If you were the evaluating athletic trainer, would you have performed this test? If so, why? If not, what other test might you have performed?

11.4 / 6. Clearly Ika'aka was extremely upset and annoyed by Al's decision to place him on the injured reserve list. If this were your athlete and he did not return for treatment or a follow-up evaluation, how would you handle this situation?

CASE 11.5

C arrie, an avid golfer, had been experiencing pain in her lower leg and ankle ever since the golfing season began. By the eighteenth hole on this particular day, she was experiencing not only pain while walking but also pain during her long game, particularly on the follow-through. The next morning, she could no longer tolerate the pain and reported to her employer's rehabilitation clinic before beginning her shift at a local factory. After Carrie completed the necessary paperwork, the receptionist escorted her to the examination room where Emma, a certified athletic trainer, was reviewing Carrie's paperwork.

HISTORY

Carrie walks into the room limping and in apparent pain with each step. Emma begins her examination by gathering some general information. She determines that Carrie is a 42-year-old sedentary office worker with no known health issues. Every spring, Carrie actively participates in golf a minimum of 70 holes per week and attempts to walk each hole for exercise because she is 30 lbs over her ideal body weight for her height (5'5"). She had put on 15 lbs since last summer and is trying to lose that weight.

Emma says, "So tell me what happened?" Carrie replies, "I started golfing again three weeks ago. I was golfing five days per week; however, over the last two weeks I started experiencing pain here [Figure 11.5.1], and the last time I golfed not only did I have pain walking but I began to have pain during my tee shot."

When asked about whether she remembers suffering a specific injury, Carrie cannot recall any event; rather, the pain has progressively gotten worse as she plays more golf. She does have a history of hallux valgus on the involved limb but no other history of injury. Current pain is rated at 6/10 at rest and 8/10 with activity.

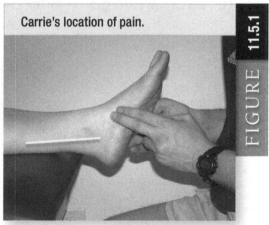

Carrie's location of pain.

FIGURE 11.5.1

Pain is also found along the length of the line.

PHYSICAL EXAMINATION

Upon physical examination, Carrie is alert and oriented. She presents with an elastic wrap around her left ankle, which Emma removes. Emma notes minimal swelling under the medial malleolus and pes planus on the involved foot when viewed from behind. There is also palpable tenderness directly behind the medial malleolus up to the distal calf and from the sustentaculum tali to the navicular. An attempt to rise on her toes produces severe pain. Slight swelling under the medial malleolus

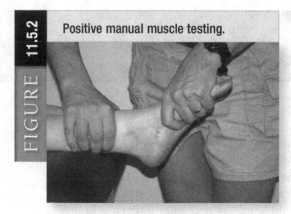

FIGURE 11.5.2

Positive manual muscle testing.

Direction of resistance is dorsiflexion and eversion.

is visible when viewed from the rear and compared with the other foot. Inversion and plantarflexion AROM are diminished on the left side, with increased pain. Eversion and dorsiflexion PROM end-feels are abnormal and produce pain. Isometric break testing is 3+/5 with plantarflexion and inversion. Muscle testing reveals moderate weakness against gravity (Figure 11.5.2). A neurovascular examination is unremarkable.

When the physical examination is complete, Emma discusses her findings with Carrie. She recommends RICE and NSAIDs (following the manufacturer's recommendations). She also recommends the use of LowDye taping, followed by orthotics if the LowDye taping alleviates her symptoms. After Carrie leaves, Emma puts her notes into injury tracking software, including the ICD-9-CM code 726.72.

Please answer the following questions based on the above case information.

11.5 / **1.** Based on the information presented in the case, determine (a) the differential diagnoses and (b) the clinical diagnosis.

11.5 / **2.** During the observation component of the physical examination, Emma apparently performed a posterior evaluation of Carrie's posture and noted pes planus. If you were the evaluating clinician, what other lower extremity postural deviations, if any, would you want to note?

11.5 / **3.** Emma noted palpable tenderness directly behind the medial malleolus up to the distal calf and from the sustentaculum tali to the navicular. (a) What structure is located between the sustentaculum tali and the navicular? (b) What is the clinical significance of this structure?

11.5 / **4.** Do you believe that Figure 11.5.2, the positive manual muscle testing, demonstrates the proper procedure for evaluating manual muscle strength of the ankle plantar flexors and foot invertors against gravity? If not, what if anything would you do differently?

11.5 / **5.** Why did Emma apply a LowDye taping procedure? If you were the treating clinician, how would you perform the taping procedure?

CASE

11.6

Hancock is a 40-year-old father of triplet teenage boys. He was out playing a pick-up game of two-on-two basketball Saturday morning when suddenly he felt an intense pain in his left calf. After getting up from the court with the boys' help, Hancock limped into the house and called his next door neighbor, James, who was an athletic trainer at the local university. James told Hancock that he was on his way to work to cover a soccer match but would be glad to take a look at his leg if he came down to the soccer field. When Hancock arrived, James noted that he was using crutches, and he appeared to be in moderate discomfort.

HISTORY

James immediately believes that he knows what he is dealing with and asks Hancock, "So what happened old man?" Hancock states, "I was out playing ball with the boys, when I went on a fast break. As I approached for the lay-up, I went to jump off my left leg when—wham—I felt like I got kicked in the left calf. I fell to the ground and had a hard time getting up. In fact, I got a knot still in the middle of my calf." James asks, "When was the last time you played ball with the boys?" Hancock replies, "I think the last time I played ball was about a month ago. I have been real consumed with the new gaming software my company is getting ready to release. In fact, I really have not had much time for any exercise over the last three months. Today was the first Saturday I didn't have to work." Further questioning reveals difficulty ambulating, particularly when trying to stand on his tiptoes. Hancock's pain is 8/10.

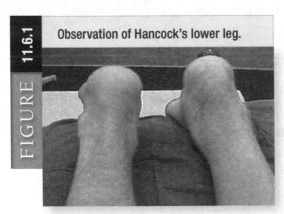

FIGURE 11.6.1

Observation of Hancock's lower leg.

Used with permission of University of Wisconsin-Eau Claire, Department of Kinesiology, Athletic Training.

PHYSICAL EXAMINATION

Upon examination, Hancock presents with evidence of swelling (+1.5 in) of the posterior aspect of the distal calf, ecchymosis, and deformity (Figure 11.6.1). He is unable to bear weight on the left limb. Upon palpation, James notes a step deformity in the continuity of the Achilles tendon, approximately 4 cm from the malleolus border, and elicits mid-substance gastrocnemius-soleus pain; however, the swelling is making it difficult to palpate. A test for a calcaneus fracture is unremarkable. Dorsal pedis and posterior tibial pulses are unremarkable. Deep tendon reflex testing is not attempted because of the pain. Dermatome and peripheral nerve assessment is unremarkable. Figure 11.6.2 reveals a positive special test. Results of Hancock's ROM and muscle testing are found in Table 11.6.1.

James discusses the results of the physical examination with Hancock. He explains that he will need to see an orthopedic surgeon for confirmation of a clinical diagnosis. James places Hancock in a Bledsoe Boot (Bledsoe Brace Systems, Grand Prairie, TX) and provides home care instructions.

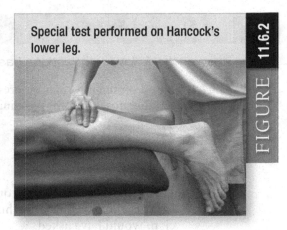

Special test performed on Hancock's lower leg.

FIGURE 11.6.2

TABLE	11.6.1	Hancock's range of motion results.

| | | FINDINGS | |
MOTION	JOINT MOTION	RIGHT	LEFT
AROM	Talocrural plantarflexion	50°	10°
	Talocrural dorsiflexion	21°	12°
	Subtalar inversion	35°	20°
	Subtalar eversion	35°	20°
PROM	Talocrural plantarflexion	Firm end-feel	
	Talocrural dorsiflexion	Increased pain mid-to-end-range motion, abnormal end-feel	
	Subtalar inversion	Firm end-feel	
	Subtalar eversion	Hard end-feel	
RROM	Talocrural plantarflexion	3/5	
	Talocrural dorsiflexion	4/5	
	Subtalar inversion	4/5	
	Subtalar eversion	4/5	

? Q U E S T I O N S   CASE 11.6

Please answer the following questions based on the above case information.

11.6 / **1.** Based on the information presented in the case, determine (a) the differential diagnoses and (b) the clinical diagnosis.

11.6 / **2.** James asked several history questions to guide his physical examination. Identify three or four other history questions you, as the evaluating clinician, would have asked.

11.6 / **3.** (a) If you were the evaluating clinician, how would you assess plantarflexion strength based on the muscle strength grade found in the physical examination? (b) How do you explain Hancock's muscle strength, given the clinical diagnosis?

11.6 / **4.** What is the name of the special test performed in Figure 11.6.2? What is considered a positive finding?

11.6 / **5.** During the physical examination, James assessed Hancock's dermatome patterns, which were unremarkable. What are dermatomes? If you were the evaluating clinician, what levels would you have assessed? Identify the location of these dermatome levels.

CASE 11.7

ieutenant (Lt.) Commander Logan is working as an athletic trainer at the United States Naval Academy after completing an ROTC program as an undergraduate. He is a certified athletic trainer and the sports medicine medical director at the Naval Academy. Lt. Commander Logan was in his office first thing Monday, as was his normal routine. He was busy completing medical documentation from the previous week and determining the status of the current week. During a break between classes, Midshipman Brady, a junior lacrosse defenseman, reported to the athletic training facility complaining of heel pain. Lt. Commander Logan pulled up Midshipman Brady's medical records before beginning the assessment, noting no previous history of ankle or foot injury.

HISTORY

Lt. Commander Logan determines that Midshipman Brady began developing right heel pain three days ago. Midshipman Brady states, "During practice on Thursday I jumped for a pass and landed on my heel pretty hard. Immediately after the injury, I really had a hard time walking. I iced after practice, but the pain began to get really bad last night after completing my marching tour (12 h). Walking to class this morning, I could feel pain each time I landed on the right heel. The worst pain is located here." (See Figure 11.7.1.) Further questioning from Lt. Commander Logan reveals no previous history of heel pain. Pain at rest is 3/10 and 8/10 when running and jumping.

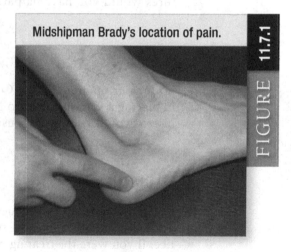

Midshipman Brady's location of pain.

FIGURE 11.7.1

PHYSICAL EXAMINATION

Midshipman Brady is alert, oriented, and in minor-to-moderate discomfort on physical examination. Logan notes swelling and warmth over the lateral aspect of the right heel. There is palpable tenderness over the plantar surface and lateral aspect of the calcaneus. Weight-bearing and gait analysis reveals an unwillingness to bear full weight upon a right-side heel strike. Active, passive, and resistive ROM are unremarkable. Tests for fracture (bump test) and neurological testing are also unremarkable. Lt. Commander Logan places an insert into Midshipman Brady's right shoe in hopes of reducing the pain experienced while walking around. He instructs Midshipman Brady to report to the athletic training room before lacrosse practice so he or another staff athletic trainer can prepare him for practice.

Please answer the following questions based on the above case information.

11.7 / **1.**   Based on the information presented in the case, determine (a) the differential diagnoses and (b) the clinical diagnosis.

11.7 / **2.**   (a) Was the MOI in this case typical for the injury? (b) What other mechanisms, if any, may exist?

11.7 / **3.**   If you were the evaluating clinician in this case, what anatomical structures would you have palpated based on the clinical presentation?

11.7 / **4.**   (a) In your opinion, did Lt. Commander Logan make the correct decision in placing a single insert into Midshipman Brady's shoe? (b) What type of inserts would you consider using based on the clinical diagnosis?

11.7 / **5.**   Lt. Commander Logan requested that Midshipman Brady return to the athletic training facility so a staff athletic trainer can prepare him for practice. If you were the treating clinician, what would you do to prepare this athlete for athletic competition?

CASE **11.8**

Jennifer, a high school athletic trainer and the Director of Outreach Sports Medicine services at Bison Medical Center, was covering a summer mountain bike racing series at the local ski resort. The day's events had been busy, and except for a fractured collar bone, the injuries had been minor. As Jennifer was talking to some of the volunteers, a call came in over the radio that one of the racers had severely injured herself, and medical personnel were needed on the other side of the mountain. Jennifer, two EMTs, and an athletic training student hopped onto a Gator and made their way over to the biker. The information provided over the radio was unclear as to the extent of the injury.

ON-SCENE ARRIVAL

When they arrive, the rider, Georgia, is laying on the ground with her helmet off. Jennifer immediately begins to calm and reassure Georgia that everything is going to be all right. The EMTs complete an initial assessment that reveals no immediate threats to Georgia's life. A rapid assessment of Georgia reveals significant trauma to her left ankle, which Jennifer begins to stabilize. The athletic training student is sent to collect the splints and backboard from the Gator.

HISTORY

Jennifer begins questioning Georgia while the EMTs complete the detailed physical examination. Georgia states, "I was coming down the hill when I tried to lift the front wheel off the drop to avoid a stump. Somehow I ended up catching some air, and when I landed, my right foot was on the peg; but my left had fallen off, and when I hit, my left foot got caught and I twisted the living crap out of it. It hurts like you wouldn't believe." Further questioning reveals that Georgia heard a crack when her left foot hit the ground.

PHYSICAL EXAMINATION

Georgia is alert, oriented, and in severe discomfort. Her vital signs are in Table 11.8.1. There is observable joint deformity at the left ankle (Figure 11.8.1) and skin

TABLE 11.8.1	Georgia's on-scene vital signs.
VITAL SIGNS	**FINDING**
Pulse	94 and strong
Respiration	15, unlabored and normal
Blood pressure	128/85
Mental status	Conscious but in severe discomfort

FIGURE 11.8.1   Observation of Georgia's foot and lower leg.

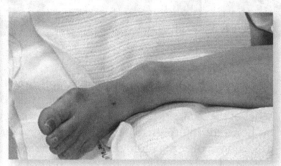

Used with permission of S. Eriksson.

puckering. The joint begins to swell immediately. Georgia has palpable tenderness around the anterior and posterior tibiotalar joint. Muscle and ROM testing are deferred because of pain.

IMMEDIATE CARE

Jennifer, the EMTs, and the athletic training student stabilize Georgia's left leg and ankle. Georgia is spine boarded and transferred to the waiting ambulance. Her vital signs on the way to the medical facility are in Table 11.8.2. However, a diminished posterior tibial pulse is noted with a whitish area around the medial malleolus. When they arrive at the medical facility, the ER physician immediately orders radiographs.

TABLE 11.8.2	Georgia's en-route vital signs.
VITAL SIGNS	**FINDING**
Pulse	74 and regular
Respiration	12 and normal
Blood pressure	118/76
Mental status	Conscious but in severe discomfort

Please answer the following questions based on the above case information.

11.8 / **1.** Based on the information presented in the case, determine (a) the differential diagnoses and (b) the clinical diagnosis.

11.8 / **2.** Based on the clinical presentation and your clinical diagnosis, identify three to five additional history questions you may have asked as the evaluating clinician.

11.8 / **3.** Do you believe Jennifer and the EMTs adequately evaluated Georgia's condition? If not, what would you have done differently as the evaluating clinician?

11.8 / **4.** (a) If you were an athletic trainer at a high school or college/university and your athlete presented with signs and symptoms similar to those presented in the case, are there any equipment or clothing complications that may make the physical examination more challenging? (b) How would you handle this situation?

11.8 / **5.** If you were the athletic trainer in this case, what type of immediate care would you have provided? Describe the steps you would have used.

CASE 11.9

Tammy, a 14-year-old gymnast, was practicing her tumbling at the local gymnastic training center. She ended her last pass with a full-twisting double back, but she missed the landing and hurt her ankle. The coach and her mother immediately went over to see if Tammy was OK. After examining Tammy for a few minutes, neither the coach nor her mother could find anything that would cause concern and figured it was a sprained ankle. Her coach instructed her to go and ice her ankle for 10 minutes every couple of hours. Over the next few weeks, Tammy complained of constant ankle pain. Finally, after three weeks, Tammy's mother brought her to see the family's orthopedic surgeon, Dr. Stewart.

On the day of the appointment, Dr. Stewart was delayed in surgery, so Jamie, his PA/ATC, was assigned to the case. After completing some paperwork, Tammy and her mother were brought into an exam room.

HISTORY

Jamie begins his evaluation by reviewing the paperwork recently completed by Tammy and notes that the initial injury occurred over three weeks ago and has only mildly improved. As Jamie questions Tammy, he learns that as she was attempting to land, she over-rotated. This forced Tammy's ankle into sudden dorsiflexion as she landed. She explains, "We originally thought it was a sprained ankle; however, during the last couple of weeks, whenever I run or jump, it feels like something is moving behind my ankle. I have been icing it and have been wearing a brace for practice, but nothing seems to help." Tammy's pain at rest is 2/10.

PHYSICAL EXAMINATION

Tammy is alert and in minor discomfort while on the table. Jamie begins by completing an inspection of the left foot and ankle in a non-weight-bearing position. He notices minor-to-moderate swelling around the lateral malleolus. There are remnants of ecchymosis around the lateral malleolus and third to fifth phalanges. Soft tissue and bony palpation reveal that most of the tenderness is posterior to the lateral malleolus, (Figure 11.9.1) with some anteriorly as well. Active ROM appears to be limited in dorsiflexion and eversion; Tammy is apprehensive moving into these directions. Passive ROM is unremarkable; however, RROM does appear to replicate Tammy's complaints of feeling "like the tendon is sliding." Jamie notes a palpable click along the lateral malleolus as Tammy moves the foot's talocrural joint through dorsiflexion and plantarflexion. Ligamentous testing about the ankle reveals 1+

FIGURE 11.9.1

Location of Tammy's tenderness.

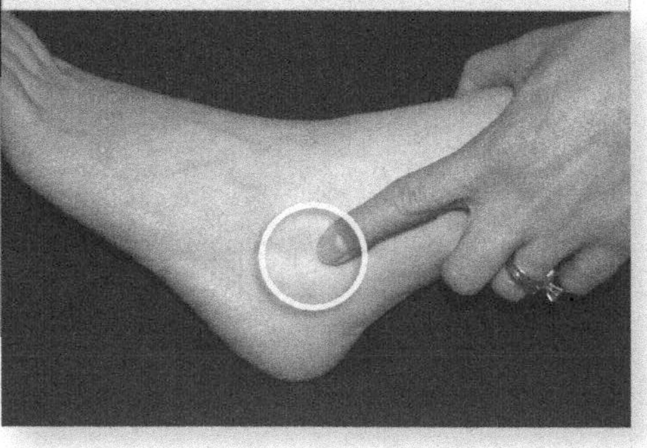

Location of tenderness is posterior to the lateral malleolus.

laxity on an anterior draw test on the involved side. Jamie performs no other special or stress tests. Neurological testing is unremarkable. Jamie discusses the result of his findings with Tammy and her mother and suggests a conservative course of care. He orders radiographs and asks to see the two again in two weeks for a follow-up visit. The tests show that plain A/P, lateral, and oblique radiographs are normal.

 QUESTIONS   **CASE 11.9**

Please answer the following questions based on the above case information.

11.9 / **1.** Based on the information presented in the case, determine (a) the differential diagnoses and (b) the clinical diagnosis.

11.9 / **2.** Jamie asked several specific history questions to guide the physical examination. However, there was one question that he did not appear to ask, which may have assisted in narrowing down the clinical diagnosis. Can you identify this question?

11.9 / **3.** (a) If Tammy had presented immediately after her injury occurred, but with her current clinical features, a careful history and physical examination would be needed to rule out what similar condition? (b) What pieces of information from the physical exam or history could have led Jamie to differentiate and determine the clinical diagnosis?

11.9 / **4.** During the physical examination, Jamie was able to reproduce Tammy's feeling that the tendon was sliding by using RROM testing. If you were the evaluating clinician, what specific motion would you muscle test, and how would you perform it?

11.9 / **5.** Given the MOI, clinical presentation, and date of initial injury, Tammy's condition appears to have progressed from an acute injury to a more recurrent chronic injury. (a) If Tammy had been treated within the first 24 hours, what type of conservative care approach would you have taken? (b) What are her options if this condition continues?

CASE 11.10

K yra, a certified athletic trainer with NASCAR, was assigned to cover the Indy 300. Kyra had been working as an athletic trainer with NASCAR for the past several years and has seen her share of accidents. During a morning training session, DJ, a 24-year-old driver in his first year on the circuit, was transitioning into curve 3 when his left passenger tire blew. The car spun out of control and eventually ended up hitting the wall head first. The firefighters and emergency medical team, which included Dr. Johnson, an emergency trauma physician, trauma nurse, and two EMTs, were called onto the scene and arrived within 30 seconds of the accident. The firefighters had DJ's door open within 1 minute of the accident. Dr. Johnson asked Tim, an EMT, to stabilize DJ's neck.

INITIAL ASSESSMENT

Dr. Johnson determines that DJ is alert and oriented to his current location, the date, and the details of his accident. Amazingly, his GCS is 15, and a rapid trauma assessment reveals only tenderness to the right foot. Pupils are equally round and reactive to light. He demonstrates no other immediate signs of secondary trauma. Vital signs include: blood pressure of 126/82; heart rate of 90; respirations of 16, unlabored and regular. The SAMPLE history reveals that as DJ hit the wall, his right foot was firmly depressed on the brake. The EMT spine boards DJ per the race track's SOP and transports him to the medical facility for further evaluation.

FIGURE 11.10.1

Location of DJ's swelling.

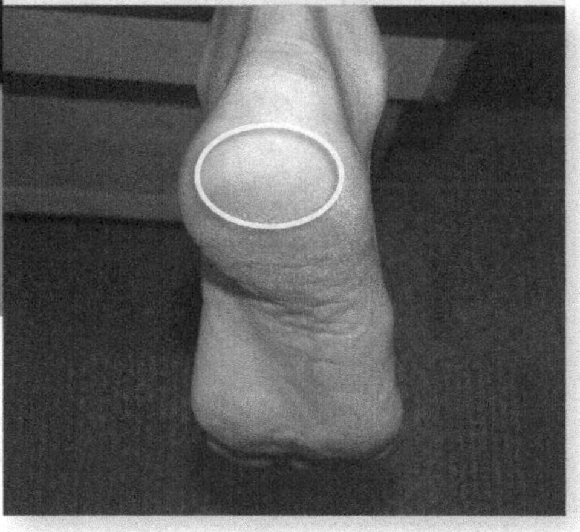

Circle indicates location of the pain and swelling.

PHYSICAL EXAMINATION

Back at the medical facility, Dr. Johnson and the trauma nurse complete a more thorough evaluation of DJ. An observation and palpation of DJ's right foot reveals immediate swelling, ecchymosis, and point tenderness (Figure 11.10.1). Range of motion is limited because of pain and swelling. Muscle testing is not performed, because of swelling and pain. Dr. Johnson orders a set of radiographs of the ankle and lower leg (A/P and lateral) to rule out bony trauma.

? QUESTIONS   CASE 11.10

Please answer the following questions based on the above case information.

11.10 / **1.** (a) Based on the information presented in the case, determine the clinical diagnosis. (b) What is the typical MOI?

11.10 / **2.** Do you believe the EMT adequately evaluated the condition in this case? If not, what would you have done differently as the evaluating clinician?

11.10 / **3.** If you were an athletic trainer at a high school or college/university and your athlete presented with signs and symptoms similar to those in the case, what other type of functional testing could you perform to assist in making the clinical diagnosis?

11.10 / **4.** If you were an athletic trainer at a high school or college/university and your athlete presented with signs and symptoms similar to those presented in the case, how would you remove the athlete from the field?

11.10 / **5.** If you were the evaluating athletic trainer in this case, how would you have removed DJ's shoe when he was in the medical facility?

L ance, a 20-year-old lacrosse player, fell to the ground after stepping into a pot-hole on the way to practice. His teammates helped him to the athletic training room. When they arrived in the athletic training room, Mike, one of the four graduate assistant athletic trainers, was cleaning whirlpools. Lance's teammates helped him to the table. It was clear to Mike that Lance was in pain.

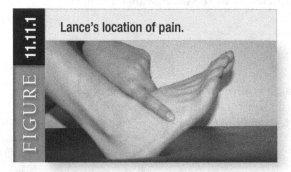

FIGURE 11.11.1

Lance's location of pain.

Pain is located at base of the fifth metatarsal.

HISTORY

Mike begins by asking Lance a series of questions about his current condition. Lance states, "I was walking to practice and joking with the guys when Pete pushed me. I lost my balance, and as I stepped down to catch myself, my right foot landed in a pothole." Mike asks Lance to describe exactly how his foot landed in the hole. Lance replies, "I think my foot turned in as I tried to catch myself." Mike further questions Lance about his current pain location. Lance states that most of his pain is on the outside of his foot, about 1-1/2 to 2 inches from the ankle (Figure 11.11.1). Lance further reports pain while bearing weight and the inability to walk more than two steps.

PHYSICAL EXAMINATION

Lance is alert and in moderate discomfort (6 or 7/10 on a numerical pain scale) while sitting during the exam. Mike begins the physical examination by observing the soft tissue around Lance's right foot and ankle. The lateral aspect of the forefoot appears swollen but non-deformed. Palpation reveals crepitus and point tenderness around the base of the fifth metatarsal. Pain is noted when Lance moves from a non-weight-bearing to a weight-bearing position. Active and passive ROM is WNL, though there is pain with active eversion (6/10). Resisted ROM (in a long sitting position) reveals weakness in eversion (3/5) and plantar flexion (3+/5). A metatarsal squeeze test elicits significant pain. Neuro-logical and circulatory tests are unremarkable. Mike decides that referral to the team's orthopedic surgeon is warranted for further evaluation and diagnostic testing. According to the Ottawa Ankle Rules for midfoot radiographs, Lance is a textbook candidate for such testing.

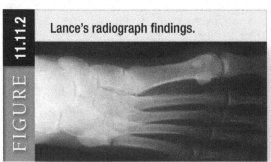

FIGURE 11.11.2

Lance's radiograph findings.

Used with permission of University of Wisconsin-Eau Claire, Department of Kinesiology, Athletic Training.

DIAGNOSTIC TESTING

The team physician agrees with Mike's decision. Lance's radiology report demonstrates osseous changes 1.5 cm distal to tuberosity of fifth metatarsal (Figure 11.11.2).

Please answer the following questions based on the above case information.

11.11 / **1.** Based on the information presented in the case, determine (a) the differential diagnoses and (b) the clinical diagnosis.

11.11 / **2.** What are the Ottawa Ankle Rules, and what information in the case led Mike to suspect the need for radiographs?

11.11 / **3.** Mike asked several history questions to guide the physical examination. (a) Based on the information presented in the case, do you believe Mike took an adequate history? (b) If not, what additional questions would you ask as the evaluating clinician?

11.11 / **4.** Based on the clinical diagnosis above, why did Lance present with decreased ankle eversion and plantarflexion strength?

11.11 / **5.** What injury should Mike suspect if Lance reported an MOI of forced inversion of the foot while the foot was plantar flexed. When does this commonly occur?

11.11 / **6.** Overall, do you believe Mike adequately evaluated Lance's condition, given the information provided in the case? If not, what would you have done differently as the evaluating clinician?

11.12

Nancy, a certified athletic trainer for a Division I volleyball team, was covering a home match with her athletic training students. During the team's warm-up, Tiffany, a 19-year-old sophomore outside hitter, was attacking when she landed awkwardly on her left foot, falling to the ground. Although she was in pain, she was able to limp over to the bench where she waited for Nancy.

HISTORY

The assessment begins with Nancy reviewing the MOI with Tiffany. Tiffany reports, "When I landed from my attack, I just came down the wrong way and landed real hard on the ball of my foot, and it hurts to put all of my weight on it now. It has been throbbing real bad too." Tiffany denies any previous history of injury to the left foot. Her pain is rated as 6/10.

PHYSICAL EXAMINATION

Tiffany is alert and oriented and is experiencing general discomfort and throbbing in her left great toe. She is able to remove her shoe and sock with minimal difficulty. An observation of Tiffany's foot reveals callus formation around the first MTPJ bilaterally but no acute signs of injury. Palpable tenderness is noted (Figure 11.12.1). Resisted plantarflexion of the hallucis interphalangeal joint is strong and painful.

Nancy is fairly certain of the clinical diagnosis and discusses the results of her physical examination and options with Tiffany. They agree the best immediate course of action would be to buddy tape the toes together and try to continue with the match.

FIGURE 11.12.1

Tiffany's location of pain.

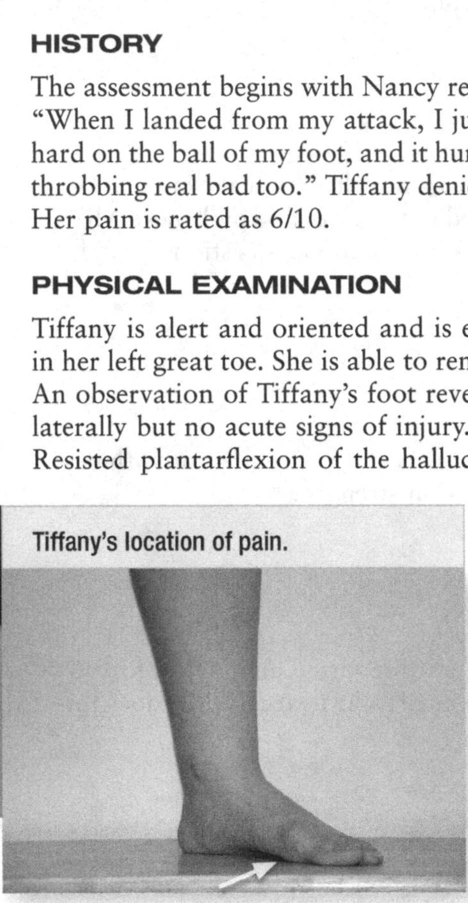

Palpable pain on the plantar surface of the first MTPJ.

FOLLOW-UP EXAMINATION

About 60 minutes after the initial physical examination Tiffany asks to be removed from the game because of increasing pain. When Nancy re-evaluates Tiffany, she now presents with great toe swelling and ecchymosis and is unable to bear weight.

Please answer the following questions based on the above case information.

11.12 / **1.** Based on the information presented in the case, determine (a) the likely differential diagnoses and (b) the clinical diagnosis.

11.12 / **2.** Based on the clinical diagnosis, is this mechanism of injury typical?

11.12 / **3.** (a) What, if anything, could a clinician add to Nancy's evaluation to assist in determining the clinical diagnosis? (b) How would you perform the evaluation?

11.12 / **4.** In your opinion, did Nancy make the correct decision in allowing Tiffany to return to play in the game? What, if anything, would you have done differently?

11.12 / **5.** What type of initial care should Nancy provide Tiffany before she leaves for home after the match?

CASE 11.13

Pvt. Cross, an 18-year-old Marine Corp recruit, reported to the Basic Marine Training Medical Center complaining of left foot pain. The on-duty triage nurse logged Pvt. Cross's personal information into the database before collecting her vital signs, which were unremarkable. The on-duty nurse forwarded her case to Steve Flower, PT/ATC, who was a civilian employee at the base. He was responsible for evaluating, diagnosing, and referring all non-life-threatening musculoskeletal injuries to the appropriate medical personnel.

HISTORY

Before speaking with Pvt. Cross, Steve reviews the complete electronic medical record from the medical center's database. Items of interest noted in her file include: (1) 18-year-old female, (2) first time reporting to the Basic Marine Training Medical Center, (3) normal blood work on her initial physical exam by the base physician, (4) no significant medical history, (5) currently taking Triphasil. Steve then asks Pvt. Cross about her medical history. She says that before her arrival at Basic Marine Training three weeks ago, she graduated from Hope High School where she participated in high school swimming and softball with little history of significant orthopedic trauma. Pvt. Cross says she did suffer a second-degree sprain during her sophomore year of high school but reports no adverse effects. Finally, Steve reviews Pvt. Cross's initial physical fitness test (PFT) (Table 11.13.1), noting her deficient areas. On this particular day, she is complaining of localized tenderness and pain. She also reports increased pain and difficulty walking after her PFT and doubletime march with a full pack. She says, "It has actually gotten worse during the past week of training even though I ice at night." She rates her pain as 6/10 or 7/10 at rest and 8/10 or 9/10 during PFT.

TABLE 11.13.1	Pvt. Cross's PFT initial assessment with points toward second-class fitness requirements.	
TEST	**TIME/NUMBER**	**POINTS**
Flexed-arm hang	55 s	70
Abdominal crunches	49	49
3-mile run	28:20	56
Weight	145 lb	
Height	70"	
Body fat	24%	
BMI	21	

PHYSICAL EXAMINATION

Pvt. Cross is alert, oriented, and in moderate discomfort at the time of the physical examination. Steve notes fusiform swelling and warmth on the dorsal aspect of the left foot. There is palpable tenderness over the dorsum of the foot (Figure 11.13.1). Inspection of Pvt. Cross's athletic shoes and boots is unremarkable; however, a weight-bearing assessment of her foot position reveals she is flatfooted on the left side. Left foot AROM appears to be WNL. Passive ROM of the third ray increases Pvt. Cross's symptoms when moved to the end range of flexion and extension. Neurological and neurovascular findings appear to be WNL. Steve decides to place her on profile and rates her as an "L" position 3 until she is reviewed by the base physician.

After completing the physical examination, Steve documents his findings and sends a copy of the report over to Maj. Weston, Chief Orthopedic Surgeon at the base. Dr. Weston agrees that Pvt. Cross warrants further diagnostic testing and immediate treatment, including the use of pharmacological agents and modification of activity.

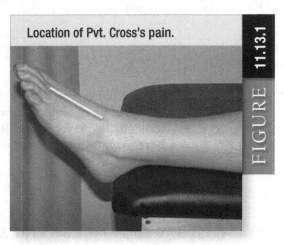

Location of Pvt. Cross's pain.

FIGURE 11.13.1

Pain falls along the line.

Please answer the following questions based on the above case information.

11.13 / **1.** (a) Based on the information presented in the case, what is the clinical diagnosis? (b) What is the common term used to describe the clinical diagnosis?

11.13 / **2.** Steve asked several history questions to guide the physical examination. (a) Based on the information presented in the case, do you believe Steve took an adequate history? If not, (b) what kinds of questions would you have asked as the evaluating clinician?

11.13 / **3.** What are Pvt. Cook's PFT deficiency areas according to Table 11.13.1?

11.13 / **4.** (a) Why did Steve assess the wear pattern of Pvt. Cook's shoes? (b) If you were the evaluating clinician, what would you hope to observe? (c) Why didn't Steve see anything?

11.13 / **5.** Given the information presented in the case, what diagnostic test would Dr. Weston most likely order first?

11.13 / **6.** As the case mentions, Steve documented his findings and sent a copy of the report to Maj. Weston. Please document your findings as if you were in Steve's position. If the case did not provide information you believe is pertinent to the clinical diagnosis, please feel free to add this information to your documentation.

J oan, a 38-year-old endurance athlete and avid soccer player, began experiencing medial lower leg pain over the past several weeks. After enduring the intense pain for about two weeks, she decided to have it evaluated. Valerie, a colleague of Joan, was an assistant athletic trainer at the university where Joan taught nutrition. She called Valerie to see if she could set up an appointment. Valerie was more than happy to see her and suggested she stop by on a day when she knew that Dr. Sharp, the university's team physician, would also be in seeing athletes.

HISTORY

After some small talk about recent events at the university, Valerie begins her examination by gathering some general information. She asks, "So tell me what's going on?" Joan says, "Well I have been training for a 100-mile run across the desert, and over the last couple of weeks, my right lower leg and foot have been really starting to bother me. At first the pain only bothered me at the beginning of training and after I finished, and the pain usually resolved with several minutes' rest; however, it is now more painful during training and while playing soccer. I have taken a couple of days off here and there, but I really need to stick to my training schedule." After some further questioning, Valerie determines that Joan has increased her mileage from 24 to 40 miles over the last two weeks and is playing three to four soccer matches per week. Joan admits she does not normally play soccer while she is training for an endurance event, but a friend convinced her to play. Joan reports eating a well-balanced diet that includes proper hydration. Her pain is rated at 7/10 during training, and she denies any previous history of foot or ankle trauma.

PHYSICAL EXAMINATION

Upon examination, Joan presents with moderate discomfort. Inspection of Joan's foot reveals callus formation under the head of the second metatarsal. Non-weight-bearing assessment of the foot and calcaneal alignment reveals right forefoot varus and what appears to be possible pes planus. Joan is point tender along the distal medial border of the tibia down into the area of the navicular. Active ROM is limited in dorsiflexion (Table 11.14.1) with crepitation on plantarflexion and inversion. Isometric break testing near the end ranges of motion demonstrates 3+/5 for ankle plantarflexion and inversion. Ligamentous stress testing is unremarkable; however, the following special test is positive (Figure 11.14.1). A neurological examination is unremarkable.

TABLE	11.14.1	Joan's active range of motion results.		

| MOTION | JOINT MOTION | FINDINGS | |
		RIGHT	LEFT
AROM	Talocrural dorsiflexion		
	Knee straight	20°	30°
	Knee flexed	12°	20°
	Talocrural plantarflexion*	45°	50°
	Subtalar inversion (forefoot)*	26°	30°
	Subtalar eversion (forefoot)	10°	15°
PROM	Talocrural dorsiflexion	Firm	
	Talocrural plantarflexion	Firm	
	Subtalar inversion	Firm	
	Subtalar eversion	Hard	

*Pain is increased.

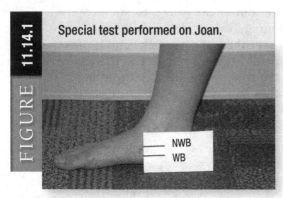

FIGURE 11.14.1

Special test performed on Joan.

NWB
WB

Joan should be standing with feet shoulder-width apart while performing the special test.

Valerie discusses the results of Joan's physical exam with Dr. Sharp. After his evaluation, Dr. Sharp sends Joan to the hospital for radiographs, which as he suspected, come back negative. He then refers her for a triple-phase bone scan. This exam demonstrates a longitudinally oriented diffuse tracer uptake around Joan's area of pain.

![?] Q U E S T I O N S   **CASE 11.14**

Please answer the following questions based on the above case information.

11.14 / 1. Based on the information presented in the case, determine the clinical diagnosis and the possible etiology.

11.14 / 2. Based on the physical examination, Valerie believed she identified a pes planus foot. Identify the common name for pes planus and describe it.

11.14 / 3. Based on the case report, Valerie performed a non-weight-bearing assessment of Joan's foot and calcaneal alignment. If you were the evaluating clinician, describe how you would perform this exam. What does the result of Valerie's exam indicate?

11.14 / 4. (a) What is the name of the special test performed in Figure 11.14.1? (b) What is considered a positive clinical finding? (c) If you were the evaluating clinician, would you have performed any other special tests?

11.14 / 5. Describe the anatomical landmarks you would use as the evaluating clinician in order to measure talocrural dorsiflexion.

CASE 11.15

evin, a certified athletic trainer for an NCAA Division I men's ice hockey team, was getting ready for practice in the university's athletic training room. This was his first year working at this level of ice hockey. Prior to this position, he was an athletic trainer at two different NCAA D-III programs. The ice hockey team had already been practicing for four weeks when one of the players, Clay, arrived to speak with Kevin. They chatted for a few minutes before beginning the evaluation.

HISTORY

Kevin begins questioning Clay as to why he is seeking out help. Clay states, "My heel is swollen. It hurts to run during dry lands and trying to skate is even worse. Just getting the skate on some days is horrible." Further questioning from Kevin reveals that the pain begins gradually each morning, increasing with the beginning of practice, and eventually diminishing as the activity continues. After practice, Clay is unable to walk without a limp. Clay denies any previous history of ankle and/or foot trauma. His pain is rated as 2/10 to 3/10 at rest and 8/10 to 9/10 when participating in athletics (i.e., skating and running).

PHYSICAL EXAMINATION

Clay is alert and oriented. An observation of Clay's gait reveals an unwillingness to put pressure on the right heel. The area around the posterior heel is red, warm, and swollen, with a noticeable deformity (Figure 11.15.1). Palpation of the posterior heel reveals localized pain at the posterior aspect of the calcaneus, particularly between the Achilles tendon and calcaneus. Active ROM is WNL; however, pain is noted at the end-range of motion (i.e., plantarflexion). Passive ROM is also positive for pain at the end-range of motion. Resistive ROM elicits pain with plantarflexion. Ligamentous stability is unremarkable, as are the results of a Thomas test.

After Kevin makes his clinical diagnosis, he recommends anti-inflammatory drugs, use of a heel cup when not practicing, and cryotherapy for now. He also instructs Clay on how to stretch his Achilles tendon. As far as practice goes, he informs Clay that he should base his decision on his pain.

FIGURE 11.15.1

Observation and location of Clay's pain.

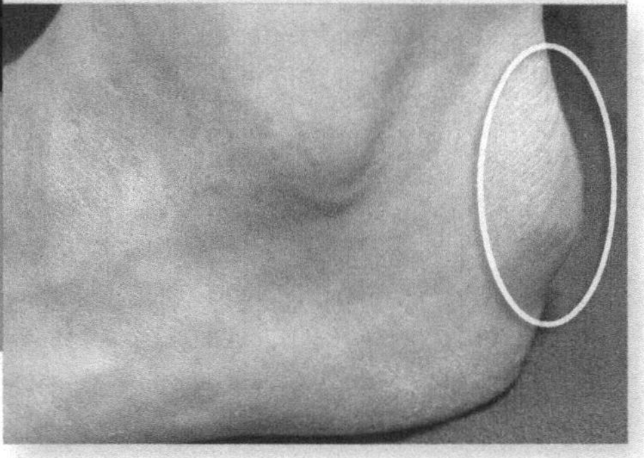

Clay's pain is located in the circle.
Used with permission from A. Kline, 2007.

FOLLOW-UP EXAMINATION

Five days later, Clay's heel pain has progressively worsened, especially wearing his skates and now his shoes. Clay stops by to see Kevin again. Kevin recommends that he see a physician, but he decides to try one more trick to alleviate the pain until then.

Please answer the following questions based on the above case information.

11.15 / **1.** Based on the information presented in the case, determine (a) the differential diagnoses and (b) the clinical diagnosis.

11.15 / **2.** Clay presented with end-range pain with PROM. (a) In what direction would you suspect the end-range pain? (b) Is there anything else that would also be palpable during AROM?

11.15 / **3.** Kevin asked several specific history questions to guide the physical examination. However, he did not appear to ask a certain question that could have assisted in determining the MOI and narrowing down the possibilities for the clinical diagnosis. Can you identify this question?

11.15 / **4.** Overall, do you believe Kevin adequately evaluated Clay's condition given the provided information? If not, what would you have done differently as the evaluating clinician?

11.15 / **5.** What "trick," or form of conservative treatment, do you think Kevin utilized on Clay during the follow-up examination?

11.16

J ennifer, a 54-year-old recreational basketball player, reported to the walk-in sports medicine clinic at St. Ogden's Sports Medicine Center. She was complaining of left ankle and foot pain. At the clinic was Kirsten, a senior athletic training student, Gena, a certified athletic trainer, and Dr. Davis, an orthopedic surgeon specializing in sports medicine. Jennifer was escorted to an examination room by Kirsten, who asked her to complete a medical history and pain profile. When all the paperwork was completed, Kirsten began the examination with the history work-up, followed with a physical examination conducted by Gena.

HISTORY

Kirsten reviews Jennifer's past medical history. Jennifer says that she suffered a left navicular fracture a year ago while playing basketball, and she just recently returned to playing basketball recreationally three days per week. Kirsten then proceeds by asking about what was going on now. Jennifer responds, "Over the past several weeks I have begun to experience diffuse pain, burning, and numbness in my foot (Figure 11.16.1). It really bothered me after I 'tweaked' my ankle at work. Working also causes an increase in pain and numbness, especially at the end of the day. However, the pain is less when I am at rest." Further questioning reveals a recently sprained ankle caused by a plantarflexion-eversion mechanism. Kirsten inquired about Jennifer's occupation and learns that she is a refuse waste collection specialist, working 10-hour days. However, she never reported the sprained ankle to her employer. Jennifer denies any history of peripheral neuropathy. The pain profile information is presented below (Figure 11.16.2).

FIGURE 11.16.1

Jennifer's location of foot and ankle pain.

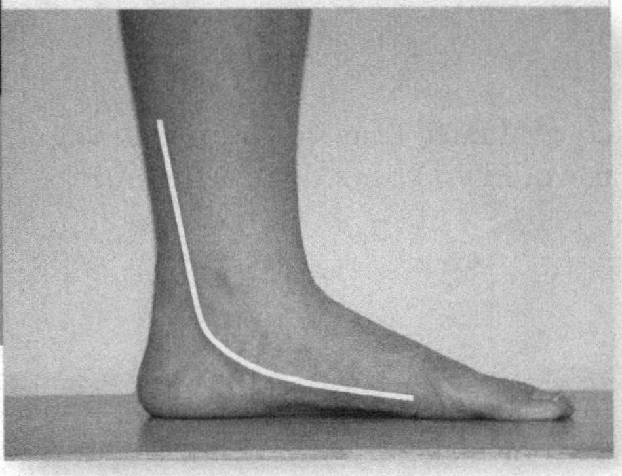

Jennifer's numbness runs along the medial portion of the ankle and plantar surface.

PHYSICAL EXAMINATION

After Kirsten finishes gathering the history, Gena walks into the exam room to begin the physical examination. Jennifer is alert, oriented, and in minimal-to-moderate discomfort according to her pain profile. A general observation of Jennifer in a non-weight-bearing position is unremarkable. Weight-bearing inspection of the lower extremity reveals, specifically, that the medial longitudinal arch demonstrates pes planus. Gena notes swelling and palpable tenderness and pain along the posteromedial aspect of the distal tibia. Active ROM of the intrinsic and extrinsic musculature is unremarkable. Jennifer does report an increase in symptoms when combined passive motion is applied to the ankle at the end-range. Resistive and manual muscle testing

| FIGURE | 11.16.2 | Jennifer's pain profiles. |

1. Please rate your current level of pain on the following scale (circle one):

0   1   2   3   ④   5   6   7   8   9   10

(no pain)   *(worst imaginable pain)*

2. Please rate your worst level of pain in the last 24 hours on the following scale (circle one):

0   1   2   3   4   5   ⑥   7   8   9   10

(no pain)   *(worst imaginable pain)*

3. Please rate your best level of pain in the last 24 hours on the following scale (circle one):

0   1   2   3   ④   5   6   7   8   9   10

(no pain)   *(worst imaginable pain)*

Note: Burning sensation is denoted by ✕.

is WNL. An anterior draw and inversion stress test are unremarkable. Eversion stress testing and Kleiger's reveals 1+ laxity on the involved side. A Tinel's sign reproduces Jennifer's symptoms inferior and distal to the medial malleolus. Gena discusses the result of her findings with Dr. Davis, and together they devise a plan of care. After instructing Jennifer about the plan, Gena dictates the results of the history and physical examination.

Please answer the following questions based on the above case information.

11.16 / **1.**   (a) Based on the information presented in the case, determine the clinical diagnosis. (b) What led you to this conclusion?

11.16 / **2.**   Jennifer presented with pain upon PROM. In which direction would you expect to find the end-range pain and why?

11.16 / **3.**   Based on the clinical diagnosis, where would you expect numbness and/or loss of function to occur?

11.16 / **4.**   Overall, do you believe Gena adequately evaluated Jennifer's condition, given the provided information? If not, what would you have done differently as the evaluating clinician?

11.16 / **5.**   What is dictation? As an experienced clinician, what pointers would you provide to Gena to improve this skill?

CASE 11.17

by William Holcomb, Ph.D., ATC, CSCS-D, University of Nevada, Las Vegas

E mma, a 29-year-old female professional soccer player, reported to the athletic training room after a preseason practice, complaining of recurring left heel pain. Adrian, the certified athletic trainer, was in the facility when she arrived. The team had been practicing for the last three weeks, and Emma's heel had been getting progressively worse. As a starting forward, Emma was worried about her place on the team, because the competitive season would begin in just three more weeks.

HISTORY

Adrian begins the examination by reviewing Emma's past medical history and gathering additional information, particularly regarding the MOI and onset. Emma reports that she began experiencing heel pain about two weeks ago. "I don't remember any particular injury, rather the pain just kinda started, and the pain has progressively worsened over the last two weeks." Adrian questions her about her chief complaint, which she reports as severe pain during the first few steps after not bearing weight, such as when she awakes in the morning, after driving long distances, or after watching a movie. She further states, "The pain started as general pain around my heel but is now most intense here (pointing to the anterior-inferior heel)." Further questioning by Adrian reveals the use of ice and OTC anti-inflammatory medication. Her pain is rated as 8/10 during training, and she denies any previous history of foot or ankle trauma.

PHYSICAL EXAMINATION

In the examination, Emma presents in moderate discomfort. Inspection of Emma's foot reveals callus formation under the head of the second and third metatarsals and excessive bilateral pronation during a tandem weight-bearing stance. She is exquisitely point tender when the calcaneus is palpated and withdraws when Adrian applies pressure over one particular area (Figure 11.17.1). Active ROM reveals a deficit in ankle dorsiflexion, but the remaining talocrural and subtalar joint motions appear WNL. Talocrural and subtalar joint RROM reveal no gross weakness, 5/5 for all movements— plantar flexion, dorsiflexion, inversion, and eversion in a non-weight-bearing position. Adrian does note pain and decreased strength with a single-leg toe raise. Passive dorsiflexion with toe extension reproduces Emma's heel pain. Feeling confident in his diagnosis, Adrian completes his evaluation and refers Emma for radiographs, according to standing orders.

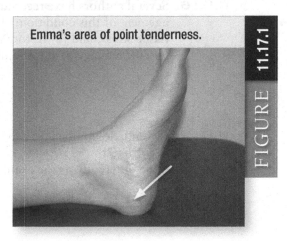

Emma's area of point tenderness.

FIGURE 11.17.1

DIAGNOSTIC IMAGING

Radiographs reveal no fractures. No further diagnostic tests were ordered.

Please answer the following questions based on the above case information.

11.17 / **1.** Based on the information provided in the case, determine (a) the differential diagnoses and (b) the clinical diagnosis.

11.17 / **2.** What do the muscles involved in the differential diagnoses and the clinical diagnosis have in common?

11.17 / **3.** Based on the results of the case, what led you to the clinical diagnosis?

11.17 / **4.** Palpation is an important part of the assessment in making the clinical diagnosis. A good understanding of the anatomy is important for successful palpation. Describe the anatomy of the structures involved in the condition and the specific location that will be point tender.

11.17 / **5.** Emma was observed to have excessive pronation during tandem weight bearing, which is implicated in roughly 80 percent of those with this condition. What other foot abnormality has been implicated and why?

11.17 / **6.** Several authors have recommended a three-step approach for the management of this condition: (1) reduce pain and inflammation, (2) reduce tissue stress, and (3) restore muscle strength and flexibility. For each, list specific management techniques that have proven effective.

11.17 / **7.** Overall, do you believe Adrian adequately evaluated Emma's condition, according to the provided information? If not, what would you have done differently as the evaluating clinician?

CASE 11.18

by Kyle Blecha, MS, ATC, Western Michigan University, Kalamazoo

Cameron, a 20-year-old collegiate club figure skater, reported to the club sports athletic trainer two months into his senior year. Cameron's CCs were right forefoot pain and numbness. Vin, a second-year graduate assistant assigned to clubs sports, was happy to evaluate his foot. Cameron was escorted to an examination room while Vin went to the back room to retrieve Cameron's medical records.

HISTORY

After some small talk about how the season was going, Vin begins his examination by asking Cameron to describe his current problem. Cameron states, "Over the past several weeks, I have begun experiencing right foot pain here (Figure 11.18.1). The pain is the worst when I am on it for long periods of time and is lots better when I get a chance to rest it. Sometimes it feels like I am walking on a pebble." Vin asks, "Is the pain sharp and occasionally burning in the forefoot?" Cameron replies, "Yes." Vin then inquires about Cameron's skates and learns they are the same ones he used last year. He also questions Cameron about any activities outside of club ice skating. He learns that Cameron works as a server in a five-star restaurant three nights per week and is required to wear wing-tipped shoes.

PHYSICAL EXAMINATION

Cameron is alert, oriented, and in minimal discomfort. Vin notices he is wearing sandals this morning. A general observation of Cameron in a non-weight-bearing position reveals a tailor bunion and Haglund's deformity of the right foot. Cameron is tender during palpation between the third and fourth metatarsal, and Vin is able to reproduce his neurological symptoms around the third and fourth digits with excessive overpressure. Active ROM is unremarkable; however, ankle dorsiflexion and toe extension PROM increases Cameron's tenderness

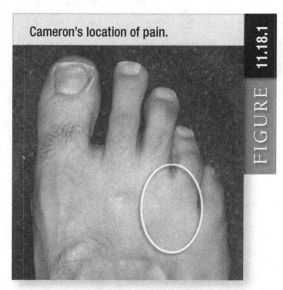

Cameron's location of pain.

FIGURE 11.18.1

Cameron's pain is located within the circle.

between the plantar surface of the third and fourth digits with palpation. Resistive and manual muscle testing is unremarkable. Distal circulation is WNL. Vin runs Cameron through some functional testing, which is limited for lack of appropriate footwear, but determines that squatting reproduces his symptoms. A Tinel's sign

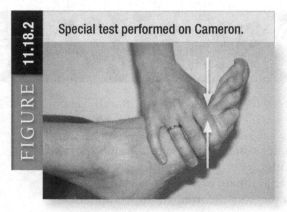

Special test performed on Cameron.

Arrows indicate direction of applied force.

over the posterior tibial nerve is unremarkable, and the test shown in Figure 11.18.2 produces pain and an audible click.

Confident in his clinical diagnosis, Vin fits Cameron with a teardrop pad and recommends anti-inflammatory drugs, cryotherapy, and a change in footwear. He asks him to return in a week for a follow-up visit. He states, "If there is no change in your symptoms, then we will need to consider referral to an orthopedic surgeon for further diagnostic testing."

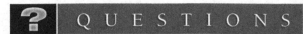

Please answer the following questions based on the above case information.

11.18 / **1.** Based on the information presented in the case, determine (a) the differential diagnoses and (b) the clinical diagnosis.

11.18 / **2.** Vin asked several different history questions to guide the physical examination. However, do you believe that his method for obtaining all of the information gathered in this case was appropriate? What would you have done differently, if anything, as the evaluating clinician?

11.18 / **3.** There is no report of the presence of any motor deficits in Cameron's right foot (i.e., intrinsic or extrinsic) or ankle. Given the clinical diagnosis, why are motor deficits not present?

11.18 / **4.** During the physical examination, Vin performed a couple of different special tests, including Figure 11.18.2. (a) What is the name of this test, and how is it performed? (b) Do you believe this test is reliable?

11.18 / **5.** If you were in Vin's position, what type of changes in footwear would you recommend and why?

CONCLUSION

As previously noted, the ankle-foot complex is structurally similar to the wrist complex, with two major exceptions. The first is that the ankle-foot complex is responsible for a great deal of weight-bearing during bipedal stance and locomotion (walking and running) and is therefore under a great deal of stress during all facets of activities of daily living. As a result, the ankle-foot complex receives much more attention from the medical community, and unlike the wrist-hand complex, the rate of injury at the ankle-foot is quite high in competitive and recreational athletes. Remember that individuals participating in competitive sports such as football, baseball, and soccer are not the only athletes. For example, young men and women in the armed services, particularly those attending basic training, place just as much stress on their ankle-foot complex and share many of the same acute and chronic injuries sustained by competitive and recreational athletes.

Traumatic injuries to the ankle-foot complex can be very easy to detect and will normally correlate well with a clinician's physical examination findings. It is the repetitive, chronic, overuse injuries such as tendinopathies, stress fractures, and neuropathies that often give a clinician the biggest challenge. The clinician must not only determine the proper clinical diagnosis but also must correctly identify and treat concurrently the intrinsic and extrinsic factors leading to the injury. This can be challenging when many of the overuse injuries are caused during running; and most sports require running as part of the activity. As you have learned in your injury evaluation courses and through some of the cases presented here, the ankle and foot are very intricate, their parts being completely intertwined with each other. Proper recognition and management require not only the taking of a thorough history, particularly of the MOI and pattern of pain, but also a strong foundation in gait and gait analysis, a concept beyond the scope of this text.

Selected Responses and Interpretations (Cases 1 and 2 of each chapter)

Refer to pages 472–476 for the references cited in these sample answers.

CASE 2.1   Orbital Blowout Fracture

2.1 / 1. *Based on the information presented in the case, determine (a) the differential diagnoses and (b) the clinical diagnosis.*

   a. Differential diagnoses: corneal abrasion/laceration, hyphema, retinal detachment, and ruptured globe[39,44]

   b. Clinical diagnosis: orbital blowout fracture

2.1 / 2. *Based on the clinical diagnosis, identify the harmful effects of being struck in the eye with a blunt force object larger than the diameter of the orbit.*

When a blunt force object larger than the orbital opening strikes the eye it compresses the floor of the orbit or the medial wall and increases the intra-orbital pressure. This increase in pressure causes the orbital bones to break at their weakest points, usually the posteriomedial portion of the orbital floor and medial orbital wall.[44,72,80] The breakage of these bones acts as a pressure valve release, preventing ruptures of the globe. When a blunt force object smaller than the orbit strikes the eye, however, unreleased compression can increase intra-ocular pressure to the point that the sclera tears and the globe ruptures.[65,72]

2.1 / 3. *If Tom had also presented with changes in visual acuity and/or vision loss, what would be the clinical implication, and how could a clinician assess these changes?*

Changes in visual acuity and/or loss of vision may indicate trauma to the optic nerve (CN II)[65] and should be assessed by using a Snellen chart and examining the patient's peripheral vision. When completing an on-field evaluation, the Snellen chart may be replaced by assessing the athlete's ability to read the scoreboard. In place of a scoreboard or a Snellen chart, Mary may also consider having the athlete identify how many fingers she is holding up.

   In cases of monocular diplopia (double vision looking through one eye) after sustaining trauma to the eye, issues such as hyphema, detached retina, or globe trauma should be suspected. Binocular diplopia (double vision looking through two eyes) may be caused by soft-tissue entrapment (zymgomatic fracture), hemorrhage, or edema.

2.1 / 4. *During Mary's observation of the eye, suppose she notices subconjunctival hemorrhaging and a shallow anterior chamber in combination with the above signs. What steps should Mary take to manage this situation?*

A teardrop-shaped or irregular pupil, subconjunctival hemorrhaging, full-thickness laceration to the cornea, or deep or shallow anterior chamber are signs of a ruptured globe. In this situation, a protective eye shield in a loose-packed position should be used to cover the eye, and the athlete should be referred to an ophthalmologist for immediate care.[65]

2.1 / 5. *Based on the information presented in the case, what if anything would you have done or added to help guide the physical examination?*

The answers to this question will vary; however, any trauma to the head requires a concussion assessment.[22] Perform a complete observation of the eye from all directions (superior, inferior, lateral, and medial). In this case, determining whether there is a zygomatic bone fracture would be warranted, as the zygomatic bone comprises infraorbital margin and floor of the orbit. Furthermore, cranial nerve testing of the optic (CN II), oculomotor (CN III), trochlear (CN IV), and abducens (CN VI) may be warranted.

2.1 / 6. *After completing the physical examination, Mary documented her findings and sent a copy of the report to the administration office. Please document your findings as if you were the treating clinician. If the case did not provide information you believe is pertinent to the clinical diagnosis, please feel free to add this information to your documentation.*

Answers will vary. Students should consider writing a SOAP note (see Appendix B) using the ABCD format when writing the short- and long-term goals.

447

CASE 2.2 Corneal Abrasion/Laceration

2.2 / 1. *Based on the information presented in the case, determine (a) the differential diagnoses and (b) the clinical diagnosis.*

   a. Differential diagnoses: conjunctivitis, corneal laceration, corneal ulceration, iritis, foreign body, and blunt trauma[10,27,35]

   b. Clinical diagnosis: corneal abrasion

2.2 / 2. *Based on the information presented in the case, what type of physician should Tamara refer Sherrie to and why?*

The physician of choice would be an ophthalmologist if available. Ophthalmologists are physicians specializing in eye and vision care. They are trained to dispense medication and provide a full spectrum of eye care, including complex and delicate eye surgery. Some ophthalmologists specialize in a certain area of eye care, such as glaucoma, refractive surgery, or retinal surgery. If an ophthalmologist is not available, a referral to the team physician or emergency room is a viable option.

2.2 / 3. *Tamara asked Sherrie several history questions to guide the physical examination. Based on the clinical diagnosis above, identify three to five specific history questions you as the evaluating clinician may have asked.*

The answers to this question will vary; however, according to the clinical diagnosis, there are several history questions a clinician could ask to assist in determining the clinical diagnosis.[27,87] These questions include but are not limited to:

   a. Did you suffer any type of acute trauma to the eye (e.g., fingers, fingernails, self-inflicted rubbing)?

   b. Do you have a sensation of a foreign body in your eye?

   c. Do you remember getting any dirt in your eye and then rubbing your eye?

   d. Do you wear contacts?

   e. How long have you been wearing this pair of contacts?

   f. When was the last time you cleaned your contacts?

   g. Did you remove your contacts last night?

2.2 / 4. *There is one mechanism of injury common to the case's clinical diagnosis that typically occurs outside of participating in athletics. Identify this mechanism of injury, and discuss how it causes the clinical diagnosis.*

Contact lenses put the wearer at greater risk of developing corneal abrasions because of the action of placing contacts into the eye. Inserting and removing contacts predisposes the wearer to corneal abrasions from fingernails.[27,87] Contacts that are dirty or damaged also increase the risk of damage to the corneas (scratch) as they move around. Contacts improperly placed in the eye also increase the risk of trauma.

2.2 / 5. *(a) Overall, do you believe Tamara adequately evaluated Sherrie's condition, given the information provided in the case? (b) What, if any, tests or procedures were omitted that could have helped in establishing the clinical diagnosis? (c) Describe how these test(s) are performed.*

   a. The answers for this question will vary.

   b. Based on the information presented, Tamara could have used a fluorescein strip and a cobalt blue. A corneal abrasion is an epithelial defect that stains when a fluorescein dye is used. In conjunction with a cobalt light in a darkened room, the defect turns greenish-yellow.[27,93]

   c. Begin the test by soaking a fluorescein strip in sterile saline. Ask the patient to look up and gently touch the inside of the lower eyelid with the moistened strip, taking care not to touch the cornea (Figure A2.1.1). Touching the cornea may cause the athlete significant discomfort. Ask the athlete to blink her eye several times, and wash the eye thoroughly with eye wash or saline to irrigate the eye. Darken the room, shine a cobalt blue light into the affected eye, and observe for a defect.

   Tamara could have also inverted the upper eyelid to identify any foreign objects. If no fluo-

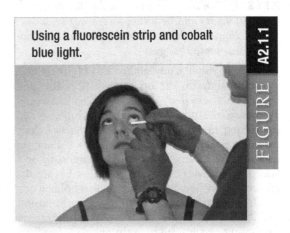

Using a fluorescein strip and cobalt blue light.

FIGURE A2.1.1

rescein strips are available, Tamara could have used a penlight angled from the lateral and medial borders at the cornea while in a dark room. Tamara could have also suggested the use of sunglasses to assist with the photosensitivity.

CASE 3.1 Vertebral Fracture with Spinal Cord Trauma (C5-C6)

3.1 / 1. *Based on the information presented in the case, determine (a) the differential diagnoses and (b) the clinical diagnosis.*

a. Differential diagnoses: cervical spine dislocation, cervical strain, cervical sprain, spinal cord shock, spinal cord trauma, vertebral artery trauma

b. Clinical diagnosis: cervical fracture, possible secondary spinal cord trauma

3.1 / 2. *Once Seth arrived at Hector's side and determined that the scene was safe, Seth should have immediately begun to assess what?*

After completing the scene survey, a primary assessment should be performed. This includes:

- Forming a general impression of the victim (i.e., CC, gender, and age)
- Assessing level of consciousness and/or mental status according to the AVPU scale or GCS

- Assessing the victim's airway, breathing, and circulation[2] and providing interventions as necessary, such as supplemental oxygen and, in this case, cervical stabilization

3.1 / 3. *Based on the case, once a medic arrived on scene, she should have been responsible for performing what?*

Based on the MOI (a fall over 15 ft or three times Hector's height), the rescuer(s) (Seth and medics) should have assumed a possible cervical spine trauma, and the second medic would have begun providing in-line stabilization in order to maintain stabilization of the cervical spine to limit secondary injury.

3.1 / 4. *Discuss the difference between the AVPU scale and the Glasgow coma scale (GCS). If you were in this situation, which scale would you prefer to use and why?*

The acronym "AVPU" stands for Alert, Verbal, Painful, and Unresponsive and is a mnemonic used to determine a trauma patient's level of consciousness during an emergency. The Glasgow Coma Scale is a clinical scoring system for objectively assessing the consciousness of a patient (Table A3.1.1). Although the GCS is limited in predicting functional outcomes, the scale is useful when

TABLE	A3.1.1	Glasgow Coma Scale.
Eye-opening response	Spontaneous, open with blinking at baseline	4 points
	Opens to verbal command, speech, or shout	3 points
	Opens to pain, not applied to face	2 points
	None	1 point
Verbal response	Oriented	5 points
	Confused conversation, but able to answer questions	4 points
	Inappropriate responses, words discernible	3 points
	Incomprehensible speech	2 points
	None	1 point
Motor response	Obeys commands for movement	6 points
	Purposeful movement to painful stimulus	5 points
	Withdraws from pain	4 points
	Abnormal (spastic) flexion, decorticate posture	3 points
	Extension (rigid) response, decerebrate posture	2 points
	None	1 point

A GCS score ranges between 3 and 15 with the total score being the sum of the scores in three categories.

making decisions about management in the acute setting, particularly for patients with traumatic brain injuries. It is composed of three sections measuring the level of consciousness, each with a maximum and minimum point value based on a patient's eye-opening response (1–4), verbal response (1–5), and motor response (1–6). The sum of each section determines a patient's classification.[37] A severe traumatic brain injury has a GCS of 3 to 8, moderate traumatic brain injury 9 to 12, and slight traumatic brain injury 13 to 15.[40] "Patients who score less than 15 need imaging or observation, and patients with scores less than 9 need to be promptly considered for definitive airway management."[45]

A study examining the variability in agreement between ER physicians and nurses found a high level of inter-rater agreement.[11] However, in 10 of the 108 cases, some GCS scores did differ more than 2 points. The authors suggest that although the agreement between the emergency room professionals was high, the disagreement indicates that clinical decisions should not be based solely on single GCS scores.

3.1 / 5. *Discuss how you would have managed this situation from scene survey to packaging and transport of Hector.*

The answers to this question will vary depending on level of training and clinical experience. However, the answers should be consistent with the recommendations established in the 2009 National Athletic Trainers' Association Position Statement on the acute management of cervical spine–injured athletes.[41] The answers should be discussed with the classroom instructor, clinical instructor, and/or approved clinical instructor (ACI). In fact, consider consulting with your athletic training medical staff and physician to determine whether this type of event has ever occurred and, if it has, how it was handled.

CASE 3.2   Brachial Plexus Trauma

3.2 / 1. *Based on the information presented in the case, determine (a) the differential diagnoses and (b) the clinical diagnosis.*

   a. Differential diagnoses: cervical disc pathology, cervical sprain, cervical strain injuries, shoulder/AC joint dislocation, shoulder impingement, thoracic outlet syndrome[44]

   b. Clinical diagnosis: brachial plexus trauma or what is commonly referred to as a "burner" or "stinger"[9,26]

3.2 / 2. *Lisa asked several specific history questions to guide the physical examination. Based on the clinical diagnosis above, identify three to five additional history questions you may have asked as the evaluating clinician.*

These answers will vary. Overall, Lisa appeared to generate an adequate history; however, there are some specific questions that could have helped guide the physical examination. These include:

   ■ Any prior history of cervical trauma or brachial plexus injury?

   ■ What position was your head in while making the tackle?

   ■ Where specifically does the pain and numbness radiate down the arm?

   ■ Are you now suffering or did you suffer any changes in sensation?

   ■ Did you hear or feel any snapping or popping of the neck?

   ■ Are you now suffering or did you ever suffer any changes in muscle function?

3.2 / 3. *If this injury were to persist during the athletic season, what type of physician would be best suited to manage Tom's case and why?*

Most clinicians would start with an orthopedic surgeon, but a neurologist would be preferred. A neurologist typically manages disorders of the nerves and nervous system, including the central nervous system (CNS) and the peripheral nervous system (PNS) (i.e., sensory and motor nerves throughout the body). In this situation, a neurologist would consider conducting an electromyography/nerve conduction velocity (EMG/NCV) tests to determine the extent of neurological damage to the brachial plexus.

A neurosurgeon may also be considered, depending on symptom severity and/or duration of symptoms. Lisa could assist the team physician in deciding which medical specialty is most appropriate for Tom's situation, based on her familiarity with the case and her medical documentation.

3.2 / 4. *Based on the results of functional and neurological exams presented in this case, which nerve roots and peripheral nerves are most likely to be involved?*

A traction force applied to the cervical nerve roots can affect any level of the nerve roots; however, the lateral and posterior cords innervated by C5 and C6 are the most commonly affected (suprascapular, lateral pectoral, musculocutaneous, and axillary nerve). Forced abduction of the arm and lateral side bending involve the C8 and T1 nerve roots.[16,18,33,37] In this case, it is likely that the C5 to C7 nerve roots were affected, along with the axillary and suprascapular peripheral nerves.

3.2 / 5. *Considering Tom's clinical diagnosis, identify the criteria Lisa should use in order to make a return-to-play decision.*

Based on the clinical diagnosis, Tom should present with full AROM of the neck and shoulder, normal upper extremity muscle strength including scapular stabilizers, paraspinal musculature (grip and strength), and a normal neurological exam (i.e., peripheral nerves, dermatomes, myotomes, and deep tendon reflexes) before he is allowed to return to play. Returning with any deficits in ROM or muscular strength places Tom at risk of further injury. The athlete should be monitored closely for re-injury upon returning to play.

3.2 / 6. *(a) What other special tests, if any, should Lisa perform to confirm her clinical diagnosis? (b) Identify how to perform these tests.*

a. Two tests commonly reported for assessing the brachial plexus are the brachial plexus traction and compression test and the Tinel's sign.[16,18,33,37]

b. To perform the brachial plexus traction and compression test, begin by placing the patient in a seated or standing position. Stand behind the patient, placing one hand on the side of the patient's head and the other over the ACJ of the ipsilateral side. Then passively laterally flex the patient's head to the contralateral side while applying a downward pressure over the ACJ (Figure A3.2.1). A positive finding may occur on either side of the neck. Pain and/or a reproduction of neurological symptoms on

the side toward the flexed head indicate a compressive force, while pain and/or a reproduction of neurological symptoms on the side away from the stretch indicate a traction force.

To perform a Tinel's sign place the patient in a seated, standing, or supine position. Gently tap the cervical neck area near Erb's point (anterior to the transverse process of C6, 2 cm superior to the clavicle). A change in sensation in the upper extremity on the ipsilateral side is considered a positive finding.

CASE 4.1 Acromioclavicular Sprain/Separation

4.1 / 1. *Based on the information presented in the case, determine (a) the differential diagnoses and (b) the clinical diagnosis.*

a. Differential diagnoses: clavicular fracture, rotator cuff pathology, shoulder dislocation, labrum lesion, deltoid contusion[42]

b. Clinical diagnosis: AC joint separation

4.1 / 2. *Based on the clinical diagnosis, describe the common grading scale used to quantify this injury.*

The degree of clavicular displacement depends on the severity of injury to the AC joint capsule, ligaments, and supporting muscles of the shoulder. Rockwood's classification quantifies AC joint injuries into six grades[38]:

- Grade or Type I: minor sprain of AC ligament, intact joint capsule, intact CC ligament, intact deltoid and trapezius

- Grade or Type II: rupture of AC ligament and joint capsule, sprain of CC ligament but CC intact, minimal detachment of deltoid and trapezius

- Grade or Type III: rupture of AC ligament, joint capsule, and CC ligament; clavicle elevated (up to 100% displacement); detachment of deltoid and trapezius

- Grade or Type IV: rupture of AC ligament, joint capsule, and CC ligament; clavicle displaced posteriorly into the trapezius; detachment of deltoid and trapezius

- Grade or Type V: rupture of AC ligament, joint capsule, and CC ligament; clavicle elevated (>100% displacement); detachment of deltoid and trapezius

- Grade or Type VI (rare): rupture of AC ligament, joint capsule, and CC ligament; clavicle displaced behind the tendons of the biceps and coracobrachialis

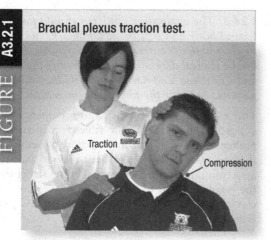

FIGURE A3.2.1

Brachial plexus traction test.

Traction

Compression

4.1 / 3. *Based on the clinical diagnosis, identify the ligaments that may be affected and their location.*

Ligamentous structures that may be affected include the inferior and superior AC ligaments and the CC ligament, specifically the conoid and trapezoid. The AC ligaments arise from between the medial facet of the acromion process of the scapula and attach to the distal clavicle; the CC ligaments attach from the coracoid process of the scapula to the inferior surface of the clavicle.

4.1 / 4. *What would be the appropriate short-term management plan for treating this type of injury?*

The most appropriate management plan for an acute AC joint injury includes applying a sling and swath to support the weight of the arm to lessen stress on the AC joint. Refer the athlete for diagnostic tests to rule out fractures and to determine the degree of displacement or laxity of the AC joint.[46]

4.1 / 5. *Overall, do you believe Tony adequately evaluated Rob's condition given the information presented in the case? If not, what would you have done differently as the evaluating clinician?*

The answers to this question will vary. Given the MOI and initial presentation, Tony should have noted a step deformity and completed ligamentous stress testing to confirm the clinical diagnosis before referring him to a physician. Ligamentous stress testing to confirm an AC joint sprain includes the piano key sign, AC joint compression test, and AC joint distraction/traction test.[7,20,26,41]

■ Step deformity: obvious displacement of the clavicle from the acromion, resulting in a gap or separation

■ Piano key: pressing on the distal end of the clavicle that results in pushing the clavicle downward and springing back up when let go

■ AC joint traction test: applying downward traction on the humerus, resulting in a step deformity or pain

■ AC joint compression test: placing both hands on either side of the AC joint, squeezing together to compress the joint, causing pain or joint movement is a positive result

4.1 / 6. *Based on the clinical diagnosis, what are some potential complications (short or long term) as a result of the injury?*

Potential complications of AC joint sprains are based on the severity of the MOI. These complications include: (1) wound abrasions or lacerations, (2) arthritis resulting from grade 2 or 3 separation, (3) development of thoracic outlet syndrome, (4) neurovascular alterations (i.e., paresthesia over the shoulder or upper arm, trapezius weakness), (5) brachial plexus injury,[39] and (6) subacromial space stenosis (SAS). Therefore, a complete examination of the shoulder joint is necessary even in the presence of an easily recognizable injury.

CASE 4.2   Sternoclavicular Sprain/Separation

4.2 / 1. *Based on the information presented in the case, determine (a) the differential diagnoses and (b) the clinical diagnosis.*

a. Differential diagnoses: clavicle fracture and dislocation, rib fracture, sternal fracture[39]

b. Clinical diagnosis: anterior sternoclavicular joint sprain

4.2 / 2. *Describe the classification of ligamentous injuries commonly associated with this type of injury.*

The degree of sternoclavicular displacement depends on the severity of injury to the SC joint capsule, ligaments, and supporting muscles of the shoulder. There are three types of SC joint injuries.

■ Type 1: ligaments (anterior and posterior SC and interclavicular ligaments) are intact with the patient usually experiencing pain and swelling of the joint

■ Type 2: rupture of the above ligaments with pain and swelling and anterior deformity

■ Type 3: complete rupture of the above ligaments and joint dislocation and asymmetry. The head may also be titled to the affected side, and the patient will experience pain, swelling, and difficulty moving the arm of the affected side.[4]

4.2 / 3. *The evaluating clinician should palpate several bony and soft tissue landmarks in order to determine the correct clinical diagnosis. Based on the clinical diagnosis above, identify the bony and soft tissue landmarks you should/would have palpated to guide the physical examination.*

The exact anatomical structures palpated will depend on the extent of the athlete's pain and apprehension. Given the information presented in the case, you would have been wise to palpate, at a minimum, the following bony structures: the jugular notch, the sternum, the SC joint, the clavicle, the acromion process, and the AC joint (Figure A4.2.1).

Clavicle
Acromion process
ACJ
Jugular notch
SCJ
Sternum

It would also be wise to palpate the following soft-tissue areas: the interclavicular, sternoclavicular, and costoclavicular ligaments, the pectoralis major and minor, the SCM, the scalene (anterior and middle), and the deltoid.

Instructors may wish to add additional structures based on their learned injury-evaluation approach.

4.2 / 4. *If this injury were a posterior dislocation as opposed to an anterior one, the injury would be classified as a potential medical emergency. Why?*

A posterior SC joint dislocation can result in a life-threatening respiratory obstruction with dyspnea, particularly in younger patients.[4,26] This occurs because of trauma to the trachea as the clavicle moves in a posterior direction and places pressure on the structure. Many times, patients with a posterior dislocation can complain of neurovascular conditions in the upper extremity (numbness, weakness, lack of blood flow), difficulty breathing, or difficulty swallowing.[4,46] Other associated complications include haemopneumothorax, tracheal damage or rupture, laceration, damage to the larynx and superior vena cava, and occlusion of the subclavian artery and/or vein.[24,39]

4.2 / 5. *As the evaluating clinician, describe how you would initially manage this injury?*

The answer to this question may vary among students. However, students should recognize

the need to place the athlete in a sling or figure-8 harness. Medical referral is required to rule out potential life-threatening complications. The athlete should initially avoid exercises or movements that cause or increase pain. The application of cryotherapy and NSAIDs (assuming no contraindication) for pain and swelling will be warranted. If the patient has a Type 3 SC joint sprain, surgical intervention may be necessary.

CASE 5.1 Ulnar Collateral Ligament Sprain

5.1 / 1. *Based on the information presented in the case, determine (a) the differential diagnoses and (b) the clinical diagnosis.*

a. Differential diagnoses: cervical disc or nerve root pathology, flexor pronator muscle tear, ulnar neuritis/ulnar nerve entrapment, medial epicondyle fracture, medial epicondylitis, valgus extension overload, medial triceps subluxation, olecranon osteophytes[40,54]

b. Clinical diagnosis: medial (ulnar) collateral ligament injury (sprain) with ulnar neuritis (caused by a traction force)

5.1 / 2. *Sean asked several history questions to guide the physical examination. Based on the information presented in the case, (a) do you believe Sean took an adequate history? If not, (b) what questions would you have asked as the evaluating clinician?*

a. According to the clinical diagnosis, there are several other questions the evaluating athletic trainer should have inquired about. Specifically, these questions should have addressed changes in training regimens or any changes in the athlete's accuracy, velocity, stamina, and strength.[17,44,54] An athletic trainer should be asking about a gradual decrease in velocity and accuracy which may be explained by a decrease in wrist flexor/pronator EMG[54] from the increased stress placed on these structures in providing stability to the medial elbow joint complex.[17]

b. Other history questions given the case should focus around changes in the neurovascular status of the athlete, including but not limited to, numbness and tingling, stiffness or heaviness in the arm, tendency to drop objects, and cold intolerance.

5.1 / 3. *The injury in this case presents as a chronic condition with an insidious onset. What piece of information obtained as part of the history could have led Sean to believe that the injury was acute in nature?*

Athletes suffering from an acute ulnar collateral ligament sprain of the elbow can normally pinpoint the exact day and pitch thrown when the injury occurred.[6] They will often report hearing and/or feeling a "pop" during the throwing phase.[44,57]

5.1 / 4. *(a) Identify the dynamic and static stabilizers of the medial elbow joint. (b) Identify the location of the static stabilizers. (c) Which structures were specifically involved in the injury and why?*

a. The static stabilizers of the medial elbow joint are the anterior bundle, posterior bundle, and transverse ligament of the ulnar collateral ligament. The dynamic stabilizers include the flexor-pronator muscle mass (particularly the flexor carpi ulnaris), flexor digitorum superficialis, triceps, anconeus, and internal rotators of the shoulder.

b. The anterior bundle of the ulnar collateral ligament originates on the inferior medial epicondyle and inserts onto the medial aspect of the coronoid process. The anterior band of the anterior bundle serves as the primary restraint to a valgus force between 30° and 90°, increasing its contribution to valgus stability as the angle increases[18,44,84] and is "subjected to near-failure tensile stress during the acceleration phase of the throwing motion."[17] At 120° of flexion, the anterior band is considered a co-primary restraint to a valgus force.[18,81,84] It is most readily palpable between approximately 50° and 70° of flexion as the medial muscle mass moves anteriorly.[17] The posterior bundle, a less-defined thickening of the posterior elbow capsule, originates on the medial epicondyle and inserts onto the olecranon process and provides stability beyond 55–60° of elbow flexion. Finally, the transverse ligament originates and inserts on the same bone and offers little to no valgus stability.

c. The primary structure involved in this injury is the anterior bundle of the ulnar collateral ligament. As previously mentioned, the anterior bundle is the prime static stabilizer against a valgus force at 30°, 60°, and 90° of elbow flexion. The combination of high valgus torque forces applied to the elbow during the late cocking phase in combination, repeated stress, and rapid elbow extension causes microtearing to the static stabilizers, which over time results in stretching and instability to the medial elbow restraints.[17,70,81] The decreased external rotation of the shoulder and the increased abduction also contributes to the increased valgus stresses at the elbow joint.

5.1 / 5. *During the assessment, Sean performed several stress and special tests. If the athlete asked you to explain why the elbow is flexed to 25°, (a) what would your response be? (b) What is the purpose of the Tinel's sign in this case?*

a. Studies have demonstrated[17] that flexing the elbow greater than 30° increases the difficulty of providing adequate stabilizing to the humerus, despite the fact that the greatest degree of medial instability occurs between 70° and 90° of elbow flexion. By placing the elbow in 20° to 30° of flexion, the olecranon tip is unlocked from the olecranon fossa while still maintaining adequate stability of the humerus.[17]

b. The ulnar nerve is relatively superficial as it crosses the elbow's joint line medially and the medial epicondyle posteriorly. The nerve is directly palpable as it passes through the cubital tunnel before entering the forearm. Because of the close relationship between the ulnar nerve and the medial elbow, excessive valgus forces cause a traction force on the ulnar nerve, predisposing the athlete with a valgus instability to ulnar neuritis. Tinel's sign is used to reproduce pain and tingling along the ulnar nerve as it passes through the cubital tunnel.

5.1 / 6. *(a) What is a moving valgus stress test, and how is it performed? (b) If you were the evaluating clinician, would you have performed this test and why? (c) If not, what other tests might you have performed?*

a. The moving valgus stress test (see Figure A5.1.1) is a provocative test used to diagnose medial elbow ligamentous instability

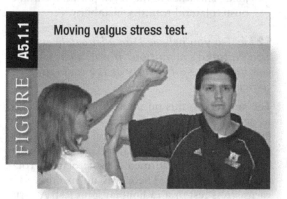

Moving valgus stress test.

FIGURE A5.1.1

(a) Involved shoulder is abducted and elbow maximally flexed.

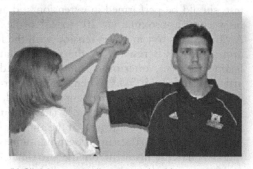

(b) Clinician externally rotates shoulder.

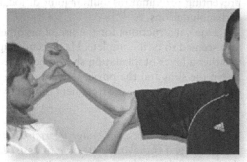

(c) Clinician maintains a valgus torque and quickly extends the elbow to 30° of flexion looking to reproduce medial elbow pain consistent with pain noted during activity.

by reproducing the stress mechanism and kinematics responsible for the signs and symptoms associated with repetitive trauma to the ulnar collateral ligament. The test is performed with the patient standing, the involved shoulder abducted to 90°, and the elbow maximally flexed. A moderate torque is applied to the elbow until the shoulder is fully externally rotated. The clinician maintains the valgus torque and quickly extends the elbow to 30° of flexion while looking for medial elbow pain consistent with the pain noted during activity. The pain should also be maximal during the late cocking (120°) and early acceleration (70°) phase of throwing[57] and may elicit an apprehension response from the patient. A positive test occurs when pain is elicited during extension and flexion of the elbow (usually to a lesser degree).

b. The moving valgus stress test has been found to have a sensitivity of 100 percent (17 of 17 patients) and a specificity of 75 percent (3 of 4 patients) when compared with surgically confirmed tears.[57] When pain from valgus stress in the physical exam was compared with the results of the intraoperative findings, sensitivity fell to 65 percent (11 of 17 patients) and specificity to 50 percent (2 of 4 patients). When the intraoperative findings were compared with joint laxity during the physical assessment, sensitivity again fell to 19 percent (3 of 16 patients), but specificity was 100 percent (4 of 4 patients). O'Driscoll[59] believes that when performed correctly, the moving valgus stress test may be a useful tool in assessing the throwing athlete.

c. Another test that could be performed is the milking sign or maneuver (Figure A5.1.2). In this test, the clinician flexes the involved elbow

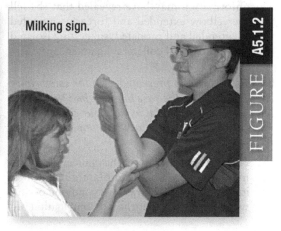

Milking sign.

FIGURE A5.1.2

80° to 100° with the forearm supinated. The patient grasps his own thumb and pulls laterally, exerting a valgus stress, thereby reproducing the stress experienced during throwing. A positive finding occurs when the patient reports pain comparable to what is experienced during throwing.[69]

CASE 5.2 Radial Collateral Ligament Sprain (RCL)

5.2 / 1. *Based on the information presented in the case, (a) what is the likely clinical diagnosis? (b) What makes this clinical diagnosis unique?*

a. Clinical diagnosis: radial collateral elbow sprain

b. Isolated injury to the radial collateral ligament complex is rare. Because the body protects the medial aspect of the elbow, there is less chance for a direct traction or for varus forces to be applied to the elbow.[76,85] Significant trauma, such as elbow dislocations and fracture dislocations, increase the risk of soft-tissue disruption to the radial collateral ligament[52] and insufficiency of the lateral soft tissue[22]; isolated injuries occur with forearm supination and elbow hyperextension.[76]

5.2 / 2. *Don asked several specific history questions to guide the physical examination. However, one question may have assisted him in narrowing down the clinical diagnosis, which he either did not ask or which may not have been answered appropriately because of a translation error. Can you identify this question?*

Don did not determine the specific MOI for this case. He determined that Natsuko fell backwards as she was backpedaling, but he never identified the position of the arm and hand when she landed. This information may have revealed that she fell with her elbow extended and forearm supinated versus extended and pronated, suggesting isolated trauma to the radial collateral ligament.

5.2 / 3. *If Natsuko presented with the same clinical findings from the case but also had weakness with wrist extension, (a) would your clinical diagnosis possibly change? (b) What would cause you to make this change?*

a. Given this information, the clinical diagnosis may now be acute posterolateral rotatory instability of the elbow. This condition occurs when a patient experiences a combination of axial compression, external rotation, and valgus force applied to the elbow, which causes a disruption of the lateral restraints and muscle origins from the lateral epicondyle.[22]

b. The lateral ulnar collateral and annular ligaments are the primary restraints against rotatory instability. With this injury, if left unchecked or misdiagnosed, gaping at the humeroulnar articulation occurs from ligamentous damage and the inability of the secondary static and dynamic stabilizers to support the joint. This leads to the development of chronic posterolateral rotatory instability.

5.2 / 4. *Do you believe Don adequately evaluated Natsuko's condition? If not, what would you have done differently as the evaluating clinician?*

The answers to this question will vary. However, recognize that Don performed one inappropriate test and failed to perform several others. He performed posteromedial rotatory instability when he should have performed a posterolateral rotatory instability test. There was no mention of a varus stress test or a radioulnar joint test. A varus stress test is used to assess the integrity of the radial collateral ligament. This test, similar to a valgus test, should be performed in extension and again between at approximately 20° to 25° of flexion. A varus stress test in full extension with the forearm supinated is resisted by the radial collateral ligament (15%), anterior capsule (30%), and the articular surface (50%).[87] When flexed, the articular surface now resists 75 percent of the load, and the radial collateral 10 percent.[87] The radioulnar stress test assesses the integrity of the annular ligament, which shares the same insertion point as the radial collateral ligament on the proximal ulna and functions to bind the radius and ulna together, preventing proximal radioulnar joint dislocations and subluxations.

Don's instructions for the use of cryotherapy also seemed to be incomplete. He does not suggest whether a layer of insulation should be placed between the skin and the physical agent. Depending on these instructions, the treatment time may need to be varied.

5.2 / 5. *In this case, a language barrier existed. Fortunately, a translator was able to assist Don during the physical examination. If you were placed in a situation in which you were unable to communicate with a patient because of a language barrier, how would you handle the situation?*

When placed in a language-barrier situation, several strategies could be employed. These include, but are not limited to, the following:

- Begin by identifying those individuals on your staff who have knowledge of the language, and use them as interpreters.

- If the patient has brought a friend who may be able to interpret, and the patient consents, use the intermediary.

- When an interpreter is not present, speak slowly and carefully in terms as simple as possible. Do not use technical jargon or terms that convey value judgments.

- Remember to ask for permission to physically examine the patient and do not touch the patient until granted permission.

- If you work in the area where this language barrier is encountered often, consider learning the necessary key phrases and terms.

- When possible, provide simple, illustrated printed materials to allow the patient to describe her situation. For example, use pain charts or images of patients falling on the ground or being struck with an object.

Good patient communication is a necessary component of a successful physical examination. Being able to interact and engage with the patient involves recognizing and responding to the patient as a whole person. When communication between the clinician and patient is unhampered, the patient feels a sense of value, and this helps improve patient satisfaction and clinical outcomes that ultimately affect the productivity and appearance of the facility. There are several models that clinicians can employ in their practices to improve clinician-patient communication. One area in need of development is cultural competency. In many parts of the country, clinicians must learn to effectively communicate with non–English speaking patients. When dealing with a non–English speaking patient, remember to be aware of your own cultural biases and preconceptions, and respect the patient's cultural beliefs. In some situations, the patient's view of you may be defined by ethnic or cultural stereotypes, so do not take things personally.

CASE 6.1 Ulnocarpal and Ulnar Collateral Sprain

6.1 / 1. *Based on the information presented in the case, determine (a) the differential diagnoses and (b) the clinical diagnosis.*

a. Differential diagnoses: ulna styloid fracture, carpal fracture, midcarpal instability, triangular fibrocartilage lesions, distal ulna joint arthritis, and wrist strain[51]

b. Clinical diagnosis: ulnocarpal/ulnar carpal sprain

6.1 / 2. *Ray presented with tenderness along the palmar and medial wrist joint surface as shown in textbook Figure 6.1.1. Identify the structures responsible for providing palmar and medial joint stability.*

Joint stability is provided by extrinsic and intrinsic ligaments of the wrist, which when damaged can lead to chronic wrist pain and carpal instability. The palmar (volar) extrinsic ligaments are the most important ligaments responsible for wrist stability (Table 6.2 in the Ch. 6 Introduction); the intrinsic ligaments serve as a restraint to rotational movements. Medial joint stability is provided by the ulna collateral ligament (UCL). The UCL arises from ulna styloid process running distally to the medial aspect of the dorsal triquetrum and the pisiform palmarly. This ligament becomes taut during the end ranges of flexion and extension and is responsible for limiting radial deviation.[61,90]

6.1 / 3. *As part of the physical examination, Genki performed a wrist glide that was positive. Which wrist glide do you think he used and how would you perform it?*

An posterior-anterior (PA) glide would be the position demonstrating the greatest amount of translation. The PA glide is used to examine wrist extension mobility. To perform the PA glide, the athlete should be placed in a seated position with the wrist and hand over the end of the table in a pronated position. The athletic trainer will need to stabilize the distal forearm while grasping the proximal carpal row. A downward force is then applied to the proximal carpal row.[87]

6.1 / 4. *Genki decided that referral to the UST-FA's orthopedic surgeon was warranted in this case. Do you believe this was an appropriate decision? Why or why not?*

The answers to this question will vary among students. Referring an athlete such as Ray to an orthopedic surgeon, particularly one specializing in the wrist and hand would be an appropriate action given the information provided in the case. Injuries to the wrist and hand are often treated as minor or inconsequential injuries. In fact, trauma to the wrist is often diagnosed as a wrist sprain in the absence of gross injury. Injuries such as radial fractures and carpal fracture are sometimes misdiagnosed as wrist sprains and strains by ER physicians.[33,34] With this in mind, it would be best for Ray to be seen by a professional who can properly diagnosis and treat his injury.

6.1 / 5. *Describe how to properly apply a volar splint.*

The answers to this question will vary because volar splints can be applied many different ways. However, regardless of which method students choose, they need to check for signs of circulation, sensation, and movement before and after immobilization of the extremity; cover all open wounds with a sterile dressing; and apply cryotherapy in and around the area to decrease edema formation and to control pain.

To apply a volar splint using a SAM SPLINT (Figure A6.1.1):

- Stabilize and support the extremity.
- Assess the distal neurovascular status.
- Roll the edge in order to allow the hand to assume a position of function, and create a C-curve.
- Using your arm as a model, mold the splint in the position of function.
- Apply the splint to the athlete from the proximal forearm to the distal palmar crease, and secure the splint using elastic wrap, cravat, or roller bandage.
- Place a gauze pad between the sling and swathe knots for comfort.
- Reassess the distal neurovascular status, and document findings.

To apply a rigid volar splint:

- Stabilize and support the extremity.
- Assess the distal neurovascular status.
- Place a padded rigid splint on the volar surface of the involved forearm.

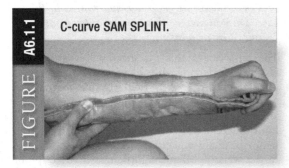

FIGURE A6.1.1

C-curve SAM SPLINT.

- Place a roller bandage in the athlete's hand so the hand assumes a position of function.
- Secure the splint using elastic wrap, cravat, or roller bandage.
- When dealing with a trauma to the bone, be sure to immobilize the wrist to limit flexion and extension.
- Provide additional support by using a sling and swathe with the forearm in a slightly elevated position, if comfortable.
- Place a gauze pad between the sling and swathe knots for comfort.
- Reassess the distal neurovascular status, and document findings.

CASE 6.2   Volar Plate Rupture

6.2 / 1. *Based on the information presented in the case, determine (a) the differential diagnoses and (b) the clinical diagnosis.*

a. Differential diagnoses: dislocated PIPJ, subluxed PIPJ, volar plate avulsion, collateral ligament sprain, phalange fracture[17,85]

b. Clinical diagnosis: distal volar plate injury

6.2 / 2. *Given the MOI, why did Nadal find increased laxity when she performed an anterioposterior glide of the proximal interphalangeal joint?*

The volar plate lies on the volar aspect of phalange's PIPJ, forming the floor of the joint and separating the joint space from the flexor tendons. It is ligamentous at the proximal origin and cartilaginous at the distal insertion,[85] and that allows the flexor tendon to glide past the joint without catching.[17] According to Combs and Schultz, Houlgum, and Perrin,[17,87] the volar plate may be damaged two different ways. The volar plate can be detached from the proximal attachment, resulting in a pseudo-boutonniere deformity. Rupture from the distal attachment results in a swan-neck deformity; an avulsion from its distal bony attachment from the base of the middle phalanx results in a "chip fracture." An anterioposterior glide of the PIPJ therefore increases the stress applied to the volar plate, similar to the hypertension MOI in this case, resulting in an increase in joint laxity and/or pain.

6.2 / 3. *Do you believe Nadal adequately evaluated Carter's condition? If not, what would you have done differently as the evaluating clinician?*

The answers to this question will vary among students. However, there is no report of Nadal palpating Carter's PIPJ. This could be clinically significant, because an injury to the volar plate often results in a dorsal dislocation or subluxation of the middle phalanx. Although an acute dislocation would have been observable, an athlete may instinctively reduce a PIPJ[17] dislocation by applying longitudinal traction (Figure A6.2.1), making it more difficult to recognize the extent of the injury and increasing the index of suspicion for PIPJ injuries.[65] Had Nadal palpated the PIPJ, she would have recognized that Carter was extremely tender on the volar surface of the PIPJ, indicating possible damage to the volar plate of the PIPJ.

6.2 / 4. *Based on the information presented in the case, identify the types of splints the orthopedic surgeon may have recommended for Carter.*

Patients suffering from volar plate injuries can be splinted in different ways. When an injury is stable, it is often treated symptomatically and can be splinted using an anatomical splint, normally for six weeks.[65] Unstable injuries, which are normally associated with joint fracture/avulsion and dislocation, are treated using a dorsal extension block splint.[17,65] A dorsal blocking splint prevents full PIPJ extension during the first few weeks by initially blocking extension to 30° allowing full flexion.[13] The amount of extension is increased incrementally during the next three to four weeks, followed by approximately three months of anatomical splinting.[17] These splints can be bought commercially or fabricated using a thermoplastic and Velcro™.[13]

6.2 / 5. *(a) Do you believe Nadal made the correct decision by referring Carter to the orthopedic surgeon? If this had been an athlete, would you have treated him differently? Why, or why not?*

a. The answers to this question may vary. However, given the fact that Carter was hurt performing his assigned job duties, he may be entitled to workers' compensation benefits. Athletic trainers working in an industrial setting should become familiar with their individual state's laws, rules, and statutes governing workers' compensation. In the state of Utah, for example, an employer is required to file "Employer's First Report of Injury—Form 122" within seven days of the accident, injury, or occupational disease. The form is used for reporting accidents, injuries, or occupational diseases.[91]

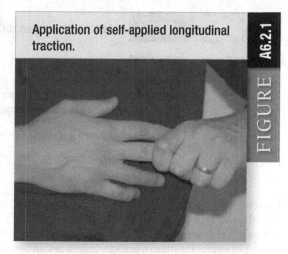

Application of self-applied longitudinal traction.

FIGURE A6.2.1

This form also serves as notice to OSHA. In conjunction with form 122, form 123, "Physician's Initial Report of Work Injury or Occupational Disease," must also be filed. This form is used by physicians and chiropractors to report their initial treatment of an injured employee.[91]

b. If this had been an athlete, the correct decision would still have been to refer the athlete to an orthopedic surgeon, particularly for radiographs. All too often, finger injuries are ignored because they are "just fingers." In this case, radiographs would be warranted because of the risk of chip fractures[17,65] and secondary damage occurring with a possible subluxation of the PIPJ.

CASE 7.1 Lumbar Strain

7.1 / 1. *Based on the information presented in the case, determine (a) the differential diagnoses and (b) the clinical diagnosis.*

a. Differential diagnoses: lumbosacral disc injuries, lumbosacral discogenic pain syndrome, lumbosacral facet syndrome, lumbosacral radiculopathy, lumbosacral acute bony trauma, lumbosacral spondylolysis and spondylolisthesis, sacroiliac joint injury[35,50]

b. Clinical diagnosis: lumbar strain

7.1 / 2. *Based on Coach Post's age and clinical presentation, do you believe Caroline's history was appropriate? If not, what would you have done differently as the evaluating clinician?*

The answers to this question will vary. Given his low-back injury, questioning further into

TABLE A7.1.1	Acute lumbar pain red flag questions specific to Coach Post.
RED FLAGS	**QUESTIONS**
Cancer	Ask about the patient's age (>50 or <20 years), history of cancer or strong suspicion of cancer, unexplained weight loss, progressive motor or sensory deficits, unrelenting night pain, failure to improve after 6 weeks of conservative therapy
Fracture	Ask about the patient's age, significant trauma, history of osteoporosis, chronic oral steroid use, and substance abuse

Coach Post's related medical history is warranted to rule out serious systemic diseases and potential surgical emergencies. This is accomplished by asking specific red-flag questions, such as those shown earlier in Table 7.1.[3,27,35] Two of the red-flag questions specific to Coach Post are shown in Table A7.1.1. Historical red-flag questions should center on the patient's risk of cancer, spinal infection, fracture, ankylosing spondylitis, and cauda equina syndrome.

Coach Post's age would raise a concern because being over 50 is considered a red flag[35] for both cancer and fracture and would warrant further medical evaluation.

7.1 / 3. *If Coach Post also presented with neurological symptoms such as sensory changes over the anterior middle-thigh, over the patella, and the medial lower-leg to the great-toe, along with weakness in ankle dorsiflexion, (a) what could you conclude about the injury? (b) What deep-tendon reflex should be assessed with this clinical presentation?*

a. If sensory change over the anterior middle thigh, patella, and the medial lower leg to great toe were present, along with weakness in ankle dorsiflexion, this would suggest compression of the L4 nerve root, probably as a result of intervertebral disc injury (herniation).[27]

b. Assessment of the L4 or quadriceps deep-tendon reflex would be indicated in this case and would be decreased. The presence of dermatome, myotome, and deep-tendon reflex deficits requires referral to a physician for further diagnostic testing.[2]

7.1 / 4. *Based on the clinical presentation, Caroline rated Coach Post's thoracolumbar extension strength as 3/5. Describe the test position required to make this determination.*

A muscle strength grade of 3/5 indicates that Coach Post is able to lift the head and sternum so that the xiphoid process is off the table with the hands held behind the back. Figure A7.1.1 shows the test position for this determination. Note, resistance does not need to be applied to the upper back as you are testing against gravity only.

7.1 / 5. *If you were the treating clinician, besides providing basic conservative therapy (i.e., cryotherapy, OTC anti-inflammatory medicine, muscle strengthening), what information should be included as part of Coach Post's rehabilitation plan?*

For all patients, regardless of the type of injury sustained, patient education (oral information or booklet information) is a vital component of the patient's recovery and prevention of further injury.[3,28,35,61] Patient education should be evidence-based and focus on the:

- Injury sustained
- MOI and aggravating factors to avoid
- Expected time course for improvement
- Modification in home, work, and recreational activities to reduce pain, speed recovery, and prevent chronic injury[9,28,35]

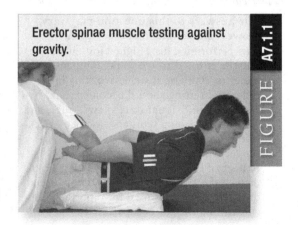

Erector spinae muscle testing against gravity.

FIGURE A7.1.1

Patient educational booklets developed to provide evidence-based information and medical advice consistent with current clinical guidelines have been shown to have a positive effect on patients' beliefs and clinical outcomes.[9] Similarly, Undermann[61] found that half of chronic low-back patients who read the educational book *Treat Your Own Back* had improvements in their pain immediately and at 9-month and 18-month follow-ups.

CASE 7.2 Lumbar Intervertebral Disc Pathology

7.2 / 1. *Based on the information presented in the case, determine (a) the differential diagnoses and (b) the clinical diagnosis.*

a. Differential diagnoses: lumbosacral disc injuries, lumbosacral discogenic pain syndrome, lumbosacral facet syndrome, lumbosacral radiculopathy, lumbosacral acute bony trauma, lumbosacral spondylolysis and spondylolisthesis, sacroiliac joint injury[33,35,50]

b. Clinical diagnosis: posterior disc herniation

7.2 / 2. *The injury in this case is typically seen in the adult population, often as a result of twisting of the trunk while carrying or lifting weight. For adolescent athletes, (a) what is the likelihood of this injury? (b) What would be the MOI?*

a. As mentioned in the chapter introduction, ruptures of the lumbar intervertebral disc in the general population are very common; however, a herniated nucleus pulposus in children and adolescents appears to account for less than 2 to 6 percent of all reported cases of lumbar disc herniations,[31,46] though the actual incidence rate is not known.[46]

b. The MOI in children and adolescents appears to be slightly different from the MOI in adults. Typically, patients in the younger age group have a history of mechanical stress applied to the lumbar spine, normally as a result of a specific traumatic event or sports injury.[32,34,46]

7.2 / 3. *During the physical examination, Kendrick notes that Eric is constantly shifting in his chair. As the evaluating clinician, what conclusion can you draw regarding this behavior?*

The direction of listing and rotation demonstrated by a patient is determined by the direction of disc herniation and may cause the body to bend toward or away from the side of involvement in order to alleviate symptoms. Because most disc herniations extrude posterolaterally, as a consequence of the relatively weak posterior longitudinal ligament,[20,21] pain is worse in positions such as sitting (flexion) that produce increased pressure on the annular fibers.[33] Increases in intradiscal pressure were reported to be higher in patients assuming a seated position or a seated position with flexion than in patients standing upright or assuming a recumbent position.[45] In fact, a more recent in vivo study found that the intradiscal pressure while sitting relaxed without a backrest was 90 percent of the pressure while standing; walking led to intradiscal pressure peaks of up to 130 percent, and flexion of the upper part of the body while standing demonstrated an intradiscal pressure at 216 percent when there is 36° of flexion between the thoracolumbar junction and the sacrum.[54] It is this increased disc pressure that probably exacerbated Eric's symptoms during sitting.

7.2 / 4. *(a) What is the difference between lumbar and thoracolumbar motion? (b) How would you as the evaluating clinician assess lumbar motion? (c) Thoracolumbar motion?*

a. Lumbar motion, particularly flexion and extension, is isolated movement of the five lumbar vertebrae. Thoracolumbar flexion and extension involve combined movements of the lumbar and thoracic spine.

b. Lumbar flexion is assessed using a tape measure with the patient in a standing position. The starting point is S2 and 10 cm above the spinous process of S2 (mark the position). The patient is instructed to flex to the limit of motion, and the difference between the two points is recorded. Extension is measured in the prone position from the table to the suprasternal notch.

   Lumbar flexion can also be measured with single and dual inclinometers. To measure lumbar ROM using a single inclinometer, place the inclinometer on the level of L1, and zero the instrument. The patient then flexes, and the measurement is taken. The patient then returns to the upright position. The inclinometer is placed on the sacrum, and the instrument is zeroed. The patient is then asked to flex again. The sacral measurement is subtracted from the L1 measurement to determine the lumbar flexion ROM. The same technique is used for extension ROM. To measure lumbar ROM using two inclinometers, place the inclinometer on the level of L1 and the sacrum, and zero both instruments. The patient then flexes the spine. The sacral reading is then subtracted from the L1 reading, giving the clinician the measurement of the lumbar flexion. The same method is performed for extension and lateral flexion, except that the inclinometer is placed on the T12 level for lateral flexion.

c. Thoracolumbar motion is assessed with the patient in a standing position and the clinician using a tape measure. In this case S2 is still the beginning position; however, the C7 spinous process is now the landmark. The patient flexes and extends the thoracolumbar spine while the clinician notes the differences between the starting and ending motions. Normal ROM is approximately 10 cm in flexion and 2.5 cm in extension.

An alternative method is to use single or dual inclinometers if available. Using a single inclinometer, follow the same technique as previously discussed with lumbar flexion ROM. This time, however, place the inclinometer on C7 and zero the instrument. The patient then performs the motion, and the measurement is taken. The inclinometer is then placed on the sacrum, the instrument is zeroed, and the patient performs the motion. The measurement is recorded. The sacral measurement is subtracted from the C7 measurement to determine thoracolumbar ROM. When using dual inclinometers, place an inclinometer on the level of C7 and the other on the sacrum. The inclinometers are then zeroed, and the patient is asked to flex or extend. The sacral inclinometer measurement is subtracted from the C7 measurement.

7.2 / 5. *As part of the physical examination, Kendrick performed a neurological examination. Complete Table 7.2.1, which shows the sensory and motor deficits associated with nerve root involvement at each lumbar and sacral level identified in the chart.*

A completed version of Table 7.2.1 (see below) is provided in Table A7.2.1 (p. 463).

7.2 / 6. *(a) Why is Eric's pain worse in the morning and improved after exercise? (b) If you were treating Eric, what activities would you have him perform during his exercise phase to reduce his discomfort?*

a. Patients with disc herniations will typically experience an increase in pain upon wakening in the morning. This occurs because the nucleus pulposus is a semi-gelatinous substance composed mainly of water. During the day, constant movement, disc compression, and dehydration cause the disc to lose fluid, thereby decreasing the size of the disc. This results in less pressure on the nerve root. Periods of rest and inactivity cause the disc to rehydrate, allowing the nuclear material to increase pressure on the nerve roots again.

b. Many physicians recommend McKenzie exercises during rehabilitation to centralize the nucleus pulposus.[21] A recent systematic review suggests that McKenzie therapy results in more of a short-term decrease (<3 months) in

TABLE	A7.2.1	Sensory and motor deficits in association with nerve root involvement at individual lumbar and sacral levels.

DISC LEVEL	LOCATION OF DERMATOME SYMPTOMS	MOTOR DEFICITS
L1	Back, over greater trochanter and groin	
L2		Hip flexion and adductors, diminished patellar tendon reflex
L3		Knee extension, diminished patellar tendon reflex
L4	Anterior medial lower leg	
L5		Great toe extension
S1	Lateral side and plantar surface of the foot	
S2		Knee flexion and great toe flexion

TABLE	A7.2.1	Sensory and motor deficits in association with nerve root involvement at individual lumbar and sacral levels.

DISC LEVEL	LOCATION OF DERMATOME SYMPTOMS	MOTOR DEFICITS
L1	Back, over greater trochanter and groin	Hip flexion
L2	Back, wrapping around to anterior superior thigh and medial thigh above knee	Hip flexion and adductors, diminished patellar tendon reflex
L3	Back, upper gluteal, anterior thigh, medial knee, and lower leg	Knee extension, diminished patellar tendon reflex
L4	Medial gluteals, lateral thigh and knee, anterior medial lower leg, dorsomedial aspect of foot and big toe	Ankle dorsiflexion and inversion (anterior tibialis), diminished patellar tendon reflex
L5	Lateral knee and upper lateral lower leg, dorsum of foot	Great toe extension
S1	Buttock, posterolateral thigh, lateral side and plantar surface of the foot	Ankle plantarflexion and eversion, diminished or absent Achilles reflex
S2	Buttock, posteromedial thigh, posterior, medial heel	Knee flexion and great toe flexion

pain and disability for LBP patients than other standard treatments, such as nonsteroidal anti-inflammatory medication, back massage with back care advice, strength training with supervision, and spinal mobilization.[10,14] The long-term effects of McKenzie rehabilitation programs are unclear, and no studies have attempted to examine this question.[10]

CASE 8.1 Traumatic Pneumothorax

8.1 / 1. *Based on the information presented in the case, determine (a) the differential diagnoses and (b) the clinical diagnosis.*

a. Differential diagnoses: clavicle fracture, rib fracture, scapular fracture, sternal fracture, punctured lung, heart contusion

b. Clinical diagnosis: traumatic pneumothorax

8.1 / 2. *What is the immediate management for this condition?*

If the athletic trainer suspects a pneumothorax, immediate oxygen supplementation and immediate referral to the hospital is the best course of action. To confirm the diagnosis, a posteroanterior (PA) chest radiograph, or an expiratory or lateral decubitus film if the condition is relatively small, would be indicated. Usually, a pulmonologist will diagnosis a pneumothorax as a percentage of the lung affected, such as 20 to 30 percent pneumothorax. Depending on the severity, re-expansion of

the lung with a chest tube (Heimlich chest valve drain) or thoracostomy is warranted,[3,6] along with monitoring in the hospital.

8.1 / 3. *(a) What other signs and symptoms may be presented with this injury? (b) What precautions should an athletic trainer take?*

a. Traumatic pneumothorax may present with tachycardia, decreased breath sounds, tracheal deviation, distended neck veins, hypotension, breathing difficulties, pain radiating to the shoulder and neck on the affected side, pain in the chest with exertion, or tachypnea.[3,6,8]

b. Approximately 10 percent of traumatic pneumothorax conditions can be asymptomatic,[26] and systematic monitoring of the athlete is paramount. In addition, because symptoms may take hours or days to develop, any possible rib fracture or contusion should be followed up with X-rays, especially if symptoms do not appear to resolve or decrease over time.

8.1 / 4. *After Billy is diagnosed and treated appropriately, (a) when should he be allowed to return to play? (b) Should any other restrictions be put in place?*

a. Because of the low incidence of this condition, return-to-play guidelines are speculative. It is recommended that return to play begin after full resolution of symptoms[8] or up to three weeks for a full contact-sport athlete.[3]

b. Air travel should also be restricted because of the potential for exacerbating or enlarging the pneumothorax through pressure changes when flying, but no specific guidelines are published.

8.1 / 5. *This condition often is classified by two separate causes: one is spontaneous; the other traumatic. Please describe both.*

A spontaneous pneumothorax usually affects younger individuals between the ages of 20 and 40. The suspected cause is rupture of subpleural blebs or bullae as a result of family history; being tall and thin; smoking history; or sports activities involving pressure fluctuations, such as scuba diving, weight lifting, or jogging.[8]

A traumatic pneumothorax usually results from a blunt force that can cause a rib/sternal/clavicle fracture by pushing the rib inward to puncture the lung (rib fractures are not always associated with pneumothorax).

CASE 8.2   Sudden Cardiac Arrest

8.2 / 1. *Based on the information presented in the case, identify the clinical diagnosis.*

The athlete died as a result of sudden cardiac arrest. There are only about 100 cases of sudden cardiac arrest per year in athletics.[18] Although it occurs in low numbers, in the athletic population, sudden death from cardiac arrest is considered the leading cause of death among young athletes,[11,16,17,19,20,25] despite pre-participation physical exam screenings and emergency planning, including the availability of AEDs at athletic events.[11]

8.2 / 2. *Andrew and Tara initiated immediate medical care, as identified in textbook Figure 8.2.1, after the primary assessment. Looking at the figure, (a) what is the name of this procedure? (b) Do they appear to be performing the procedure correctly?*

a. The procedure performed in textbook Figure 8.2.1 is two-rescuer cardiopulmonary resuscitation (CPR).

b. After the primary assessment that determined the need for CPR, Andrew and Tara did not correctly perform the procedure (at least based on the photos). The first and biggest error was the hand placement for chest compressions. The hands appear to be at the level of the xiphoid process rather than on the center of the chest (shown correctly in Figure A8.2.1). Another incorrect or improper action is the lack of personal protective

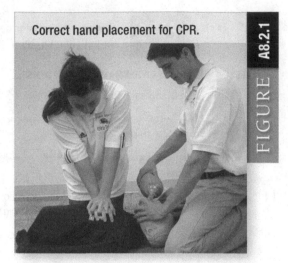

Correct hand placement for CPR.

FIGURE A8.2.1

equipment (i.e., gloves). Personal protective equipment should be used at all times and is required, according to the Bloodborne Pathogens Standard (29 CFR 1910.1030) outlined by the Occupational Safety and Health Administration (OSHA).[22] Finally, remember that during two-rescuer CPR, the cycles should continue for 2 minutes, or five total cycles, before changing positions, in order to prevent fatigue and poor mechanics.

8.2 / 3. *(a) Did Andrew and Tara handle the situation appropriately? (b) Outline the management steps you would employ in this same situation.*

a. The athletic trainers should have requested before the event that an AED be available on site or brought one with them in case of medical emergencies. If an AED was available, the athlete should have been connected, and these steps followed: One shock followed by immediate chest compressions and rescue breathing (30:2) to help improve oxygen flow and to avoid interruptions of chest compressions while waiting for rhythm analysis.[11] In addition, CPR can be initiated while the second rescuer is connecting the AED.

b. A proper emergency action plan (EAP) should have been reviewed before Andrew and Tara covered the event. Specific elements should have included:

- Lines of communication (which was correctly done in this scenario)

- Pre-event review of other emergency responders at the event; location of all emergency medical equipment (especially an AED)

- Pre-event practice run of all trained medical personnel for such emergencies

- Identification of person(s) for initiating and conducting different parts of the EAP[11]

8.2 / 4. *What are some associated medical conditions that may be involved in the outcome of the above scenario?*

Of the cardiovascular diseases that are most prevalent, hypertrophic cardiomyopathy and congenital coronary artery anomalies account for approximately 36 percent and 17 percent, respectively, of the athletes who experience sudden cardiac death (or survived cardiac arrest).[14,18] Blunt trauma to the chest (commotio cordis) is one of the leading causes of death from sudden cardiac arrest or ventricular arrhythmia. Hypertrophic cardiomyopathy (HCM) is a congenital disorder characterized by abnormal thickening of the left ventricle wall that develops before the age of 20. The thickened ventricle wall (normally >1 cm) leads to electrical problems and arrhythmia, including ventricular fibrillation. Congenital coronary artery anomalies such as congenital variations in right or left coronary anatomy are often associated with structural forms of congenital heart disease. The most common abnormality is a wrong origin of the left main coronary artery. Other conditions include Marfan syndrome, myocarditis, aortic stenosis, mitral valve prolapsed, long-QT syndrome.

8.2 / 5. *It has been postulated that pre-participation examinations (PPE) should screen for heart-related irregularities. What are some screening questions and tests that should be used to help detect abnormalities? When should an athlete be restricted from athletic participation?*[14]

Questions should be asked to determine the presence of the following conditions:

- Syncope (fainting) during or after exercise

- Pain, pressure, or discomfort in chest while exercising

- Heart skipping beats during exercise

- High blood pressure, high cholesterol, murmur, heart infection

- Family history of cardiovascular disease

- Family history of Marfan syndrome

Screening tests

- Listen for a murmur that changes in sound with squatting or standing during a Valsalva maneuver.

Suspicions raised by screening questions are grounds for restricting participation until further diagnosis. Athletes with stage 2 hypertension (higher than 160/100) should be restricted until the condition is controlled.

CASE 9.1 Sacroiliac Joint Sprain

9.1 / 1. *Based on the information presented in the case, determine (a) the differential diagnoses and (b) the clinical diagnosis.*

a. Differential diagnoses: lumbar disc pathology, facet syndrome, erector spinae or quadrates lumborum strain, sciatica, spondylosis, spondylolisthesis

b. Clinical diagnosis: sacroiliac (SI) joint sprain

9.1 / 2. *The area in question has multiple ligamentous support structures. Please identify the major ligament structures and their function in the sacral region.*

- Pubic symphysis: This ligament is comprised of three bands/ligaments called the superior, arcuate, and interpubic that connect the pubis bones together anteriorly. They function to resist shear stresses, enable superior movements of the sacrum, and prevent pubis joint separations.[26,65]

- Sacrotuberous ligament: This structure attaches on the posterior superior and inferior iliac spines, the sacrum, and coccyx and runs downward and inserts onto the ischial tuberosity.[66] It functions to limit sacral rotation.

- Anterior SI ligament: This ligament functions to limit movement of the sacrum superiorly or inferiorly and limits joint separation.[26] It is part of the anterior joint capsule and well defined.

- Posterior SI ligament: This ligament arises from the posterior aspect of the sacrum and attaches to the posterior aspect of the ilium. It limits joint separation.

- Sacrospinous ligament: This triangular shaped ligament originates on the ischial spine and inserts onto the sacrum and coccyx and lies in front of the sacrotuberous ligament. It helps to form the greater sciatic foramen and lesser sciatic foramen. Its function is to limit sacral rotation.[26]

- Iliolumbar ligament: The iliolumbar ligament runs from L4 and L5 to the iliac crest, merging with the interosseous ligament. It is designed to limit motion between the lumbar spine and the sacrum.[26]

9.1 / 3. *What are the most common pain-referral sites for this injury?*

According to Slipman,[57] patients with SI joint pain have several pain referral sites. Pain can be associated with subsequent trauma to the sciatic nerve and L5 nerve root, and pain intensity and referral patterns are highly variable, depending on severity and SI joint location. See Table A9.1.1 for pain-referral sites.

9.1 / 4. *What are some of the provocative or diagnostic tests used to differentiate this pathology? Are these tests valid and reliable?*

There are a number of tests[11] used in diagnosing or differentiating SI joint pain (Table A9.1.2). However, the thigh thrust test, compression test, and three or more positive stress tests have the better discrimination power for an appropriate SI joint diagnosis.[60] Other diagnostic tests, such as an MRI and/or CT scan are often used but may not be able to adequately diagnosis SI

TABLE A9.1.1

Sacroiliac pain-referral sites and percentage of patients reporting pain.

PAIN-REFERRAL SITE	PERCENTAGE OF PATIENTS WHO FELT PAIN AT THIS SITE
Buttock	91
Lower lumbar region	72
Posterior thigh	30
Lateral thigh	10
Posterior lower leg	18
Lateral lower leg	12
Groin	12
Lateral foot	8
Abdomen	2

TABLE A9.1.2   Provocative tests used to diagnose sacroiliac joint pathology.[35,53,60]

PROVOCATIVE TEST	TESTING PROCEDURES
Static palpation	Palpate SI joint for pinpoint tenderness.
Gillet standing flexion test	Ask the patient to stand. Place one thumb directly over the second sacral tubercle and the other thumb over left PSIS. Ask the patient to flex at the hip to 90°. If joint dysfunction is present, the left thumb will move in the cephalad direction.
Anterior distraction/Gapping	Ask the patient to lie supine. Place heels of the hands on the ASIS in a cross pattern and place pressure on heels of the hand in a downward and outward direction. If there is pain or discomfort, SI joint pathology is present.
Gaenslen's	Place patient in a supine position with knee of affected side up to the chest and opposite leg fully extended. If the test is positive, this should increase stress and elicit pain. A positive test will result in pain.
Iliac crest compression	Place patient on his side, and apply downward pressure on the iliac crest. Pain may indicate SI joint pathology.
Single leg stand	Ask the patient to stand on the leg of the affected side with opposite leg flexed at 90° at the hip and knee. After 30 to 60 seconds, stress on the leg of the affected side may produce SI joint pain.
Patrick's/FABER	Ask the patient to lie supine and place foot of test leg on opposite knee (in a "figure 4" position). In a positive test, the bent knee does not fall below the height of opposite leg and may cause SI joint pain.
Thigh thrust	Ask the patient to lie supine, place the hip at 90° of flexion with the knee bent. Place posterior shearing stress on the SI joint through the femur of the flexed leg. Pain may indicate SI joint pathology.

joint pathology.[57] Fluoroscopically guided SI joint intra-articular injection with an anesthetic has also become a popular diagnostic test used in diagnosing SI joint pathology.[57]

9.1 / 5. *Do you think Shaun should have removed Tracey's leotard for inspection of the area?*

The answers will vary. Inspection of the area required removal of clothing, but Shaun should have taken Tracey to a private location or back to the designated athletic training room for evaluation. Although Tracey may be accustomed to frequent changes of clothing in front of others, especially during performances or shows, the evaluation of an injury warrants medical privacy, confidentiality, and consent.

CASE 9.2   Quadriceps Strain

9.2 / 1. *Based on the information presented in the case, determine (a) the differential diagnoses and (b) the clinical diagnosis.*

a. Differential diagnoses: quadriceps tendon rupture, patella avulsion fracture, contusion
b. Clinical diagnosis: quadriceps femoris muscle strain

9.2 / 2. *Judy discussed some immediate treatment care for the injury. Based on the information provided, what immediate care do you think she recommended to Sumpta?*

The answers will vary. Many acute muscle injuries are best treated with rest, ice, compression, and elevation (RICE)[6,53] and NSAIDs to block prostaglandin formation and to control edema, bleeding, and pain. Keep in mind that prolonged use of NSAIDs can adversely affect muscle recovery.[1]

9.2 / 3. *Based on the clinical diagnosis, what section of muscle(s) does this type of injury usually affect and why?*

The most common site for muscular strains such as a quadriceps strain is at the myotendinous junction. This is because this transitional area between the muscle belly and tendon is subject to the greatest stress from transmitted forces directly applied to the tissue, based on its surface area, fiber orientation, and function.[6]

9.2 / 4. *Based on the clinical diagnosis, what type of muscles and muscle actions are usually associated with this type of injury?*

Muscles most at risk are those that cross two joints, because of the angular positions of the muscle fibers and the velocity that these muscles can produce. Most of the injuries occur during eccentric action, when a muscle is attempting to decelerate joint motion.[6]

9.2 / 5. *Sumpta reluctantly agreed to the immediate course of action. When she asked about returning to play, what factors did Judy need to consider before allowing her to return to play?*

The answers will vary based on a variety of factors, including extent of trauma, location of injury, sport/activity, pain tolerance, and other factors. Many clinicians require strength and flexibility comparable to the non-injured side (90%) and require functional field tests of acceleration/deceleration and changes in direction to ensure that the athlete is not placing herself at risk for further injury.

CASE 10.1   Unhappy Triad

10.1 / 1. *Based on the information presented in the case, determine (a) the clinical diagnosis and (b) the common name for this condition.*

a. Clinical diagnosis: ACL, MCL, and medial meniscus damage
b. Common name: unhappy triad or "terrible triad," typically involving a valgus stress to the knee[40]

10.1 / 2. *(a) Identify the bony and soft tissue structures that should have been palpated as part of the physical examination. Then (b) identify two or three other observations Tyler could have made during the initial assessment. (c) Why was the flexed carrying position noted sometime later during the evaluation and not initially?*

a. Possible bony and soft tissue structures that can be palpated include:
   ■ Bony: proximal tibia and fibula, distal femur, patella, condyles, joint line
   ■ Soft: MCL, LCL, patella tendon, gastrocnemius, biceps femoris, semimembranosus, semitendinosus
b. Other observations may include deformity, redness, patella alignment, gait, and symmetry of the knee.
c. The flexed carrying angle was noticed later because increased joint effusion causes the knee to flex to its open-pack position to al-

low for the greatest accumulation of the effusion. Immediate gross effusion (within 2 hours), which limits function, may indicate significant knee trauma and may suggest some degree of ACL trauma.[19,67]

10.1 / 3. *Based on Jim's MOI and his signs and symptoms, identify at least three ligamentous tests that could have been performed to assist in determining the clinical diagnosis. Describe how to perform each test.*

There are several ligamentous testing procedures that could be used in determining the clinical diagnosis. These may include, but are not limited to, the anterior draw, Lachman's test, lateral pivot shift, Solcum and Hughston's test, and valgus stress test.

10.1 / 4. *According to the evidence-based literature, which ligamentous tests used by clinicians is the most accurate in diagnosing this condition?*

According to Scholten,[82] examination of the accuracy of diagnostic testing for assessing trauma to the anterior cruciate ligament found the Lachman's test a more accurate overall test for assessing the ACL, followed by the lateral pivot shift test. The anterior draw test, according to authors, appears to be of little value due to guardin gof the hamstring muscles. The position of the anterior draw test places the knee in less of an open-pack position during the test.

10.1 / 5. *Jim questions you as to why the doctor wants to see him tomorrow and why he needs an MRI. How do you answer him?*

The answer should focus on the need for further evaluation by a medical physician. In states where an athletic trainer works under the direct supervision of a licensed physician, it will often be necessary for a physician to determine the final medical diagnosis and assess the need for, as well as order, the appropriate diagnostic imaging.

In this case, the MRI is used to detect soft tissue lesions (i.e., ligaments). As a diagnostic modality, an MRI uses a powerful magnetic field and radiofrequency waves to visualize anatomical structures (e.g., joint, tendons, ligaments). A patient is placed within a magnetic field as radiowaves are introduced, absorbed, and released by the tissues. The intensity of the signals differs, based on the make-up of the involved tissues, and the signals are then converted into a set of tomographic images by using field gradients in the magnetic field, all of which permits a three-dimensional localization of the point sources of the signals.[75,87]

CASE 10.2 Lateral Collateral Ligament Sprain with Secondary Peroneal Nerve Damage

10.2 / 1. *Based on the information presented in the case, determine (a) the potential differential diagnoses and (b) the clinical diagnosis.*

a. Differential diagnoses: osteochondral fracture, tibial plateau fracture, extensor mechanism rupture, patellofemoral injury

b. Clinical diagnosis: lateral collateral ligament sprain with secondary peroneal nerve damage

10.2 / 2. *Textbook Figure 10.2.1 demonstrated a positive knee ligamentous test. The test revealed instability at 0° and 20° of knee flexion. What is the name of the test performed, and what is the diagnostic accuracy of this test?*

The name of the test is a varus stress test, which assesses the stability of the lateral collateral ligament. Positive findings included increased laxity, decreased quality of the end point, and increased pain compared with the uninvolved knee.

According to McConagy,[58] there is no data examining the accuracy of the medial or lateral collateral ligamentous tests.

10.2 / 3. *What is the clinical significance of varus ligamentous instability at both 0° and 20° of knee flexion?*

The lateral collateral ligament (LCL) is the primary static stabilizer of the lateral knee. Damage to the LCL is typically sustained when a varus force is applied to the knee. Ligamentous testing for the stability of the LCL is accomplished through a varus stress test. Laxity or a decreased end-point when the knee is in 15°–20° indicates damage to the LCL, while significant laxity in full extension may indicate concomitant injury to the joint capsule, posterior cruciate ligament, and possibly, the anterior cruciate ligament[46] and other related soft-tissue structures.[49,86]

10.2 / 4. *Why was a deficit in ankle dorsiflexion and eversion noted?*

Concomitant common peroneal nerve injury can occur with an LCL injury because of a traction force[54] applied to the nerve as it wraps around the fibula head. As the LCL is stretched, so is the common peroneal nerve. The traction injury can result in drop foot (from weakness of the dorsiflexor muscles of the foot, which are enervated by the deep peroneal nerve) and numbness in the dorsum of the foot, as well as other neurological issues.[54]

10.2 / 5. *How would you respond to Sam if he asks, "How is the doctor going to determine exactly what is wrong with me?"*

The answers to this question will vary. The answer should include a statement that initially the physician will correlate the findings of the history and physical examination. From there, the physician will determine the need for further diagnostic testing if the history and physical examination do not clearly determine the clinical diagnosis. In this case, a physician would most likely order diagnostic testing, such as an MRI or electrophysiological testing (electromyography and nerve conduction study). Consult your team physician to determine how she would manage this patient in her medical practice.

CASE 11.1 ATF and CF Ligament Sprain with Peroneal Tendon Strain

11.1 / 1. *Based on the information presented in the case, determine (a) the differential diagnoses and (b) the clinical diagnosis.*

a. Differential diagnoses: ankle fracture, foot fracture, peroneal tendon subluxation, Achilles tendon rupture, tendonitis, tenosynovitis[93]

b. Clinical diagnosis: sprain of the anterior talofibular ligament (ATFL) and calcaneofibular ligament (CFL) with concomitant peroneal strain (caused by an excessive eccentric force)

11.1 / 2. *Based on the information presented in the case, do you believe Josh took an adequate history? If not, what, if any, additional questions would you ask as the evaluating clinician?*

Answers will vary. Remember that when assessing an acute lateral ankle sprain, determining the MOI and position of the joint at the time of injury is really the first step in a good clinical assessment.[4,151] It is often easier for the patient to demonstrate the position of the involved ankle with the uninvolved ankle rather than trying to explain the position. As the evaluating clinician, remember to phrase the questions as open-ended, rather than forced-choice (e.g., Ask, "Can you explain what position your foot was in?" instead of, "Was your foot turned inward?"). Also, determine if the injury was unprovoked or if it occurred in a situation that normally does not result in ankle injury, because the patient's condition may be the result of another pathology, such as tarsal coalition, osteochondritis, or peroneal tendon dislocation.[4] The history should include the location of pain, presence of swelling, and functional capacity, including the ability to bear weight, walk, run, and jump. Additional questions that should be asked include ones about any prior injuries, treatments, impairments,[59] or joint weaknesses. If there was a feeling that the ankle gave way,[127] age, general health status, occupation (e.g., in the setting outside of collegiate or high school sports), and leg dominance should be ascertained.

11.1 / 3. *Overall, do you believe Josh adequately evaluated Jasmine's condition given the clinical presentation? If not, what would you have done differently as the evaluating clinician?*

The answers to this question will vary. Overall, Josh appeared to perform an adequate clinical examination; however, one issue of concern is related to Figure 11.1.2. Assessment textbooks commonly recommend placing the ankle in a plantarflexed position between 15° and 20° when performing an anterior drawer.[69,106,124,131] However, Josh decided to place the ankle in a neutral position, which can yield questionable results, even though in this case it was reported as a positive finding.

The ability of stress tests such as the anterior draw and talar tilt to differentiate between specific ligaments has been reported as debatable.[47] A cadaver biomechanical analysis aimed at quantifying the instability of the hindfoot complex during the anterior displacement of the hindfoot by five clinicians under three conditions (intact ligaments, after sectioning the ATF ligament in an isolated ATFL injury, then after sectioning the CF ligament in a combined ATFL/CFL injury) found greater anterior displacement in the neutral position (Table A11.1.1).[47] It is believed, however, that when the foot is in plantarflexion, the ATFL orients itself parallel to the long axis of the fibula, acting as the main collateral ligament.[24] This then supports the result of Bahr,[9] who found greater force application to intact cadaver ATFL when in 20° of plantarflexion (Table A11.1.2). Bahr also noted a small increase in anterior translation between the intact and cut ATFL in 10° and 20° of plantarflexion. When both ligaments were transected, cadaveric anterior translation increased at all flexion angles used during testing.[9] In a more recent study, researchers found that knee and ankle position influences anterior drawer laxity and stiffness of the ankle complex.[71] Specifically, they found that anterior drawer testing of the ankle complex with the

TABLE A11.1.1	ATFL and CFL displacement under three conditions.[47]

CONDITION	NEUTRAL POSITION	20° PLANTARFLEXION
Intact ATFL	15.1 mm (± 4.0 mm)	8.3 mm (± 4.0 mm)
Sectioned ATFL	19.0 mm (± 3.0 mm)	10.3 mm (± 4.4 mm)
Combined ATFL and CFL section	19.2 mm (± 3.2 mm)	10.9 mm (± 3.8 mm)

TABLE A11.1.2	ATFL and CFL force during 80-Newton anterior drawer testing with foot at different flexion angles.

POSITION	ATFL IN NEWTONS	CFL IN NEWTONS
10° Dorsiflexion	33 (SE, 6)	40 (SE, 6)
Neutral	23 (SE, 5)	15 (SE, 5)
10° Plantar flexion	34 (SE, 6)	6 (SE, 3)
20° Plantar flexion	53 (SE, 24)	−3 (SE, 2)

knee positioned at 90° of flexion and 10° of ankle plantarflexion produced the most laxity and the least stiffness. This suggests that this position permits better isolation of the ankle ligamentous structures than knee extension or a neutral ankle position. Clinically, these three studies provide very different results; however, two of the three studies used cadaver sections of the lower leg, while Kovaleski[71] used human subjects. This fact suggests that other factors may affect the sensitivity of the test, including (1) variations in individual tissue properties and bony structures, (2) torque and axial load application by a clinician, (3) joint position (knee and ankle), and (4) the effects of other structures such as the gastrocnemius-Achilles tendon complex.[47,48,71,75]

11.1 / 4. (a) What is the name of the ligamentous stress test performed in textbook Figure 11.1.3? (b) Why is it used, and what is considered a positive finding?

a. The stress test performed in textbook Figure 11.1.3 is commonly referred to as the talar tilt or inversion stress maneuver.

b. It is commonly used to evaluate injuries of the lateral ligaments of the ankle joint,[48,78] particularly the stability of the CFL. The test is typically performed with the patient lying supine or side-lying, with the foot relaxed.

The ankle is held in a neutral position while the clinician supports the calcaneus and tries to invert the calcaneus with respect to the tibia.[78] The difficulty with the test is that there ". . . is no standardized value for the degree of talar tilt, which indicates instability" and that the test cannot evaluate isolated pathologies of the lateral ankle ligaments (i.e., CFL).[48] Gaebler found that reports of talar tilt values more than 5° greater than those of the involved side indicate significant injury, even though a tilt of 15° to 30° indicates only moderate instability.[48] Lynch sites reports that talar tilt values between 5° and 23° are normal, but a 10° difference between ankles is considered abnormal.[78]

11.1 / 5. Josh assessed active and passive ROM as part of the on-field assessment; however, his clinical findings do not list any specific ROM limitations. (a) Why do you believe this is the case? (b) If you were doing the evaluation, how could you quantify AROM, particularly ankle dorsiflexion? (c) How much active dorsiflexion is considered normal during a walking gait?

a. The most probable explanation for a lack of quantitative ROM findings as part of the physical examination is a lack of a goniometer.

b. Goniometry is typically used to assess PROM, but it can be used to asses AROM as well. To assess ankle dorsiflexion, the patient is placed in short-sitting or long-sitting with the knee flexed 20° to 30° to reduce gastrocnemius tension. The axis of the goniometer is placed inferior to the lateral malleolus while the stationary arm is parallel to the long axis of the fibula and the movable arm is parallel to the sole of the foot.

c. During a normal walking gait, a patient should be able to produce 10° of ankle dorsiflexion from mid-stance to terminal stance.

CASE 11.2 Deltoid Sprain with Fibula Fracture

11.2 / 1. *Based on the information presented in the case, determine (a) the differential diagnoses and (b) the clinical diagnosis.*

a. Differential diagnoses: fibula fracture, medial malleolus fracture, talus fracture, calcaneus fracture, syndesmosis sprain, lateral ankle sprain, peroneal strain

b. Clinical diagnosis: deltoid sprain concomitant fibula fracture

11.2 / 2. *Mary presented with tenderness over and inferior to the distal medial malleolus. Identify the structures responsible for providing medial ankle joint stability.*

The medial "deltoid" ligament is a fan-shaped (delta), broad complex with an apical attachment above to the medial malleolus and to the talus, calcaneus, and navicular bone and spring ligament.[123] Although clinicians commonly refer to the ligament as a single unit, it is composed of superficial and deep fibers and is divisible into separate anatomical parts.[118,123] The superficial fibers are comprised of the tibiocalcaneal (TC) ligament (apex of the medial malleolus to the calcaneus directly below the medial malleolus) and tibionavicular (TN) ligament (runs beneath and slightly posterior to the anterior tibiotalar ligament, inserting onto the medial navicular surface).[87,118] The deep fibers are composed of the anterior tibiotalar (ATT) (anteromedial medial malleolus to the superior medial talus) and posterior tibiotalar (PTT) (posterior medial malleolus to the posterior talus) ligaments. During maximum ankle dorsiflexion (10°–20°), the TC and PTT are taut; the ATT and TN are taut during 30°–40° of ankle plantarflexion.[118,131]

11.2 / 3. *Based on the clinical presentation and the MOI, what is one pertinent history question Nichole could have asked to guide the physical examination?*

In this case, based on the MOI (forced ankle eversion) and the injury pattern (especially the medial popping sensation), Nichole would have been wise to ask about any other unusual sounds or sensations, such as cracking or snapping. A cracking or snapping sensation would correspond with trauma (fracture) to the distal fibula. The lower position of the lateral malleolus (distal fibula) limits eversion ankle injuries. However, in situations in which excessive eversion forces have been applied and there is direct trauma to the distal fibula, concomitant injury such as fibula fracture, or a bimalleolar fracture should be suspected with a medial ankle sprain.

11.2 / 4. *As the evaluating clinician, in addition to the obvious anatomical landmarks (e.g., malleoli), what other bony anatomical landmarks would you have assessed to guide the physical examination?*

The answers to this question will vary. However, emphasis should be placed on structures such as the tibia, fibula (particularly the distal end), talus, calcaneus, navicular, cuneiforms, cuboid, and metatarsals.

11.2 / 5. *Overall, do you believe Nichole made the correct decision by removing Mary from the ice after completing her on-ice evaluation? If not, why? What would you have done differently?*

The answers to this question will vary. However, a review of the vital signs (blood pressure 126/90; radial pulse 124 bpm, rapid, weak; and respiration 21, shallow, labored) may suggest shock. Even though the pulse and respiration rate appear normal, given the case's clinical presentation (participating in athletics), the rhythm and quality are abnormal. The vital signs in this case mandate immediate medical intervention, including supplemental oxygen and activation of EMS.

11.2 / 6. *As a new certified athletic trainer, how would you respond to the assistant coach's request for playing status? If a difference of opinion occurred, how and when should the situation be handled?*

This answer to this question will vary because there is not necessarily only one correct answer. Certainly, the actions of the coach were at best inappropriate and could have been handled much differently.

REFERENCES   Cited in the Selected Responses

(Only those items cited in the selected answers are included here; thus, items are not sequential.)

Chapter 2

10. Buglisi JA, Knoop KJ, Levsky ME, Euwema M. Experience with bandage contact lenses for the treatment of corneal abrasions in a combat environment. *Mil Med.* 2007; 172(4):411–413.

22. Guskiewicz KM, Bruce SL, Cantu RC, et al. National Athletic Trainers' Association Position Statement: management of sport-related concussion. *J Athl Train.* 2004; 39(3):280–297.

27. Heimmel MR, Murphy MA. Ocular injuries in basketball and baseball: what are the risks and how can we prevent them? *Cur Sports Med Rep.* 2008; 7(5):284–288.

35. Khan FH, Silverberg MA. Corneal abrasion [electronic version]. *eMedicine.* 2009. Available from: http://www.emedicine.com/emerg/topic 828.htm. Accessed December 29, 2009.

39. Kwitko GM. Orbital fracture, floor [electronic version]. *eMedicine.* 2009. Available from: http://www.emedicine.com/oph/topic229.htm. Accessed May 15, 2009.

44. Levine MR. How to manage orbital fractures. *Rev Ophthalmol.* 2000; 7(3):70–73.

65. Petrigliano FA, Williams R. Orbital fractures in sport: a review. *Sprts Med.* 2003; 33(4):317–322.

72. Rodriguez JO, Lavina AM. Prevention and treatment of common eye injuries in sports. *Am Fam Physician.* 2003; 67:1481–8,1494–6.

80. Smith B, Regan W. Blowout fracture of the orbit: mechanism repair. *Am J Ophthalmol.* 1957; 44: 733–739.

87. Torok PG, Mader TH. Corneal abrasions: diagnosis and management. *Am Fam Physician.* 1996; 63(8):2521–2529.

93. Wilson SA, Last A. Management of corneal abrasions. *Am Fam Physician.* 2004; 70(1):123–128.

Chapter 3

2. American Red Cross. *Emergency Response.* Yardley, PA: Staywell; 2001.

9. Gallaspy JB, May JD. *Signs and Symptoms of Athletic Injuries.* St. Louis, MO: Mosby; 1996.

11. Holdgate A, Ching N, Angonese L. Variability in agreement between physicians and nurses when measuring the Glasgow coma scale in the emergency department limits its clinical usefulness. *Emerg Med Australas.* 2006; 18(4):379–384.

16. Konin JG, Wiksten D, Isear JA, Brader H. *Special Tests for Orthopedic Examination* (3rd ed.). Thorofare, NJ: Slack; 2006.

18. Magee DJ. *Orthopedic Physical Assessment* (5th ed.). Philadelphia, PA: WB Saunders; 2007.

26. Prentice WE. Arnheim's Principles of Athletic Training: A Competency-Based Approach (13th ed.). Boston, MA: McGraw Hill Publishing; 2009.

33. Schultz SJ, Houglum PA, Perrin DH. *Examination of Musculoskeletal Injuries* (2nd ed.). Champaign, IL: Human Kinetics; 2005.

37. Starkey C, Ryan J. Evaluation of Orthopedic and Athletic Injuries (2nd ed.). Philadelphia, PA: FA Davis; 2002.

40. Swartz EE, Floyd RT, Cendoma M. Cervical spine functional anatomy and the biomechanics of injury due to compressive loading. *J Ath Train.* 2005; 40(3):155–161.

41. Swartz EE, Nowak J, Shirley C, Decoster LC. A comparison of head movement during back boarding by motorized spine-board and log-roll techniques. *J Athl Train.* 2005; 40(3):162–168.

44. Trojian TH, Vaca FE, Young O. Brachial plexus injury [electronic version]. *eMedicine.* 2006. Available from: http://www.emedicine.com/sports/topic13.htm. Accessed April 30, 2007.

45. Wiese MF. British hospitals and different versions of the Glasgow coma scale: telephone survey. *BMJ.* 2003; 327(7418):782–783.

Chapter 4

4. Asplund C. Posterior sternoclavicular joint dislocation in a wrestler. *Mil Med.* 2004;169:134–136.

7. Bergfeld J, Andrish P, Clancy W. Evaluation of the acromioclavicular joint following first and second degree sprains. *Am J Sports Med.* 1978; 6:153–159.

20. Konin JG, Wiksten D, Isear JA, Brader H. *Special Testsnfor Orthopedic Examination* (3rd ed.). Thorofare, NJ: Slack; 2006.

24. Marker L, Klareskov B. Posterior sternoclavicular dislocation: an American football injury. *Br J Sports Med.* 1996;30:71–72.

26. Mirza A, Alam K, Ali A. Posterior sternoclavicular dislocation in a rugby player as a cause of silent vascular compromise: a case report [electronic version]. *Br J Sports Med.* 2005;39:e28–e30. Available from: http://www.bjsportmed.com/cgi/content/full/39/5/e28. Accessed June 4, 2009.

38. Rockwood C, Young D. Disorders of the acromioclavicular joint. In: Rockwood C, Matsen F, eds. *The Shoulder.* Philadelphia, PA: WB Saunders; 1990:413–476.

39. Rudzki J, Matava M, Paletta G. Complications of treatment of acromioclavicular and sternoclavicular joint injuries. *Clin Sports Med.* 2003;22:387–405.

41. Schultz SJ, Houglum PA, Perrin DH. *Examination of Musculoskeletal Injuries* (2nd ed.). Champaign, IL: Human Kinetics; 2005.

42. Seade E, Bartz R, Josey R. Acromioclavicular joint injury [electronic version]. *eMedicine.* 2008. Available from: http://emedicine.medscape.com/article/92337-overview. Accessed June 4, 2009.

46. Starkey C, Ryan J. *Evaluation of Orthopedic and Athletic Injuries* (2nd ed.). Philadelphia, PA: FA Davis; 2002.

Chapter 5

6. Azar FM, Andrews JR, Wilk KE, Groh D. Operative treatment of ulnar collateral ligament injuries of the elbow in athletes. *Am J Sports Med* [electronic version]. 2000; 28:16–23. Available from: http://ajs.sagepub.com/cgi/content/abstract/28/1/16. Accessed June 19, 2007.

17. Cain EL, Dugas JR, Wolf RS, Andrews JR. Elbow injuries in throwing athletes: a current concepts review. *Am J Sports Med* [electronic version]. 2003; 31:621–635. Available from: http://ajs.sagepub.com/cgi/content/abstract/31/4/621. Accessed July 7, 2007.

18. Callaway GH, Field LD, Deng XH, Torzilli PA, O'Brien SJ, Altchek DW, et al. Biomechanical evaluation of the medial collateral ligament of the elbow. *J Bone Joint Surg [Am].* 1997; 79-A (8):1223–1231.

22. Cohen MS, Bruno RJ. The collateral ligaments of the elbow: anatomy and clinical correlation. *Clin Orthop.* 2001; (383):123–130.

40. Kacprowicz RF, Chumbley E. Ulnar collateral ligament injury. *eMedicine* [electronic version]. 2007. Available from: http://www.emedicine.com/sports/topic139.htm. Accessed June 4, 2009.

44. Langer P, Fadale P, Hulstyn M. Evolution of the treatment options of ulnar collateral ligament injuries of the elbow. *Br J Sports Med* [electronic version]. 2006; 40:499–506. Accessed July, 31, 2007.

52. McKee MD, Schemitsch EH, Sala MJ, O'Driscoll SW. The pathoanatomy of lateral ligament disruption in complex elbow in stability. *Journal of Shoulder and Elbow Surgery.* 2003; 12:391–396.

54. Nassab PF, Schickendantz MS. Evaluation and treatment of medial ulnar collateral ligament injuries in the throwing athlete. *Sports Medicine and Arthroscopy Review.* 2006; 14:221–231.

57. O'Driscoll SWM, Lawton RL, Smith AM. The "Moving Valgus Stress Test" for medial collateral ligament tears of the elbow. *Am J Sports Med* [electronic version]. 2005; 33:231–239. Available from: http://ajs.sagepub.com/cgi/content/abstract/33/2/231. Accessed June 18, 2007.

59. Otsuka NY, Kasser JR. Supracondylar fractures of the humerus in children. *J Am Acad Orthop Surg.* 1997; 5:19–26.

69. Rettig AC. Managing elbow problems in throwing athletes. Journal of Musculoskeletal Medicine. 2007; 24:129–135.

70. Rettig AC, Sherrill C, Snead DS, Mendler JC, Mieling P. Nonoperative treatment of ulnar collateral ligament injuries in throwing athletes. *Am J Sports Med* [electronic version]. 2001; 29: 15–17. Available from: http://ajs.sagepub.com/cgi/content/abstract/29/1/15. Accessed June 18, 2007.

76. Schultz SJ, Houglum PA, Perrin DH. *Examination of Musculoskeletal Injuries* (2nd ed.). Champaign, IL: Human Kinetics; 2005.

81. Singh H, Osbahr DC, Wickham MQ, Kirkendall DT, Speer KP. Valgus laxity of the ulnar collateral ligament of the elbow in collegiate athletes. Am J Sports Med [electronic version]. 2001; 29: 558–561. Available from: http://ajs.sagepub.com/cgi/content/abstract/29/5/558. Accessed June 18, 2007.

84. Sojbjerg JO, Ovesen J, Nielsen S. Experimental elbow instability after transection of the medial collateral ligament. *Clin Orthop.* 1987; 218: 186–190.

85. Starkey C, Ryan J. *Evaluation of Orthopedic and Athletic Injuries* (2nd ed.). Philadelphia, PA: F.A. Davis; 2002.

87. Stirmont TJ, An KN, Morrey BF. Elbow joint contact study: comparison of technique. *J Biomech.* 1985; 18:329–336.

Chapter 6

13. Chan DY. Management of simple finger injuries: the splinting regime. *Hand Surg.* 2002; 7(2):223.

17. Combs JA. It's not "Just A Finger". *J Athl Train.* 2000; 35(2):168–178.

33. Guly HR. Diagnostic error in an accident and emergency department. *Emerg Med J.* 2001; 18:263–271.

34. Guly HR. Injuries initially misdiagnosed as sprained wrist (beware the sprained wrist). *Emerg Med J.* 2002; 19(1):41–42.

51. Lichtman DM, Joshi A. Ulnar-sided wrist pain. *eMedicine* [electronic version]. 2009. Available from: http://emedicine.medscape.com/article/1245322-overview#DifferentialDiagnosis. Accessed December 29, 2009.

61. Moore K, Dalley A. *Clinically Oriented Anatomy* (5th ed.). Baltimore, MD: Lippincott Williams & Wilkins; 2005.

65. Morgan WJ, Slowman LS. Acute hand and wrist injuries in athletes: evaluation and management. *J Am Acad Orthop Surg.* 2001;9(6):389–400.

85. Robinson M. Jammed fingers *eMedicine* [electronic version]. 2007. Available from: http://emedicine. medscape.com/article/98081-overview. Accessed May 19, 2009.

87. Schultz SJ, Houglum PA, Perrin DH. *Examination of Musculoskeletal Injuries* (2nd ed.). Champaign, IL: Human Kinetics; 2005.

90. Starkey C, Ryan J. *Evaluation of Orthopedic and Athletic Injuries* (2nd ed.). Philadelphia, PA: F.A. Davis; 2002.

91. State of Utah Labor Commission. Labor Commission, Industrial Accidents. Available from: http://www.rules.utah.gov/publicat/bulletin/2005/20050601/27900.htm. Accessed May 20, 2008, May 19, 2009.

Chapter 7

2. Anderson M, Parr G, Hall S. *Foundations of Athletic Training: Prevention, Assessment, and Management* (4th ed.). Baltimore, MD: Lippincott Williams & Wilkins; 2008.

3. Atlas S, Deyo R, Keller R, et al. The Maine Lumbar Spine Study, part III, 1-year outcomes of surgical and nonsurgical management of lumbar spinal stenosis. *Spine.* 1996; 21:1787–1794.

9. Burton A, Waddell G, Tillotson K, Summerton N. Information and advice to patients with back pain can have a positive effect: a randomized controlled trial of a novel educational booklet in primary care. *Spine.* 1999; 24(2484–2491).

10. Busanich B, Verscheure S. Does McKenzie therapy improve outcomes for back pain? *J Athl Train.* 2006; 41(1):117–119.

14. Clare H, Adams R, Maher C. A systematic review of efficacy of McKenzie therapy for spinal pain. *Aust J Physiother.* 2004; 50:209–216.

20. Ebraheim NA, Hassan A, Lee M, Xu R. Functional anatomy of the lumbar spine. *Semin Pain Med.* 2004; 2(3):131–137.

21. Eddy D, Congeni J, Loud K. A review of spine injuries and return to play. *Clin J Sports Med.* 2005; 15:453–458.

27. Heck JF, Sparano JM. A classification system for the assessment of lumbar pain in athletes. *J Athl Train.* 2000; 35(2):204–211.

28. Henrotin Y, Cedraschi C, Duplan B, Bazin T, Duquesnoy B. Information and low back pain management: a systematic review. *Spine.* 2006; 31:E326–E334.

31. Hoffman H. Childhood and adolescent lumbar pain: differential diagnosis and management. *Clin Neurosurg.* 1980; 27:553–576.

32. Hood-White R, Lowdon JD. Herniated nucleus pulposus with radiculopathy in an adolescent: successful nonoperative treatment. *South Med J.* 2002;95(8):932–933.

33. Humphreys SC, Eck JC. Clinical evaluation and treatment options for herniated lumbar disc. *Am Fam Physician.* 1999; 59(3):575–582.

34. Kazemi M. Adolescent lumbar disc herniation in a Tae Kwon Do martial artist: a case report. *J Can Chiropractic Assoc.* 1999;43(4):236.

35. Kinkade S. Evaluation and treatment of acute low back pain. *Am Fam Physician.* 2007; 75:1181–1188, 1190–1182.

45. Nachemson A. Disc pressure measurements. *Spine.* 1981;6:93–97.

46. Ozgen S, Konya D, Toktas OZ, Dagcinar A, Ozek MM. Lumbar disc herniation in adolescence. *Pediatr Neurosurg.* 2007; 43(2):77–81.

50. Radebold A. Lumbosacral spine sprain/strain injuries. *eMedicine* [electronic version]. 2007. Available from: http://www.emedicine.com/sports/topic69.htm. Accessed August 10, 2008.

54. Rohlmann A, Claes L, Bergmann G, Graichen F, Neef P, Wilke HJ. Comparison of intradiscal pressures and spinal fixator loads for different body positions and exercises. *Ergon.* 2001; 44(8):781–794.

61. Udermann B, Spratt K, Donelson R, Mayer J, Graves J, Tillotson J. Can a patient educational book change behavior and reduce pain in chronic low back pain patients? *Spine J.* 2004; 4(4):425–435.

Chapter 8

3. Blecha K. Managing a traumatic pneumothorax. *Athl Ther Today.* 2006; 11(5):51–53.

6. Ciocca M. Pneumothorax in a weight lifter: the importance of vigilance. *Physician SportsMed.* 2000; 28(4):97–103.

8. Curtin SM, Tucker AM, Gens DR. Pneumothorax in sports: issues in recognition and follow-up care. *Physician SportsMed.* 2000;28(8):23–32.

11. Drezner J, Courson R, Roberts W, Mosesso V, Link M, Maron B. Inter-Association Task Force recommendations on emergency preparedness and management of sudden cardiac arrest in high school and college athletic programs: a consensus statement. *J Athl Train.* 2007; 42(1):143–158.

14. Giese EA, O'Connor FG, Brennan FH, et al. The athletic preparticipation evaluation: cardiovascular assessment. *Am Fam Physician.* 2007; 75(7):1008–1014.

16. Maron BJ. Heart disease and other causes of sudden death in young athletes. *Curr Probl Cardiol.* 1998; 23(9):480–529.

17. Maron BJ. Sudden death in young athletes. *N Engl J Med.* 2003; 349(11):1064–1075.

18. Maron BJ, Doerer JJ, Haas TS, Tierney DM, Mueller FO. Sudden deaths in young competitive athletes: analysis of 1866 deaths in the United States, 1980–2006. *Circulation.* 2009; 119(8): 1085–1092.

19. Maron BJ, Maron MS, Lesser RL, et al. Sudden cardiac arrest in hypertrophic cardiomyopathy in the absence of conventional criteria for high risk status. *Am J Cardiol.* 2008; 101:544–547.

20. Maron BJ, Roberts W, McAllister H, Rosing D, Epstein S. Sudden death in young athletes. *Circulation.* 1980; 62(2):218–229.

22. Occupational Safety and Health Administration. Bloodborne pathogens.-1910.1030. United States Department of Labor. Available from: http://www.osha.gov/pls/oshaweb/owadisp. show_document?p_table=STANDARDS&p_ id=10051. Accessed July 19, 2009.

25. Van Camp S, Bloor C, Mueller F, Cantu R, Olson H. Nontraumatic sports death in high school and college athletes. *Med Sci Sports Exerc.* 1995;27:641–647.

26. Volk CP, McFarland EG, Hornsmon G. Pneumothorax: on-field recognition. *Physician and Sportsmedicine.* 1995; 23(10):43–46.

Chapter 9

1. Almekinders L. Anti-inflammatory treatment of muscular injuries in sport: an update of recent studies. *Sports Med.* 1999; 28:383–388.

6. Brothers A, Alamin T, Pedowitz R. Basic clinical management of muscle strains and tears. *J Musculoskel Med.* 2003; 20:303–307.

11. DeMann JL. Sacroiliac dysfunction in dances with low back pain. *Man Ther.* 1997; 29(1):2–10.

26. Harrison D, Harrison D, Troyanovich, S. The sacroiliac joint: a review of anatomy and biomechanics with clinical implications. *J Manipulative Physiol Ther.* 1997; 20(9):607–617.

53. Prentice WE. *Arnheim's Principles of Athletic Training: A Competency-Based Approach* (13th ed.). Boston, MA: McGraw Hill Publishing; 2009.

57. Slipman C, Patel R, Whyte W, et al. Diagnosing and managing sacroiliac pain. *J Musculoskel Med.* 2001; 18:325–332.

60. Szadek K, van der Wurff P, van Tulder M, Zuurmond W, Perez R. Diagnostic validity of criteria for sacroiliac joint pain: a systematic review. *J Pain.* 2009; 10(4):354–368.

65. Willard F. The anatomy of the lumbosacral connection. *Spine: State of the Art Rev.* 1995; 9:333–355.

66. Woodley S, Kennedy E, Mercer S. Anatomy in practice: the sacrotuberous ligament. *Physiother.* 2005; 33(3):91–94.

Chapter 10

19. Cutts S, Edwards A. Clinical review. *GP: Gen Pract.* 2006; 49–50.

40. Hubble MW, Hubble JP. *Principles of Advanced Trauma Care.* Clifton Park, NY: Delmar-Thompson Learning; 2002.

46. Kakarlapudi TK, Bickerstaff DR. Knee instability: isolated and complex. *Br J Sports Med.* 2000; 34(5):395–400.

49. Konin JG, Wiksten D, Isear JA, Brader H. *Special Tests for Orthopedic Examination* 3rd ed. Thorofare NJ: Slack; 2006.

54. Lorei MP, Hershman EB. Peripheral nerve injuries in athletes: treatment and prevention. *Sports Med.* 1993; 16(2):130–147.

58. McConaghy JR. What is the diagnostic accuracy of the clinical examination for meniscus or ligamentous knee injuries? *J Fam Pract.* 2002 Jan; 51(1):85.

67. Noyes FR, Bassett RW, Grood ES, Butler DL. Arthroscopy in acute traumatic hemarthrosis of the knee: incidence of anterior cruciate tears and other injuries. *J Bone Joint Surg Am.* 1980; 62-A(5):687–695,757.

75. Prentice WE. *Arnheim's Principles of Athletic Training: A Competency-Based Approach.* 13th ed. Boston MA: McGraw Hill Publishing; 2009.

82. Scholten RJ, Opstelten W, van der Plas CG, Bijl D, Deville WL, Bouter LM. Accuracy of physical diagnostic tests for assessing ruptures of the anterior cruciate ligament: a meta-analysis. *J Fam Pract.* 2003 Sep; 52(9):689–94.

86. Starkey C, Ryan J. *Evaluation of Orthopedic and Athletic Injuries.* 2nd ed. Philadelphia PA: F.A. Davis; 2002.

87. Steadman's Concise Medical Dictionary. *Steadman's Medical Dictionary.* Philadelphia PA: Lippincott Williams & Wilkins; 2001.

Chapter 11

4. Anderson SJ, Harmon KG, Rubin A. Acute ankle sprains. *Physician Sportsmed.* 2002; 30(12):29.

9. Bahr R, Pena F, Shine J, Lew W, Conrad L, Tyrdal S, et al. Mechanics of the anterior drawer and talar tilt tests: a cadaveric study of lateral ligament injuries of the ankle. *Acta Orthop.* 1997; 68(5):425–441.

24. Burks R, Morgan J. Anatomy of the lateral ankle ligaments. *Am J Sports Med.* 1994; 22;72–7.

47. Fujii T, Luo ZP, Kitaoka HB, An KN. The manual stress test may not be sufficient to differentiate ankle ligament injuries. *Clin Biomech*. 2000; 15(8):619–623.

48. Gaebler C, Kukla C, Breitenseher M, Nellas Z, Mittlboeck M, Trattnig S, et al. Diagnosis of lateral ankle ligament injuries: comparison between talar tilt, MRI and operative findings in 112 athletes. *Acta Orthop Scand*. 1997; 68(3): 286–290.

59. Ivins D. Acute ankle sprain: an update. *Am Fam Physician*. 2006; 74:1714–1720, 1723–1714, 1725–1716.

71. Kovaleski J, Norrell P, Heitman RJ, Hollis JM, Pearsall IV, Albert W. Knee and ankle position, anterior drawer laxity, and stiffness of the ankle complex. *J Athl Train*. 2008; 43(3):242–248.

75. Liu W, Maitland M, Nigg B. The effect of axial load on the in vivo anterior drawer test of the ankle joint complex. *Foot Ankle Int*. 2000; 21(5):420–426.

78. Lynch S. Assessment of the injured ankle in the athlete. *J Athl Train*. 2002; 37(4):406–412.

87. Moore K, Dalley A. *Clinically Oriented Anatomy*. 5th ed. Baltimore MD: Lippincott Williams & Wilkins; 2005.93. Muresanu M, Quinn A. Ankle injury, soft tissue. *eMedicine* [electronic version]. 2009. Available from: http://emedicine.medscape.com/article/822378-overview. Accessed May 20, 2010.

118. Rubin A, Sallis R. Evaluation and diagnosis of ankle injuries. *Am Fam Physician*. 1996; 54(5): 1609–1618.

123. Schneck CD, Mesgarzadeh M, Bonakdarpour A, Ross GJ. MR imaging of the most commonly injured ankle ligaments. Part I. Normal anatomy. *Radiology*. 1992; 184(2):499–506.

127. Sharma D, Harris A. Clinical: management of ankle sprains. *GP: Gen Pract*. 2005; 53–55.

131. Starkey C, Ryan J. *Evaluation of Orthopedic and Athletic Injuries*. 2nd ed. Philadelphia PA: F. A. Davis; 2002.

151. Wolfe MW. Management of ankle sprains. *Am Fam Physician*. 2001; 63(1):93.

BOC Standards of Professional Practice

Introduction

The mission of the Board of Certification Inc. (BOC) is to provide exceptional credentialing programs for healthcare professionals. The BOC has been responsible for the certification of Athletic Trainers since 1969. Upon its inception, the BOC was a division of the professional membership organization the National Athletic Trainers' Association. However, in 1989, the BOC became an independent non-profit corporation.

Accordingly, the BOC provides a certification program for the entry-level Athletic Trainer that confers the ATC® credential and establishes requirements for maintaining status as a Certified Athletic Trainer (to be referred to as "Athletic Trainer" from this point forward). A nine member Board of Directors governs the BOC. There are six Athletic Trainer Directors, one Physician Director, one Public Director and one Corporate/Educational Director.

The BOC is the only accredited certification program for Athletic Trainers in the United States. Every five years, the BOC must undergo review and re-accreditation by the National Commission for Certifying Agencies (NCCA). The NCCA is the accreditation body of the National Organization for Competency Assurance.

The BOC Standards of Professional Practice consists of two sections:

  I. Practice Standards

  II. Code of Professional Responsibility

I. Practice Standards

Preamble

The Practice Standards (Standards) establish essential practice expectations for all Athletic Trainers. Compliance with the Standards is mandatory.

The Standards are intended to:

- assist the public in understanding what to expect from an Athletic Trainer
- assist the Athletic Trainer in evaluating the quality of patient care
- assist the Athletic Trainer in understanding the duties and obligations imposed by virtue of holding the ATC® credential

The Standards are NOT intended to:

- prescribe services
- provide step-by-step procedures
- ensure specific patient outcomes

The BOC does not express an opinion on the competence or warrant job performance of credential holders; however, every Athletic Trainer and applicant must agree to comply with the Standards at all times.

Standard 1: Direction

The Athletic Trainer renders service or treatment under the direction of a physician.

Standard 2: Prevention

The Athletic Trainer understands and uses preventive measures to ensure the highest quality of care for every patient.

Standard 3: Immediate Care

The Athletic Trainer provides standard immediate care procedures used in emergency situations, independent of setting.

Standard 4: Clinical Evaluation and Diagnosis

Prior to treatment, the Athletic Trainer assesses the patient's level of function. The patient's input is considered an integral part of the initial assessment. The Athletic Trainer follows standardized clinical practice in the area of diagnostic reasoning and medical decision making.

Standard 5: Treatment, Rehabilitation and Reconditioning

In development of a treatment program, the Athletic Trainer determines appropriate treatment, rehabilitation and/or reconditioning strategies. Treatment program objectives include long and shortterm goals and an appraisal of those which the patient can realistically be expected to achieve from the program. Assessment measures to determine effectiveness of the program are incorporated into the program.

Standard 6: Program Discontinuation

The Athletic Trainer, with collaboration of the physician, recommends discontinuation of the athletic training service when the patient has received optimal benefit of the program. The Athletic Trainer, at the time of discontinuation, notes the final assessment of the patient's status.

Standard 7: Organization and Administration

All services are documented in writing by the Athletic Trainer and are part of the patient's permanent records. The Athletic Trainer accepts responsibility for recording details of the patient's health status.

II. Code of Professional Responsibility

Preamble

The Code of Professional Responsibility (Code) mandates that BOC credential holders and applicants act in a professionally responsible manner in all athletic training services and activities. The BOC requires all Athletic Trainers and applicants to comply with the Code. The BOC may discipline, revoke or take other action with regard to the application or certification of an individual that does not adhere to the Code. The *Professional Practice and Discipline Guidelines and Procedures* may be accessed via the BOC website, www.bocatc.org.

Code 1: Patient Responsibility

The Athletic Trainer or applicant:

1.1 Renders quality patient care regardless of the patient's race, religion, age, sex, nationality, disability, social/economic status or any other characteristic protected by law

1.2 Protects the patient from harm, acts always in the patient's best interests and is an advocate for the patient's welfare

1.3 Takes appropriate action to protect patients from Athletic Trainers, other healthcare providers or athletic training students who are incompetent, impaired or engaged in illegal or unethical practice

1.4 Maintains the confidentiality of patient information in accordance with applicable law

1.5 Communicates clearly and truthfully with patients and other persons involved in the patient's program, including, but not limited to, appropriate discussion of assessment results, program plans and progress

1.6 Respects and safeguards his or her relationship of trust and confidence with the patient and does not exploit his or her relationship with the patient for personal or financial gain

1.7 Exercises reasonable care, skill and judgment in all professional work

Code 2: Competency

The Athletic Trainer or applicant:

2.1 Engages in lifelong, professional and continuing educational activities

2.2 Participates in continuous quality improvement activities

2.3 Complies with the most current BOC recertification policies and requirements

Code 3: Professional Responsibility

The Athletic Trainer or applicant:

3.1 Practices in accordance with the most current BOC Practice Standards

3.2 Knows and complies with applicable local, state and/or federal rules, requirements, regulations and/or laws related to the practice of athletic training

3.3 Collaborates and cooperates with other healthcare providers involved in a patient's care

3.4 Respects the expertise and responsibility of all healthcare providers involved in a patient's care

3.5 Reports any suspected or known violation of a rule, requirement, regulation or law by him/herself and/or by another Athletic Trainer that is related to the practice of athletic training, public health, patient care or education

3.6 Reports any criminal convictions (with the exception of misdemeanor traffic offenses or traffic ordinance violations that do not involve the use of alcohol or drugs) and/or professional suspension, discipline or sanction received by him/herself or by another Athletic Trainer that is related to athletic training, public health, patient care or education

3.7 Complies with all BOC exam eligibility requirements and ensures that any information provided to the BOC in connection with any certification application is accurate and truthful

3.8 Does not, without proper authority, possess, use, copy, access, distribute or discuss certification exams, score reports, answer sheets, certificates, certificant or applicant files, documents or other materials

3.9 Is candid, responsible and truthful in making any statement to the BOC, and in making any statement in connection with athletic training to the public

3.10 Complies with all confidentiality and disclosure requirements of the BOC

3.11 Does not take any action that leads, or may lead, to the conviction, plea of guilty or plea of nolo contendere (no contest) to any felony or to a misdemeanor related to public health, patient care, athletics or education; this includes, but is not limited to: rape; sexual abuse of a child or patient; actual or threatened use of a weapon of violence; the prohibited sale or distribution of controlled substance, or its possession with the intent to distribute; or the use of the position of an Athletic Trainer to improperly influence the outcome or score of an athletic contest or event or in connection with any gambling activity

3.12 Cooperates with BOC investigations into alleged illegal or unethical activities; this includes but is not limited to, providing factual and non-misleading information and responding to requests for information in a timely fashion

3.13 Does not endorse or advertise products or services with the use of, or by reference to, the BOC name without proper authorization

Code 4: Research

The Athletic Trainer or applicant who engages in research:

4.1 Conducts research according to accepted ethical research and reporting standards established by public law, institutional procedures and/or the health professions

4.2 Protects the rights and well being of research subjects

4.3 Conducts research activities with the goal of improving practice, education and public policy relative to the health needs of diverse populations, the health workforce, the organization and administration of health systems and healthcare delivery

Code 5: Social Responsibility

The Athletic Trainer or applicant:

5.1 Uses professional skills and knowledge to positively impact the community

Code 6: Business Practices

The Athletic Trainer or applicant:

6.1 Refrains from deceptive or fraudulent business practices

6.2 Maintains adequate and customary professional liability insurance

* * *

See also **Professional Practice and Discipline Guidelines and Procedures,** available at http://www.bocatc.org/images/stories/multiple_references/disciplinaryguidelines.pdf

SOAP Note

Mandy Manning, 22 y.o. female soccer player
DOI: October 21, 2010
DOE: October 21, 2010

Subjective:

Demographic: Pt.: 22 y.o. Caucasian female, R-handed, college senior.

Current Condition/CC: Pt. indep amb from field was supporting L-elbow in a flexed position complaining of severe pn. Pt. stated pn was sharp and burning immediately after trauma, now feels like an "intense burning with pn", rating a 9/10; Pn: centrally located around the medial ulna-humeral joint, denies any radiating pn.

Mechanism of Injury: Pt. states her & the opposing player became aggressive, a tussle ensued and Pt. fell on an outstretched arm, experienced a valgus force as opposing player fell across Pt.'s lateral elbow while hyperextended and supinated. Pt. heard and felt an extremely loud and unusual pop from her elbow.

History: Pt. denies past Hx of trauma to UE.

General Health: healthy female with no known medical conditions, NKA and NKDA.

Social/Health Habits: Pt. plays college soccer & recreational soccer during offseason, practices 5 x wk, games 1–2 x/wk, does not drink or smoke.

Family Health Hx: No complications.

Functional Status: Pt. c/o severe pn & has not indep moved L-elbow since amb off field.

Medication: No current medication usage.

Objective:

Observation: Pt. indep amb off field cradling L-elbow in a flexed position. No observable gross deformities. Ecchymosis & edema occurring rapidly.

Palpation: No palpable deformities. Elbow warm to the touch, point tender to proximal 1/3 of ulna, medial epicondyle, UCL, and wrist flexor muscle mass. Palpation limited secondary to Pt. pn. Girth measurement 1" distal to the medial epicondyle demonstrated 1" difference compared to uninvolved arm.

ROM: AROM R-elbow: 0°–135°, AROM L-elbow: 3°–90° secondary to pn, PROM was WNL for R-elbow, L-elbow lacked 10° flexion secondary to excessive swelling & pn (9/10). Pt. unwilling to perform supination after flexion due to pn.

Special Tests: Valgus stress test: positive with excessive pn 10/10. Varus and radioulnar stress test: negative.

Peripheral Nerve: Pt. failed to discriminate between sharp and dull sensations accurately x 2 to ulnar nerve. L-side weakness (3+/5) noted with resisted fifth phalange abduction, wrist flexion & ulnar deviation.

Assessment:

Dx: Possible grade 2 or 3 UCL sprain with concomitant ulnar n. irritation due to altered sensation and slight muscle weakness. In addition, due to the Pt.'s level of pn, a fracture or subluxation is possible.

- *Short-term goals:* Decrease Pt.'s pn to 4/10 within 3 days of RX to increase Pt. ability to begin AROM exercises. Increase L-elbow flexion 0°–120° within 7 days to enable Pt. to begin RROM exercises.

- *Long-term goals:* Pt. will regain full L-AROM with 3 weeks to enable Pt. to RTP with elbow bracing.

Plan:

Treatment: Crushed ice applied to Pt.'s L-medial elbow with a circumferential compression wrap. Pt. instructed in home application of cryotherapy for 20 minutes. L-elbow placed in a sling & swath to allow for rest. Referred Pt. to the emergency room for further evaluation.

F/U: Pt. will follow up on October 22, 2010.

Home program: Based on hospital recommendations.

SCAT2

 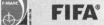

Sport Concussion Assessment Tool 2

Name _____

Sport/team _____

Date/time of injury _____

Date/time of assessment _____

Age _____ Gender ☐ M ☐ F

Years of education completed _____

Examiner _____

What is the SCAT2?[1]

This tool represents a standardized method of evaluating injured athletes for concussion and can be used in athletes aged from 10 years and older. It supersedes the original SCAT published in 2005[2]. This tool also enables the calculation of the Standardized Assessment of Concussion (SAC)[3,4] score and the Maddocks questions[5] for sideline concussion assessment.

Instructions for using the SCAT2

The SCAT2 is designed for the use of medical and health professionals. Preseason baseline testing with the SCAT2 can be helpful for interpreting post-injury test scores. Words in Italics throughout the SCAT2 are the instructions given to the athlete by the tester.

This tool may be freely copied for distribtion to individuals, teams, groups and organizations.

What is a concussion?

A concussion is a disturbance in brain function caused by a direct or indirect force to the head. It results in a variety of non-specific symptoms (like those listed below) and often does not involve loss of consciousness. Concussion should be suspected in the presence of **any one or more** of the following:
- Symptoms (such as headache), or
- Physical signs (such as unsteadiness), or
- Impaired brain function (e.g. confusion) or
- Abnormal behaviour.

Any athlete with a suspected concussion should be REMOVED FROM PLAY, medically assessed, monitored for deterioration (i.e., should not be left alone) and should not drive a motor vehicle.

Symptom Evaluation

How do you feel?

You should score yourself on the following symptoms, based on how you feel now.

	none	mild		moderate		severe	
Headache	0	1	2	3	4	5	6
"Pressure in head"	0	1	2	3	4	5	6
Neck Pain	0	1	2	3	4	5	6
Nausea or vomiting	0	1	2	3	4	5	6
Dizziness	0	1	2	3	4	5	6
Blurred vision	0	1	2	3	4	5	6
Balance problems	0	1	2	3	4	5	6
Sensitivity to light	0	1	2	3	4	5	6
Sensitivity to noise	0	1	2	3	4	5	6
Feeling slowed down	0	1	2	3	4	5	6
Feeling like "in a fog"	0	1	2	3	4	5	6
"Don't feel right"	0	1	2	3	4	5	6
Difficulty concentrating	0	1	2	3	4	5	6
Difficulty remembering	0	1	2	3	4	5	6
Fatigue or low energy	0	1	2	3	4	5	6
Confusion	0	1	2	3	4	5	6
Drowsiness	0	1	2	3	4	5	6
Trouble falling asleep (if applicable)	0	1	2	3	4	5	6
More emotional	0	1	2	3	4	5	6
Irritability	0	1	2	3	4	5	6
Sadness	0	1	2	3	4	5	6
Nervous or Anxious	0	1	2	3	4	5	6

Total number of symptoms (Maximum possible 22) ▢

Symptom severity score
(Add all scores in table, maximum possible: 22 x 6 = 132) ▢

Do the symptoms get worse with physical activity? ☐ Y ☐ N
Do the symptoms get worse with mental activity? ☐ Y ☐ N

Overall rating
If you know the athlete well prior to the injury, how different is the athlete acting compared to his / her usual self? Please circle one response.

no different	very different	unsure

Cognitive & Physical Evaluation

1 Symptom score (from page 1)

22 **minus** number of symptoms | of 22

2 Physical signs score

Was there loss of consciousness or unresponsiveness?   Y   N
If yes, how long?   minutes
Was there a balance problem/unsteadiness?   Y   N

Physical signs score (1 point for each negative response)   of 2

3 Glasgow coma scale (GCS)

Best eye response (E)

No eye opening	1
Eye opening in response to pain	2
Eye opening to speech	3
Eyes opening spontaneously	4

Best verbal response (V)

No verbal response	1
Incomprehensible sounds	2
Inappropriate words	3
Confused	4
Oriented	5

Best motor response (M)

No motor response	1
Extension to pain	2
Abnormal flexion to pain	3
Flexion/Withdrawal to pain	4
Localizes to pain	5
Obeys commands	6

Glasgow Coma score (E + V + M)   of 15

GCS should be recorded for all athletes in case of subsequent deterioration.

4 Sideline Assessment – Maddocks Score

"I am going to ask you a few questions, please listen carefully and give your best effort."

Modified Maddocks questions (1 point for each correct answer)

At what venue are we at today?	0	1
Which half is it now?	0	1
Who scored last in this match?	0	1
What team did you play last week/game?	0	1
Did your team win the last game?	0	1

Maddocks score   of 5

Maddocks score is validated for sideline diagnosis of concussion only and is not included in SCAT 2 summary score for serial testing.

5 Cognitive assessment

Standardized Assessment of Concussion (SAC)

Orientation (1 point for each correct answer)

What month is it?	0	1
What is the date today?	0	1
What is the day of the week?	0	1
What year is it?	0	1
What time is it right now? (within 1 hour)	0	1

Orientation score   of 5

Immediate memory

"I am going to test your memory. I will read you a list of words and when I am done, repeat back as many words as you can remember, in any order."

Trials 2 & 3:

"I am going to repeat the same list again. Repeat back as many words as you can remember in any order, even if you said the word before."

Complete all 3 trials regardless of score on trial 1 & 2. Read the words at a rate of one per second. Score 1 pt. for each correct response. Total score equals sum across all 3 trials. Do not inform the athlete that delayed recall will be tested.

List	Trial 1	Trial 2	Trial 3	Alternative word list		
elbow	0 1	0 1	0 1	candle	baby	finger
apple	0 1	0 1	0 1	paper	monkey	penny
carpet	0 1	0 1	0 1	sugar	perfume	blanket
saddle	0 1	0 1	0 1	sandwich	sunset	lemon
bubble	0 1	0 1	0 1	wagon	iron	insect
Total						

Immediate memory score   of 15

Concentration

Digits Backward:

"I am going to read you a string of numbers and when I am done, you repeat them back to me backwards, in reverse order of how I read them to you. For example, if I say 7-1-9, you would say 9-1-7."

If correct, go to next string length. If incorrect, read trial 2. One point possible for each string length. Stop after incorrect on both trials. The digits should be read at the rate of one per second.

		Alternative digit lists		
4-9-3	0 1	6-2-9	5-2-6	4-1-5
3-8-1-4	0 1	3-2-7-9	1-7-9-5	4-9-6-8
6-2-9-7-1	0 1	1-5-2-8-6	3-8-5-2-7	6-1-8-4-3
7-1-8-4-6-2	0 1	5-3-9-1-4-8	8-3-1-9-6-4	7-2-4-8-5-6

Months in Reverse Order:

"Now tell me the months of the year in reverse order. Start with the last month and go backward. So you'll say December, November ... Go ahead"

1 pt. for entire sequence correct

Dec-Nov-Oct-Sept-Aug-Jul-Jun-May-Apr-Mar-Feb-Jan   0   1

Concentration score   of 5

---

[1] This tool has been developed by a group of international experts at the 3rd International Consensus meeting on Concussion in Sport held in Zurich, Switzerland in November 2008. The full details of the conference outcomes and the authors of the tool are published in British Journal of Sports Medicine, 2009, volume 43, supplement 1.
The outcome paper will also be simultaneously co-published in the May 2009 issues of Clinical Journal of Sports Medicine, Physical Medicine & Rehabilitation, Journal of Athletic Training, Journal of Clinical Neuroscience, Journal of Science & Medicine in Sport, Neurosurgery, Scandinavian Journal of Science & Medicine in Sport and the Journal of Clinical Sports Medicine.

[2] McCrory P et al. Summary and agreement statement of the 2nd International Conference on Concussion in Sport, Prague 2004. British Journal of Sports Medicine. 2005; 39: 196-204

[3] McCrea M. Standardized mental status testing of acute concussion. Clinical Journal of Sports Medicine. 2001; 11: 176-181

[4] McCrea M, Randolph C, Kelly J. Standardized Assessment of Concussion: Manual for administration, scoring and interpretation. Waukesha, Wisconsin, USA.

[5] Maddocks, DL; Dicker, GD; Saling, MM. The assessment of orientation following concussion in athletes. Clin J Sport Med. 1995;5(1):32–3

[6] Guskiewicz KM. Assessment of postural stability following sport-related concussion. Current Sports Medicine Reports. 2003; 2: 24-30

6 Balance examination

This balance testing is based on a modified version of the Balance Error Scoring System (BESS)[6]. A stopwatch or watch with a second hand is required for this testing.

Balance testing

"I am now going to test your balance. Please take your shoes off, roll up your pant legs above ankle (if applicable), and remove any ankle taping (if applicable). This test will consist of three twenty second tests with different stances."

(a) Double leg stance:
   "The first stance is standing with your feet together with your hands on your hips and with your eyes closed. You should try to maintain stability in that position for 20 seconds. I will be counting the number of times you move out of this position. I will start timing when you are set and have closed your eyes."

(b) Single leg stance:
   "If you were to kick a ball, which foot would you use? [This will be the dominant foot] Now stand on your non-dominant foot. The dominant leg should be held in approximately 30 degrees of hip flexion and 45 degrees of knee flexion. Again, you should try to maintain stability for 20 seconds with your hands on your hips and your eyes closed. I will be counting the number of times you move out of this position. If you stumble out of this position, open your eyes and return to the start position and continue balancing. I will start timing when you are set and have closed your eyes."

(c) Tandem stance:
   *"Now stand heel-to-toe with your **non-dominant foot** in back. Your weight should be evenly distributed across both feet. Again, you should try to maintain stability for 20 seconds with your hands on your hips and your eyes closed. I will be counting the number of times you move out of this position. If you stumble out of this position, open your eyes and return to the start position and continue balancing. I will start timing when you are set and have closed your eyes."*

Balance testing – types of errors
1. Hands lifted off iliac crest
2. Opening eyes
3. Step, stumble, or fall
4. Moving hip into > 30 degrees abduction
5. Lifting forefoot or heel
6. Remaining out of test position > 5 sec

Each of the 20-second trials is scored by counting the errors, or deviations from the proper stance, accumulated by the athlete. The examiner will begin counting errors only after the individual has assumed the proper start position. **The modified BESS is calculated by adding one error point for each error during the three 20-second tests. The maximum total number of errors for any single condition is 10.** If a athlete commits multiple errors simultaneously, only one error is recorded but the athlete should quickly return to the testing position, and counting should resume once subject is set. Subjects that are unable to maintain the testing procedure for a minimum of **five seconds** at the start are assigned the highest possible score, ten, for that testing condition.

Which foot was tested: Left   Right
(i.e. which is the **non-dominant** foot)

Condition	Total errors
Double Leg Stance (feet together)	of 10
Single leg stance (non-dominant foot)	of 10
Tandem stance (non-dominant foot at back)	of 10
Balance examination score (30 **minus** total errors)	of 30

7 Coordination examination

Upper limb coordination
Finger-to-nose (FTN) task: *"I am going to test your coordination now. Please sit comfortably on the chair with your eyes open and your arm (either right or left) outstretched (shoulder flexed to 90 degrees and elbow and fingers extended). When I give a start signal, I would like you to perform five successive finger to nose repetitions using your index finger to touch the tip of the nose as quickly and as accurately as possible."*

Which arm was tested: Left   Right

Scoring: 5 correct repetitions in < 4 seconds = 1

Note for testers: Athletes fail the test if they do not touch their nose, do not fully extend their elbow or do not perform five repetitions. Failure should be scored as 0.

Coordination score	of 1

8 Cognitive assessment

Standardized Assessment of Concussion (SAC)

Delayed recall
"Do you remember that list of words I read a few times earlier? Tell me as many words from the list as you can remember in any order."

Circle each word correctly recalled. Total score equals number of words recalled.

List		Alternative word list	
elbow	candle	baby	finger
apple	paper	monkey	penny
carpet	sugar	perfume	blanket
saddle	sandwich	sunset	lemon
bubble	wagon	iron	insect

Delayed recall score	of 5

Overall score

Test domain	Score
Symptom score	of 22
Physical signs score	of 2
Glasgow Coma score (E + V + M)	of 15
Balance examination score	of 30
Coordination score	of 1
Subtotal	**of 70**
Orientation score	of 5
Immediate memory score	of 5
Concentration score	of 15
Delayed recall score	of 5
SAC subtotal	**of 30**
SCAT2 total	**of 100**
Maddocks Score	**of 5**

Definitive normative data for a SCAT2 "cut-off" score is not available at this time and will be developed in prospective studies. Embedded within the SCAT2 is the SAC score that can be utilized separately in concussion management. The scoring system also takes on particular clinical significance during serial assessment where it can be used to document either a decline or an improvement in neurological functioning.

Scoring data from the SCAT2 or SAC should not be used as a stand alone method to diagnose concussion, measure recovery or make decisions about an athlete's readiness to return to competition after concussion.

Athlete Information

Any athlete suspected of having a concussion should be removed from play, and then seek medical evaluation.

Signs to watch for

Problems could arise over the first 24-48 hours. You should not be left alone and must go to a hospital at once if you:

- Have a headache that gets worse
- Are very drowsy or can't be awakened (woken up)
- Can't recognize people or places
- Have repeated vomiting
- Behave unusually or seem confused; are very irritable
- Have seizures (arms and legs jerk uncontrollably)
- Have weak or numb arms or legs
- Are unsteady on your feet; have slurred speech

Remember, it is better to be safe.
Consult your doctor after a suspected concussion.

Return to play

Athletes should not be returned to play the same day of injury. When returning athletes to play, they should follow a stepwise symptom-limited program, with stages of progression. For example:

1. rest until asymptomatic (physical and mental rest)
2. light aerobic exercise (e.g. stationary cycle)
3. sport-specific exercise
4. non-contact training drills (start light resistance training)
5. full contact training after medical clearance
6. return to competition (game play)

There should be approximately 24 hours (or longer) for each stage and the athlete should return to stage 1 if symptoms recur. Resistance training should only be added in the later stages.
Medical clearance should be given before return to play.

Tool	Test domain	Time	Score			
		Date tested				
		Days post injury				
SCAT2	Symptom score					
	Physical signs score					
	Glasgow Coma score (E + V + M)					
	Balance examination score					
	Coordination score					
SAC	Orientation score					
	Immediate memory score					
	Concentration score					
	Delayed recall score					
	SAC Score					
Total	SCAT2					
Symptom severity score (max possible 132)						
Return to play			Y N	Y N	Y N	Y N

Additional comments

Concussion injury advice (To be given to concussed athlete)

This patient has received an injury to the head. A careful medical examination has been carried out and no sign of any serious complications has been found. It is expected that recovery will be rapid, but the patient will need monitoring for a further period by a responsible adult. Your treating physician will provide guidance as to this timeframe.

If you notice any change in behaviour, vomiting, dizziness, worsening headache, double vision or excessive drowsiness, please telephone the clinic or the nearest hospital emergency department immediately.

Other important points:

- Rest and avoid strenuous activity for at least 24 hours
- No alcohol
- No sleeping tablets
- Use paracetamol or codeine for headache. Do **not** use aspirin or anti-inflammatory medication
- Do **not** drive until medically cleared
- Do **not** train or play sport until medically cleared

Clinic phone number

Patient's name

Date/time of injury

Date/time of medical review

Treating physician

Contact details or stamp

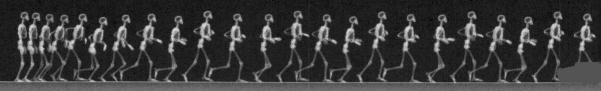

A&O *alert and oriented;* assessment of level of consciousness.

A/P or AP *anterior-posterior.*

AAJ *atlanto-axial joint.*

ABC *airway, breathing, circulation;* basic functions of life.

ABD *abdomen.*

AC joint (ACJ) *acromioclavicular joint;* articulation between the acromion process and the distal clavicle.

ACI *approved clinical instructor;* a BOC-certified athletic trainer or other qualified health care professional (with a minimum of one year of work experience in their respective academic or clinical area) who provides direct supervision during a clinical education experience and provides formal instruction and evaluation of clinical competencies and proficiencies and the ability of the students to integrate their clinical skills into professional practice.

ACL *anterior cruciate ligament;* major knee ligament extending from the anteromedial intercondylar eminence of the tibia to the posterior aspect of the medial surface of the lateral condyle of the femur.

ADL *activities of daily living;* activities that an average person performs routinely in the course of a day, such as bathing, dressing, and meal preparation.

AED *automated external defibrillator;* portable device that diagnoses and treats cardiac events.

AIIS *anterior inferior iliac spine.*

Amb *ambulate.*

ANS *autonomic nervous system;* part of the nervous system which represents the motor innervation of smooth muscle, cardiac muscle, and gland cells.

antalgia pain.

antalgic gait pattern of walking (limping); altered secondary walk used to avoid pain.

AOJ *atlanto-occipital joint;* articulation between the atlas (C1) and occiput (skull).

AROM *active range of motion;* the range of movement a patient can actively (without assistance) move a joint using the adjacent muscles.

ASIS *anterior superior iliac spine.*

ATFL *anterior talofibular ligament;* major lateral ankle ligament extending anteromedially from lateral malleolus to the talar neck.

auscultation listening to internal body sounds, usually with a stethoscope.

avascular necrosis death or decay of tissue due to local ischemia in the absence of infection.

AVPU *alert, verbal, painful, unconscious;* mnemonic used when assessing a patient's level of consciousness.

bilat or (B) *bilateral.*

BMI *body mass index;* method of assessing nutritional status; correlates with risk of disease and death due to causes associated with obesity; because it does not distinguish excess adiposity from excess lean body mass, it is not useful in competitive athletes, body builders, pregnant women, or children.

BP *blood pressure;* vital sign which measures the pressure or tension of the blood within the systemic arteries.

C/O or c/o *complains of;* patient report of symptoms or issues related to the condition.

CC or C/C *chief complaint;* primary symptom reported by a patient.

CC ligament (CCL) *coracoclavicular ligament;* ligament uniting the clavicle to the coracoid process; it is subdivided into the conoid ligament and the trapezoid ligament.

cephalad toward the head.

CFL *calcaneofibular ligament;* major lateral ankle ligament passing posteroinferiorly from the tip of lateral malleolus to the lateral surface of the calcaneus.

CMC joint (CMCJ) *carpometacarpal joint;* articulation between the carpals and metacarpals.

CN *cranial nerves;* 12 paired nerves emerging from, or entering, the skull, includes; CN I - olfactory, CN II - optic, CN III - oculomotor, CN IV - trochlear, CN V - trigeminal, CN VI - abducens, CN VII - facial, CN VIII - vestibulocochlear, CN IX - glossopharyngeal, CN X - vagus, CN XI - accessory, and CN XII - hypoglossal nerves.

CNS *central nervous system;* the brain and the spinal cord.

CSF *cerebrospinal fluid;* a fluid secreted by ventricles of the brain, filling the ventricles and the subarachnoid cavities of the brain and spinal cord.

CSI *cervical spine injury.*

CT scan *computerized tomography scan;* X-ray technique producing overlapping cross-sectional images of internal structures of your body.

cyanotic dark bluish or purplish coloration of the skin, nail beds, lips, or mucous membranes due to deficient oxygenation of the blood.

DF *dorsiflexion.*

DIP joint (DIPJ) *distal interphalangeal joint;* articulation between the distal and middle phalange on the hands and feet.

diplopia double vision.

DJD *degenerative joint disease;* arthritis characterized by erosion of articular cartilage, resulting in pain and loss of function; affecting weight-bearing joints.

DOE *date of evaluation.*

DOI *date of injury.*

DOTS *deformity, open wounds, tenderness, and swelling;* mnemonic used when performing a rapid assessment of an injured patient during the secondary assessment.

DTR *deep tendon reflex;* a tonic contraction of the muscles in response to a stretching force, due to stimulation of muscle proprioceptors.

DVT *deep vein thrombosis;* blood clot forming in a vein deep in the body. Clots occur when blood thickens and clumps together.

Dx *diagnosis.*

dyspnea shortness of breath.

EAP *emergency action plan.*

EBV *Epstein-Barr virus;* a virus of the herpes family and one of the most common viruses in humans, can cause infectious mononucleosis.

ecchymosis a purplish patch caused by extravasation of blood into the skin; a bruise.

EMG *electromyography;* diagnostic test which records the electrical activity of muscles. Used to test for muscle disorders, including muscular dystrophy.

EMS *emergency medical services.*

EMT *emergency medical technician;* allied healthcare worker providing pre-hospital care for injured and ill patients.

ER or E.R. *emergency room.*

EVA *ethyl vinyl acetate;* elastic material commonly used in the formation of athletic mouthguards.

F/U *follow-up.*

fluorescein nontoxic, water-soluble indicator used diagnostically to trace water flow and to visualize corneal abrasions.

FOOSH *fall on out stretched hand;* mechanism of injury for many different types of injures to the upper extremity.

FX or fx fracture.

GCS *Glasgow Coma Scale;* scale used to measure level of consciousness, especially after head trauma in which level of consciousness is determined by summing three factors; amount of eye opening, verbal responsiveness, and motor responsiveness.

GH joint (GHJ) *glenohumeral joint;* articulation between the glenoid fossa of the scapula and the humeral head.

GI *gastrointestinal.*

HCM *hypertrophic cardiomyopathy;* congenital disorder characterized by abnormal thickening of the left ventricle.

hematuria blood in the urine.

hemothorax blood in the pleural cavity of the lungs.

HIPS *history, inspection, palpation, special tests;* mnemonic used when performing an injury assessment.

HO *heterotopic ossification;* the process of bony tissue formation outside of the skeleton.

HOPS *history, observation, palpation, special tests;* mnemonic used when performing an injury assessment.

Hx *history.*

ICC *intraclass correlation coefficient.*

ICD–9 CM *International Classification of Disease, Ninth Revision, Clinical Modification;* diagnostic and procedure used in medicine.

indep *independent.*

innominate pelvic bone consisting of the ilium, ischium, and pubis.

ITB *iliotibial band;* thickening of the fascia latae in the lateral thigh.

ITBFS *iliotibial band friction syndrome;* common knee injury that usually presents as lateral knee pain caused by inflammation of the distal portion of the iliotibial band.

IV *intravenous.*

Jones fracture transverse stress fracture of the proximal shaft of the fifth metatarsal.

kyphotic relating to kyphosis; a normal anteriorly concave curvature of the vertebral column.

LLE *left lower extremity.*

L or Ⓛ *left.*

LBP *low back pain;* common musculoskeletal symptom that may be either acute or chronic. Caused by a variety of diseases and disorders affecting the lumbar spine.

LCL *lateral collateral ligament;* ligament providing restraint against a varus force, located throughout the body at various joint articulations.

LCPD *Legg-Calve-Perthes disease;* condition when the femoral head of the femur does not receive adequate blood flow, resulting in bone death.

LE *lower extremity.*

LLQ *left lower quadrant;* term used to describe 1 of the 4 quadrants of the abdomen.

LOC *level of consciousness;* a measure of an individual's arousability and responsiveness to stimuli from the environment.

lordotic relating to lordosis; a normal anteriorly convex curvature of the vertebral column.

LUQ *left upper quadrant;* term used to describe 1 of the 4 quadrants of the abdomen.

malocclusion any deviation from a physiologically acceptable contact of opposing dentitions.

MCL *medial collateral ligament;* ligament providing restraint against a valgus force, located throughout the body at various joint articulations.

MCP joint (MCPJ) *metacarpophalangeal joint;* articulation between the metacarpal and the proximal phalange.

min *minute.*

MMT *manual muscle test;* evaluation of the function and strength of individual muscles and muscle groups based on effective performance of a movement in relation to the forces of gravity and manual resistance.

MOI *mechanism of injury.*

MRI *magnetic resonance imaging;* diagnostic modality where the magnetic nuclei (especially protons) of a patient are aligned in a strong, uniform magnetic field, absorb energy from tuned radiofrequency pulses, and emit radiofrequency signals as their excitation decays to create three-dimensional images of a patient's organs and tissues. MRIs do not use ionizing radiation or carry risk of causing cancer.

MTPJ *metatarsophalangeal joint;* any joint located between the metatarsal and the proximal phalange.

mucopurulent exudate containing pus and a relatively conspicuous proportion of mucous material.

myocarditis inflammation of the heart muscle.

NCAA *National Collegiate Athletic Association.*

NCS *nerve conduction study;* test to determine if a nerve is functioning normally.

NCV *nerve conduction velocity.*

neurapraxia an injury to a nerve that interrupts conduction causing temporary paralysis but not degeneration and that is followed by a complete and rapid recovery.

neuroma non-cancerous tumor that develops on a nerve.

NKA *no known allergies.*

NKDA *no known drug allergies.*

NPS *numeric pain scale;* scale used to measure pain from 0–10.

NSAID *non-steroidal anti-inflammatory drug;* medicines used to treat inflammation and reduce fevers from a variety of medical conditions.

NWB *non–weight-bearing;* inability to apply weight to a joint, normally the lower leg.

OPQRTS *onset, provocation, quality, radiating, time, severity;* mnemonic used when assessing a patient's symptoms.

ORIF *open reduction-internal fixation;* surgical procedure where plates, screws, and wires are use to correct a musculoskeletal trauma/disorder.

otalgia   earache.

OTC   *over-the-counter.*

otorrhea   discharge from the ear.

p   *after.*

P   *pulse;* vital sign producing a palpable rhythmic expansion of an artery as the heart contracts.

PA   *posterior-anterior;* also *physician's assistant.*

paresthesia   altered sensation.

PCL   *posterior cruciate ligament;* major knee ligament extending from the posterior intercondylar area of the tibia to the anterior part of the lateral surface of the medial condyle of the femur.

PCS   *post-concussive syndrome* or *post-concussive symptoms.*

PE   *physical examination* or *pulmonary embolus.*

PEARRL   *pupils equal, round, reactive to light and accommodation.*

pes cavus   condition where the arch is an excessively raised arch, opposite of pes planus.

pes planus   condition where the arch or instep of the foot collapses and comes in contact with the ground during ambulation; opposite of pes cavas.

PF   *plantarflexion.*

PFP   *patellofemoral pain.*

PFPS   *patellofemoral pain syndrome;* retropatellar or peripatellar pain resulting from physical and biochemical changes in the patellofemoral joint.

PIIS   *posterior inferior iliac spine.*

PIP joint (PIPJ)   *proximal interphalangeal joint;* articulation between the proximal and middle phalange on the hands and feet.

pn   *pain.*

PNF   *proprioceptive neuromuscular facilitation;* technique using passive muscle stretching and resisted muscular contractions to reduce resting tension mediated by Golgi tendon organs and muscle spindles.

PNS   *peripheral nervous system;* part of the nervous system external to the brain and spinal cord from their roots to their peripheral terminations.

PPM   *policy and procedure manual;* document describing the rules and regulations and procedures of an organization.

PRICE   *protect, rest, ice, compression, elevation;* acronym summarizing common treatments for skeletal and soft-tissue injuries.

PROM   *passive range of motion;* range of movement performed by someone other than the patient's muscles.

pruritus   itch, itching.

PSIS   *posterior superior iliac spine.*

Pt. or pt.   *patient.*

PT   *physical therapy.*

PTFL   *posterior talofibular ligament;* major lateral ankle ligament extending horizontally medially and slightly posteriorly from the malleolar fossa to the lateral tubercle of the posterior process of the talus.

RLE   *right lower extremity.*

R   *right.*

radiculopathy   disorder of the spinal nerve roots.

RE   *right extremity.*

rhinorrhea   discharge from the nose.

RICE   *rest, ice, compression, elevation;* mnemonic used describing the immediate care applied to an acute injury.

RLQ   *right lower quadrant;* term used to describe 1 of the 4 quadrants of the abdomen.

ROM   *range of motion;* the distance and direction of movement of a joint.

RROM   *resistive range of motion;* range of movement performed by the patient's muscles.

RTP   *return to play.*

RUQ   *right upper quadrant;* term used to describe 1 of the 4 quadrants of the abdomen.

SAC   *standardized assessment of concussion;* objective sideline measurement tool used to assess neurocognitive deficits in athletes immediately following an injury.

SAMPLE   *symptoms, allergies, medications, past pertinent history, last oral intake, event leading to the situation;* mnemonic used as part of the secondary assessment of an ill or injured patient.

SC joint (SCJ)   *sternoclavicular joint;* articulation between the sternum and the proximal clavicle.

SAS   *subacromial space stenosis.*

SC ligament (SCL)   *sternoclavicular ligament;* the ligament attaching the proximal clavicle to the sternum.

SCAT2   *Sport Concussion Assessment Tool 2;* standardized clinical assessment tool used to evaluate and document an acute concussion.

SCFE *slipped capital femoral epiphysis.*

SCM *sternocleidomastoid.*

SDH *subdural hematoma;* acute or chronic extravasation of blood between the dural and arachnoidal membranes.

SI *sacral iliac.*

SLAP *superior labral tear from anterior to posterior;* traumatic tear of the superior part of the glenoid labrum, beginning posteriorly and extending anteriorly.

SLR *straight leg raise;* exercise used to rehabilitate the hip and lower extremity.

SOAP acronym; *(S) subjective;* information received from the patient during a physical examination; *(O) objective;* results of the tests and measures performed and observation by the clinician during the physical examination; *(A) assessment;* summary of the patient's main symptoms/diagnosis and may include excepted outcomes and anticipated goals; and *(P) plan;* may include excepted outcomes and anticipated goal, intervention plan, and discharge plan.

spinal stenosis narrowing of the spinal canal that occurs congenitally or as a result of trauma.

spondylolisthesis condition in which a vertebra in the lower part of the spine slips forward and onto a vertebra below it.

spondylosis any of various degenerative diseases of the spine.

STJN *subtalar joint neutral;* position in which the forefoot is locked on the rearfoot with maximum pronation of the midtarsal joint.

Sx *symptoms.*

tachypnea rapid breathing.

TBI *traumatic brain injury.*

TENS *transcutaneous electrical neural stimulation;* form of therapy where an electrical current is introduced to the body producing a desirable physiological effect, normally for pain management.

TFCC *triangular fibrocartilage complex;* segment of cartilage in the wrist joint, often considered the 'wrist meniscus.'

tid or t.i.d. *three times a day.*

Tietze syndrome an inflammation of the costochondral junction.

TMJ *temporomandibular joint;* articulation between the mandible and the mandibular fossa and articular tubercle of the temporal bone.

TOS *thoracic outlet syndrome.*

UE *upper extremity.*

VA *vertebral artery;* first branch of the subclavian artery, divided into four parts; the prevertebral part, before it enters the foramen of the transverse process of the sixth cervical vertebra; the transverse part, in the transverse foramina of the first six cervical vertebrae; the atlas, running along the posterior arch of the atlas; and the intracranial part, within the cranial cavity to unite with the artery from the other side to form the basilar artery.

valgus characterized by an abnormal outward turning of a bone.

valsalva forcible exhalation against a closed airway.

varus characterized by an abnormal inward turning of a bone.

VAS *visual analog scale;* tool to rate the intensity of certain sensations and feelings, such as pain using a 10 cm straight line with one end meaning no pain and the other end meaning the worst pain imaginable.

VBI *vertebrobasilar insufficiency;* conditions in which blood supply to the back of the brain is disrupted.

VMO *vastus medialis oblique.*

Volkmann's ischemic contracture a deformity of the hand, fingers, and wrist caused by injury to the muscles of the forearm.

VS *vital signs;* objective measurements of a patient's general health and cardiorespiratory function, includes temperature, pulse, respirations, blood pressure, and pupils.

wk *week.*

WNL *within normal limits.*

y.o. or y/o *years old.*

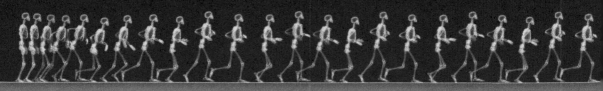

Photo Credits

Photos are by authors Leisha and David Berry unless otherwise noted.

Chapter 2

Figures 2.7.1; 2.13.2; 2.13.3 by Landon Deru, Weber State University, Ogden, UT.

Figure 2.6.1 Retrieved from http://www.uwec.edu/Kin/diglib/ATvid/images/cauliflowerear_1.JPG. Used with permission.

Chapter 3

Figures 3.2.1; 3.2.2; A3.2.1; 3.3.1; 3.5.2 by Landon Deru.

Chapter 4

Figures 4.1.1; 4.2.1; 4.7.1; 4.7.2; 4.8.1; 4.9.1 by Nikki Pappas, Weber State University, Ogden, UT.

Chapter 5

Figure 5.6.1, University of Wisconsin Eau Claire AT Digital Library. Used by permission. Retrieved from http://www.uwec.edu/kin/majors/AT/aidil/images/elbowdisact.jpg

Figure 5.9.2; 5.9.3 by Joel Bass, Weber State University, Ogden, UT.

Figure 5.13.1 by Dr. Charles Goldberg, MD. Copyright © 2005 The Regents of the University of California. All Rights Reserved. Used by permission. Retrieved from: http://meded.ucsd.edu/clinicalimg/upper_septic_bursitis.htm

Chapter 6

Figure 6.6.1 by Millikin University Athletic Training Program.

Figure 6.7.3, Used with persmission by Learning Radiology.com. Retrieved from http://www.learningradiology.com/notes/bonenotes/perilunate dislocatepage.htm

Figure 6.4, 6.11.2, 6.14.3 by Joel Bass, Weber State University, Ogden, UT.

Chapter 7

7.4.3 Used with persmission by Learning Radiology. com. Image avilable at: http://www.learningradiology.com/caseofweek/caseoftheweekpix2006/cow204lg.jpg

7.8.1; 7.8.2; 7.8.3; 7.8.4 by Joel Beam, University of North Florida, Jacksonville, FL.

Chapter 9

Figures 9.3.1; 9.4.1; 9.8.1 by Nikki Pappas.

Figure 9.3.2 Sloan, R. (1998). Quadriceps contusions and hip pointers in football [Electronic Version]. Used with permission from Hughston Health Alert. Retrieved from http://www.hughston.com/hha/a.quad.htm.

Figure 9.7.2 Used with permission by eMedicine. Retrieved from http://emedicine.medscape.com/article/87420-media

Chapter 10

Figure 10.3.1 by Michael Miller, Western Michigan University, Kalamazoo, MI.

Chapter 11

Figure 11.4.2 by Joel Bass, Weber State University, Ogden, UT.

Figure 11.6.1 Used with the permission of University of Wisconsin-Eau Claire, Department of Kinesiology, Athletic Training. Image available at: www.uwec.edu/Kin/diglib/ATvid/images/rapriortosurg_1.JPG

Figure 11.8.1 Used with permission of S. Eriksson, S. (n.d.) The ankle. *The Med Cell.* Available at: http://www.fighttimes.com/magazine/magazine.asp?article=481.

Figure 11.11.1 Used with the permission of University of Wisconsin-Eau Claire, Department of Kinesiology, Athletic Training. Image avilable at: http://www.uwec.edu/Kin/diglib/ATvid/images/jonesap_1.JPG

Figure 11.15.1 Used with permission from Kline, A. (2007). Haglund's correction with removal of retrocalcaneal spur and transverse achilles tenoplasty: 2 case reports. *Podiatry Internet Journal,* 2 (1). Available at: http://podiatry.wordpress.com/2007/01/01/haglund%E2%80%99s-correction-with-removal-of-retrocalcaneal-spur-and-transverse-achilles-tenoplasty–2-case-reports/

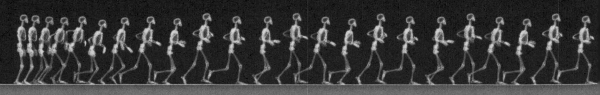

Index

Printed in the United States
by Baker & Taylor Publisher Services